ANALYZING A LONG DREAM SERIES

T0388484

Analyzing a Long Dream Series provides an extraordinary insight into the richness and variability of dreams, considering over 12,000 dreams that have been recorded for more than 30 years.

Internationally recognized dream scientist Michael Schredl opens up his own personal dream series, offering a unique window into the interplay between waking life and dreaming. The book considers a huge range of dream topics, including family, friends, schoolmates, colleagues, erotic dreams, alongside the appearance of everyday objects. It also discusses rarer themes such as pain perception, temperature perception, and typical dreams about toilets, exams, and teeth. As the author is both the dreamer and the researcher, questions like why we dream about topics we have never experienced in waking life – for example, about the pain of being shot in the stomach – can be addressed, shedding light on the creative nature of dreams. The in-depth analyses provided in this book attempt to answer the field's most profound questions: why do we dream every night, and why do we dream in such creative ways about the issues that are important to us in waking life? The dreams analyzed question existing dream theories such as simulation theories, and the author proposes a function of recalled dreams for creative problem solving and provides ideas for future research.

This fascinating book is an essential read for all dream researchers and students of the psychology of dreams.

Michael Schredl is Head of Research at the Sleep Laboratory, Central Institute of Mental Health, Medical Faculty Mannheim/Heidelberg University, Germany.

ANALYZING A LONG DREAM SERIES

What Can We Learn About How Dreaming Works?

Michael Schredl

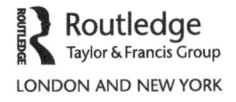
Routledge
Taylor & Francis Group

LONDON AND NEW YORK

Designed cover image: © Getty

First published 2024
by Routledge
4 Park Square, Milton Park, Abingdon, Oxon OX14 4RN

and by Routledge
605 Third Avenue, New York, NY 10158

Routledge is an imprint of the Taylor & Francis Group, an informa business

British Library Cataloguing-in-Publication Data
A catalogue record for this book is available from the British Library

ISBN: 978-1-032-29178-9 (hbk)
ISBN: 978-1-032-28749-2 (pbk)
ISBN: 978-1-003-30037-3 (ebk)

DOI: 10.4324/9781003300373

Typeset in Sabon
by Apex CoVantage, LLC

CONTENTS

PRELUDE

This book is about a long dream series: 12,679 dreams, recorded over a period of more than 30 years. As these dreams were recorded by myself, I have two different roles: being the dreamer and being the researcher analyzing the dreams. The focus of this book is not the personal meaning of the dreams; that is, the question, what can I learn from my dreams – e.g., expand my horizon based on these dream experiences, working with dreams to foster self-actualization, and so on. This was the reason I chose to refer to the dreamer in third person; that is, take on the role of the researcher. In this framework, the questions are different: What can I learn about dreaming ("How does it work?") by studying a long dream series? An example of such a question would be: How often do persons show up in the dream, even though the dreamer has had no contact with these persons for a very long time; for example, schoolmates or former romantic partners?

Being the researcher and the dreamer has many advantages, as I (researcher) know very much about the waking life of the dreamer. This knowledge is even more accessible, as I also started to keep a diary in 1986, providing useful information; for example, regarding starting and ending dates of romantic relationships. This intimate knowledge about the waking life of the dreamer facilitates coding whether a specific dream experience – for example, pain – really occurred in the dreamer's waking life (see Chapter 6). On the other hand, one can argue that I, being the author and the dreamer, might be cautious regarding which dreams were selected as examples (like Sigmund Freud in his book *The Interpretation of Dreams*). These considerations did play a role in selecting the dream examples, not only for protecting my privacy but also the privacy of my social network. However, the analyses and the statistics include all dreams I remembered – there was no selection – including dream topics like having erotic interactions with family members.

Before I start delving into the exploration of the long dream series, I would like to outline my motivation that kept me and keeps me going (it is a lot of work to record, type, and code such a large number of dreams). As a young man, I read almost every book Erich Fromm has written; his ideas about a humanistic psychology fascinated me. One of his books, *The Forgotten Language*, deals with fairytales, dreams, and myths. At that time, I did not recall any of my dreams, with the exception of a vague recollection of childhood nightmares (falling through a slimy, green mass). Erich Fromm praised dreaming a lot, so I got curious about dreams (how is it to experience and remember dreams) and bought a book about working with dreams that also included tips to increase dream recall (Ann Faraday's book, *The Dream Game*). And, it worked. After buying a dream diary, putting in the date of the next morning prior to sleep onset, I recalled my first dream after more than ten years. This was very encouraging. Sticking to the routine, dream recall increased over the next month, and today, I recall dreams almost every night (and – as you will see – also quite often after naps). For me, the most fascinating aspect of dreams is their creativity. The first year or so, I recorded several adventure dreams; being shy in waking life, these experiences were spectacular. Later on, when I started studying psychology and got into therapy and therapeutic training, I was fascinated by how dreams can depict an inner issue with such simple but illustrative means. For example, my problems with setting boundaries in social interaction in waking life were depicted in dreams in which the walls of the room I live in has gaps to the outside; or I live in a very large room with other persons and cannot have my privacy, as the room is not partitioned off; or, in one dream, my brother takes something out of my room without asking me. I also worked with my dreams in dream groups, in therapy sessions, or for myself; however, in regard to the total number of dreams I recalled, this was only a very small portion. After more than 30 years, I still like to record my dreams; they are still creative (one dream unlike another, even though some topics, like the boundary issue, come up now and then) and enrich my waking life.

I sincerely hope you like reading this book and enjoy your own dreams like I do.

Michael Schredl

1

BASICS

1.1 What is a dream?

As this book is about dreams, the most basic question is: "What is a dream?" Reviewing the dream literature, Pagel et al. (2001) started the abstract of their article, "Definitions of dream," with the following statement: "A single definition for dreaming is most likely impossible given the wide spectrum of fields engaged in the study of dreaming, and the diversity in current applied definitions" (p. 195). Despite this rather pessimistic view, these authors agreed on a few things (see as follows). The tentative statement of the authors is based on two arguments. First, the research disciplines that study the dream phenomenon are, indeed, very diverse – psychology, neurosciences, anthropology, literature sciences, cultural sciences, to name a few. Second, theories of dreams vary a lot across cultures (Mageo, 2021; Tedlock, 1991), ranging from conceptualizing dreaming as a "real" world outside our normal waking reality to views of dreams as internally created images.

The first distinction is to be made between dream (dream report) and dreaming as a state of consciousness. Whereas psychoanalytic theories link dreaming with "unconsciousness" or "subconsciousness," the modern approach defines dreaming as a distinct state of consciousness – the "dream consciousness" (Hobson et al., 2000). Within this line of thinking, it is also important to differentiate dreaming from brain activation, comparable to the differentiation in the waking state. Research clearly indicates that brain activation in related to waking consciousness – e.g., doing math is associated with brain activity in different areas than thinking about the upcoming meal after spending so much time in the scanner (Gazzaniga et al., 2019). This is crucial to keep in mind if we talk about REM sleep physiology – e.g., high

DOI: 10.4324/9781003300373-1

activation of the limbic system (Maquet et al., 1996) – and thus, not about dreaming. Similarly, the title of the paper published by Dement (1960), "The effect of dream deprivation," is misleading, as the authors deprived the participants of REM sleep – i.e., drastically interfered with their normal sleep pattern (some of the effects they found might be attributed to this). Within the discipline of psychology, dreaming can be defined as subjective experiences that occur during sleep, and the dream report, as a recollection of these subjective experiences after waking up (Schredl, 2018b). Even though these definitions seem simple at first glance, a few aspects need closer attention. First, some authors stress the fact that dreaming is simulating the waking world (Revonsuo, 2000a; Revonsuo et al., 2015); that is, with the exception of lucid dreaming, the dreamer thinks that s/he is awake while dreaming; these subjective experiences that occur while sleeping are experienced as real as subjective experiences in the waking state. In this view, fleeting images ("I saw some bizarre faces before me") or thoughts ("I can remember that I was thinking about tomorrow's exam") would not count as dreams. However, this view might be problematic because you might get similar answers if you ask a person about his waking-life experiences – e.g., "I was just thinking about my car that is broken." In waking, you can probe and ask about more details, physical sensations, emotions, surroundings, etc., and thus, get closer to the world simulation the brain performs in waking life. In view of this line of thinking, Schredl (2018b) argues that it is most practicable to use a broad definition for dreaming, including thoughts, images, and full-blown stories – as we can never be sure whether the other aspects (see the waking-life thoughts example earlier) have simply been forgotten.

Even though it seems obvious that dreaming is only accessible via the dream report – that is, what can the dreamer remember after waking up – this poses some problems regarding the definition of dreaming. Do animals dream? Do babies dream? The studies on cats (Jouvet, 1979b) in which Michel Jouvet experimentally disabled the REM atonia with brain stem lesions and so oneiric behavior during REM sleep suggest that cats have some form of experiencing during REM sleep, but they can never report it. The question whether animals can recall dream experiences is a very interesting question that is probably impossible to study empirically. Similarly, babies have a lot of REM sleep that is quite similar to REM sleep in children and adults, so they might experience something in this state of consciousness, but we (parents and researchers alike) will never know the nature of these experiences – even though changes of face expressions that occur during the baby's sleep might, at least, provide some hints about the emotional quality of these experiences. In a rare but severe sleep disorder – the REM sleep behavior disorder – the naturally occurring muscle atonia in REM sleep is partly not functional; thus, these patients can act out their dreams (Schenck et al., 1986). In one study (Valli et al., 2012), the observed behavior during acting-out episodes in RBD patients could be linked to the dream content the patients reported upon awakening. This would allow to us determine dream content without having to rely on dream reports, but this is much simpler in theory than in practice, as complex dreams with body movements would result in real movements of the dreamer that might not be in congruence with the surroundings; for example, an RBD patient dreamed about tackling a football player of the opposite team and woke up because he ran into the bedroom dresser. This example illustrated that obtaining video recordings of full-fledged dreams with a lot of action in them is rather difficult.

In sum, dream research has to rely on dream reports in order to get a glimpse into the world of subjective experiences that occur during sleep. Therefore, dream recall is a prerequisite of dream research (Schredl, 2018b), and researchers that apply dream content analysis as a research method to dream reports should keep in mind that these dream reports are more or less accurate recollections of the original dream experiences. To give examples, many dreamers focus on describing the actions going on in the dream but do not focus in equal detail on emotions, especially if they are not intense (Sikka et al., 2014); or on thoughts that occurred in the dreams (Meier, 1993). Kahan (2012) emphasized that expertise – aka. dream-reporting skills – are necessary to obtain reliable dream reports – similar to waking-life reporting; if you want a good summary of a movie a person has just watched, you should ask persons with some skills in this area.

The next important question is: How can we be sure that dream reports are recollections of experienced during sleep? The first sleep and dream researcher explicitly asking this question was Alfred Maury (1861). He woke up from a long dream about different phases of the French Revolution; the last dream segment consisted of him lying under the guillotine to be executed. Just as the blade touched his neck, Maury woke up because a wooden part of his bed fell on his neck. As the guillotine scene was a consequence of the actions that occurred previously in the dream, he assumed that the dream was produced within seconds during the waking process. This was termed the "Goblot hypothesis" (Goblot, 1896). Even in 1981, a well-known researcher (Hall, 1981) stated "Our hypothesis is that all dreaming takes place while we are waking up" (p. 245). However, it is not clear how his empirical data (a dream series of a man who lived by the ocean) support this claim – e.g., having 20% sexual dreams or urinating in dreams – as these are clearly activities the dreamer has not carried out in the awakening process. A bed was present in 18% of the dreams, but it was not stated if this was the bed he actually slept in (Hall, 1981). (For a closer look at beds in dreams, see Chapter 8.5; the actual bed the dreamer slept in occurs relatively rarely.) Is there a way to test empirically whether dream reports must be recollections of subjective experiences during sleep? The answer is simple: yes. Guénolé and Nicolas (2010) provided a review on this topic, stressing three areas:

research on incorporating external stimuli that were presented during REM sleep into dreams but are no longer present during the awakening process, the previously mentioned REM sleep behavior disorder in which patients act out their dreams, and lucid dreaming. Let's start with even another area that provided support for the claim that dream reports are recollections of experiences that occurred during sleep.

Horikawa et al. (2013) investigated sleep-onset dreams in an fMRI scanner. Three participants were allowed to fall asleep for a very brief time and then awakened to obtain dream reports, typically from sleep stage N1 (sleep onset). In the waking state, they presented the participants pictures of different motives – e.g., cars, humans – and determined the brain activation pattern in the higher visual cortices that occurred as a response to watching these different images. Then, they looked, in the dream reports, at whether one of these topics was present. Then, they analyzed the brain activity measured by the fMRI scanner prior to the awakening of this dream report, and, indeed, found an above-chance correlation with the brain activation pattern that corresponds to this image in the waking state. However, even though the prediction level was above chance, it was very low (about 60%) (Horikawa et al., 2013); thus, "dream reading," defined as decoding the dream content based on fMRI data, is still science fiction. However, the correlation of brain activity prior to the awakening with the content of the dream clearly contradicts the Goblot hypothesis that dream reports are generated during the awakening process. Similar studies using EEG, especially high-density EEG, could confirm these findings. The EEG methodology is better suited for recording longer periods of sleep, as it is very difficult for most people to sleep more than an hour in the scanner, not because of the noise (there are sophisticated noise-cancelling systems) but because the head is fixated and is not allowed to move. Hong et al. (1996), for example, found a correlation between brain activity over the Wernicke and Broca areas if the person is talking or listening to speech – again, the brain activity measured prior to awaking and obtaining the dream report. Siclari et al. (2017) were able to replicate this finding using high-density EEG; 4 to 2 seconds prior to awakening, there was activity in the Wernicke area if the dream report included some form of speech. For other areas (fusiform face area and posterior parietal cortex), they also found a correlation to the corresponding dream contents – faces in the first case and spatial setting in the second (Siclari et al., 2017). Similarly, autonomic parameters like heart rate, galvanic skin response, or heart rate variability can be measured and linked to dream content. Paul et al. (2019) were able to demonstrate that heart rate, eye movement density, and other autonomic parameters increased prior to waking up from a nightmare – in comparison to waking up from normal, non-nightmarish dreams. This is also the case for the stress hormone cortisol (Hess et al., 2020). These studies clearly indicate that physiological activity prior to awakening is related to dream content.

Dream researchers, starting with Weygandt (1893), presented a lot of different stimuli during REM sleep in order to test whether these stimuli are incorporated into dreams (Schredl, 2018b). The event-related potential (ERP) paradigm (Ibanez et al., 2009) was able to demonstrate that the brain is processing incoming stimuli, even though the sleeper does not react to nor awaken from the stimuli. The ERP method is relatively simple: a stimulus is applied, and the subsequent changes in brain activity are measured, typically with EEG. It is often necessary to repeat this up to 50 times because the changes due to stimulus processing in the EEG are rather small compared to the background activity. If done properly, it can be shown that stimuli are definitely processed by the sleeping brain. One can even use paradigms to show that simple cognitive tasks can be carried out during sleep – e.g., the odd-ball paradigm, where the brain is recognizing that one tone is frequently occurring and the other tone occurs relatively rarely (Takahara et al., 2006). The research assistant was singing a piece of the opera Lohengrin (Richard Wagner) while Wilhem Weygandt was sleeping; he dreamed that angels descended from heaven singing exactly this tune (Weygandt, 1893). From a scientific standpoint, this first study of incorporating external stimuli can be criticized: first, he does not have the EEG measure to prove that the presentation took place during sleep, or particularly, during REM sleep; and secondly, the singing was still present when the dreamer awakened, so Weygandt's experiment could not rule out the Goblot hypothesis. However, modern studies were able to overcome these obstacles. First, they used EEG measures, typically waiting for 5 to 15 minutes of stable REM sleep, in order to apply the stimulus. In many studies, pretests were run to ensure that the stimuli did not awaken the sleeper (stimulus intensity below awakening threshold) but were also above the perceptual threshold, and thus, processed by the brain. By measuring the EEG during stimulation, the researchers could ensure that the sleeper was not waking up (otherwise, the try would be dropped from the data analysis). Second, the researcher did not awaken the participant immediately after stimulation but waited for 30 to 60 seconds and then collected the dream report. In this case, the participant does not know what was going on prior to awakening. Third, to ensure that the dreamer did not dream about the stimulus because s/he expected stimulation, most studies included a sham condition; that is, carrying out awakenings without stimulation. In the analysis, these dreams were compared with the dream reports after stimulation – serving as a kind of baseline. In the study of Schredl, Atanasova, et al. (2009), olfactory dreams were reported also in the control condition – e.g., not related to any external stimuli, but dreams also incorporate expectations, as the participants knew that they were participating in a study about olfactory stimuli. Adhering to all these methodological issues, research clearly indicated that external stimuli (tones, names, mild pain stimuli, traffic noise, water spray) can be incorporated into dreams; the incorporations rates varied from 9%

(sinus tone) to 60% (water spray), thus showing that dreams are recollections of experiences that occurred during sleep.

Another line of evidence is based on study of a specific patient group that suffers from REM sleep behavior disorder (as mentioned earlier). In healthy participants, the impulses from the motor cortex to the muscles in the body (with the exception of the eye muscles) are actively blocked by a brain center in the brain stem, but in this specific sleep disorder, the neurons responsible for this blockading are partially damaged due to neurodegenerative processes (Silber et al., 2022). This is the reason why almost all of these patients develop, after 10 to 15 years, a neurodegenerative disease like Parkinson's (Schenck et al., 1993). In a very labor-intensive study (Valli et al., 2012) using video recordings of patients with REM sleep behavior disorder, external judges were able to link the observed behavior to the dream report obtained after awakening. The main problem, in this study, was that the participants very rarely display complex behavior during REM sleep; for example, it could be only a simple hand movement. For more complex behavior seen on the video, it was relatively easy to link the video to the corresponding dream report; however, it was very difficult or even impossible for the minor movements (Valli et al., 2012). Again, as the behavior occurred prior to awakening, the idea that dream reports are generated during the process of waking up is very unlikely.

Guénolé and Nicolas (2010) also suggested that lucid dream research can contribute to the question of whether dream reports are recollections of experiences that occurred during sleep. Even though it could be demonstrated that lucid dreams (most of them) occur during REM sleep (Hearne, 1978; LaBerge, 1980b), it has also been shown that there are differences in brain activation – e.g., in the prefrontal areas (Baird et al., 2022; Dresler et al., 2012) – between REM sleep with lucid dreaming and REM sleep with normal dreaming and, thus, lucid dreaming as a state might differ from non-lucid dreaming consciousness. In lucid dreams, the dreamer is aware that s/he is dreaming while still dreaming (LaBerge, 1985); and experienced lucid dreamers can deliberately perform actions during the dream, like knee bends (Erlacher et al., 2003) or throwing darts (Schädlich et al., 2017). Especially interesting for the topic on hand is that they can perform pre-arranged (with the experimenter prior to sleep-onset) eye movements, and these dreamed eye movements are actually carried out (no REM sleep muscle atonia in the eye muscles) and can be measured with the electrooculogram (EEG) channels included in the standard polysomnography (Dresler et al., 2022). The typical paradigm is to instruct the lucid dreamer to signal whether s/he became lucid by two left-right-left-right eye movement signals, then carry out a task – e.g., counting to 10, 20, or 30 (Erlacher et al., 2014) – perform eye signals again, and then wake up (proficient lucid dreamers can wake themselves up). Then, the lucid dreamer is reporting the dream experience in as much detail as possible, like doing eye signals, the activities between the pre-arranged eye movements, and so on. A large number of studies since the pioneering efforts of Keith Hearne and Stephen LaBerge were able to demonstrate that the dream reports match the polysomnographic recordings of the eye movements (EOG channels) very well (Dresler et al., 2022). Again, the correlation between measures obtained during sleep prior to the awakenings with the dream reports clearly refute the Goblot hypothesis.

Overall, the empirical studies convincingly demonstrated that dream reports obtained after forced awakenings in the sleep lab and, most likely, dream reports upon spontaneous awakening at home are recollections of experiences that occurred during sleep; that is, reflecting dream consciousness. Given this definition, subjective experiences occurring in other states of consciousness like sleepwalking (Oudiette et al., 2009), sleep paralysis (Sharpless & Barber, 2011), or anesthesia (Mashour, 2011) are not "really" dreams. As these states are physiologically different from sleep, one might argue that one should not use the term "dreaming" or "dreams" for the experiences in these states but use something like "dream-like" experiences because it has been demonstrated that, on a phenomenological level, there are many similarities between those experiences and dreams (Idir et al., 2022; Mashour, 2011; Sharpless & Barber, 2011). Similarly, there seems to be a considerable overlap between mind-wandering ("daydreaming" is a term that was also used in the past) and dreaming (Domhoff, 2018b) regarding phenomenology, although the two phenomena occur in very different brain states (awake vs. asleep).

1.2 What do we dream about?

After defining dreams as recollections of experiences that occurred during sleep, the next questions are: "What do we dream about?" and "How is dream content related to the waking life?".

Hobson and McCarley (1977) formulated the activation-synthesis hypothesis of dreaming, arguing against the psychoanalytic view that "the interpretation of dreams is the royal road to a knowledge of the unconscious activities of the mind" (p. 769; Freud, 1900/1991). In their model, the cortex is stimulated more or less randomly by the brain stem (brain areas regulating REM sleep), and the forebrain synthesizes the dream from these activated memories into a somewhat coherent story. Interestingly, this theory does not contradict the idea that dreams reflect waking-life experiences (see as follows) but challenges the view that dreaming – defined as subjective experiences during sleep – has a specific purpose or function. Even more focused on the bizarre quality of many dreams, Crick and Mitchison (1983) hypothesized that we dream about things, especially associations between those things, that we should forget. Based on the functionality of neural networks, they outlined the idea that these networks are stimulated during REM sleep and produce unwarranted associations with the idea that the neural network can get rid of these parasitic modes ("reverse learning"). One should keep in mind that this theory is arguing on a neuronal level (see section on the functions of dreams) and not on a consciousness level. Thus, even if the neurons are doing something during REM sleep, it is far from sure that dreaming – defined as subjective experiences during sleep – is involved in this.

In contrast to these very influential neuroscientists, Bell and Hall (1971) focused on the similarities between waking and dreaming, stating: "The continuity hypothesis holds general speaking because dreams and waking behavior are both motivated by the same unfulfilled impulses" (p. 123). In a later book, Calvin S. Hall gave a more detailed description of the continuity hypothesis:

> These facts and many others obtained from the content analysis of many dream series have led us to formulate what we call the *continuity hypothesis*. This hypothesis states that dreams are continuous with waking life; the world of dreaming and the world of waking are one. The dream world is neither discontinuous nor inverse in its relationship to the conscious world. We remain the same person, the same personality with the same characteristics, and the same basic beliefs and convictions whether awake or asleep. The wishes and fears that determine our actions and thoughts in everyday life also determine what we will dream about.
>
> *(p. 104; Hall & Nordby, 1972)*

Even though these claims are very clearly formulated, these statements also raise many questions. First, does everything we experience in our waking life show up in subsequent dreams with the same probability, or are they factors that influence the chance of waking-life experiences being incorporated into a dream? Second, some dream contents – e.g., flying without any appropriate means – clearly do not reflect waking-life experience; how does the continuity hypothesis account for that?

In the following, the original continuity hypothesis formulated by Hall and Nordby (1972) will be expanded and specified. For more information, see Schredl (2003) and Schredl (2012b). One point of discussion in the literature is about the types of waking-life aspects that show up in dreams – e.g., preoccupations, conceptions, thoughts, experiences, emotions, etc. – as these have not been specified in the original formulation (Domhoff, 2017a, 2017b, 2018a; Erdelyi, 2017; Jenkins, 2018; Schredl, 2017c). One might argue that these lines of thinking do not exclude each other (Schredl, 2012b); for example, if a person is preoccupied with cars, he might spent a lot of time driving a car (experience), thinking about cars (thoughts), talking with other car-interested persons, reading about cars, and so on. So, if this person dreams more often about cars than persons without a preoccupation with cars, it cannot be determined whether the preoccupation is related to dream content and/or the number of waking-life experiences around cars – including thoughts.

An interesting expansion of the original continuity hypothesis is the differentiation between different types of continuity (see Table 1.1). The most intuitive form is thematic continuity; for example, persons who own a dog dream more often about dogs (Schredl, Bailer, et al., 2020). Thus, the topic itself is reflected in the dream. Within this context, it is important that thematic continuity does not imply that we dream about waking-life experiences exactly the way they happen; the definition of thematic continuity is broader. Dreams with exact replays of waking-life events seem to be very rare (Fosse et al., 2003; Malinowski & Horton, 2014b); more often, topics are embedded in other contexts; for example, a friend can show up in a work-related setting in the dream, even though the friend never visited the dreamer at work in waking life.

Emotional continuity claims that the waking-life emotions are incorporated into dreams, even if the content is different – e.g., a stressful job can be reflected in negative work-related dreams (thematic continuity) but also in negatively toned dreams with other topics (emotional continuity). This might help to explain – at least partially – bizarre dream topics like flying. The flying dream does not reflect a waking-life experience of flying on a thematic level but might reflect positive waking-emotions (as positive emotions are typically experienced during flying dreams). Some preliminary evidence for this line of thinking was provided by Schredl (2008c). Similarly, hobby-related dreams were more negatively toned if job-related stress (waking life) was higher (Schredl, Coors, et al., 2022). Thus, negative emotions experienced during waking can show up in dreams with topics that are completely independent from the waking-life situations the negative emotion was associated with.

The idea of the metacognitive continuity came into focus with studies reporting that meditators do more often experience lucid dreams (Reed,

TABLE 1.1 Types of continuity

Category	Description
Thematic continuity	Dream contents reflect waking life – e.g., music students dream about music.
Emotional continuity	The emotional quality of waking-life experiences is reflected in the dream emotions but not necessarily in the content.
Metacognitive continuity	Persons who are self-reflective in waking life are also more self-reflective in dreams.
Continuity of formal characteristics	Persons with bizarre thinking – for example, patients with schizophrenia – also experience more bizarre dreams.

1978; Stumbrys et al., 2015); thus, metacognitive skills in waking like mindfulness are related to the metacognitive skill of reflecting on one's own state of consciousness in dreams (Kahan & Sullivan, 2012), which is necessary for lucid dreaming (Stumbrys, 2011).

The last type of continuity focuses on formal aspects of the dreams; for example, creative persons have more creative dreams (Pagel & Kwiatkowski, 2003; Sierra-Siegert et al., 2019). Another example would be that patients with schizophrenia, whose thinking is more bizarre, also report more bizarre dreams (Schredl & Engelhardt, 2001).

The classification of different types of continuity highlights the broadness of the continuity concept; a large variety of the waking-life aspects can be reflected in dreams.

Based on the original formulation of the continuity hypothesis (Hall & Nordby, 1972), one might get the impression that everything we experience in waking life might have equally large chances to show up in subsequent dreams. But, this is not the case; empirical research supports the notion that there are factors that affect the probability of a waking-life experience being incorporated into subsequent dreams; some waking-life experiences are more likely to show up in dreams than others (Schredl, 2003). Several of these factors are presented in Table 1.2.

Sigmund Freud (1900/1991) observed that "dreams show a clear preference for the impressions of the immediately preceding days (p. 247)" – the so-called day-residue effect. This was confirmed by later studies (Blagrove et al., 2011; Botman & Crovitz, 1989; Vallat et al., 2017). From a methodological viewpoint, it has to be mentioned that it might be difficult to look at longer time intervals between waking-life experience and dreams, especially if thoughts are also included as possible instigators of dream content. Typically, there is an exponential decrease in the chance of being incorporated into the dream the longer ago the event was (Botman & Crovitz, 1989; Strauch & Meier, 1996). There are some data (Malinowski & Horton, 2021; Roussy et al., 1998; Verdone, 1965) indicating that dreams from the first part of the night are more likely to reflect recent waking-life experiences, whereas dreams of the later part of the night can also include elements with remote time references. Interestingly, the dream-lag affect, saying that

TABLE 1.2 Factors affecting continuity

Factor
Time interval between waking-life event and dream
Emotional intensity of the waking-life experience
Type of waking-life experience
Personality factors

the chance of dreaming of a waking-life event increases on days 5 to 7, compared to the days before (with the exception of day 1 [day residue]) (Blagrove et al., 2011; Nielsen & Powell, 1989), might be related to this change of time references of the night, as many dream-lag studies used dream diaries in the home setting, typically eliciting dreams of the second part of the night. The factor would describe that waking-life elements that occurred a long time ago had a smaller chance of being incorporated into a dream.

A variety of studies (see Schredl, 2018b) showed that some life events can occur in dreams even after decades – e.g., World War II-related dreams were reported 55 years after the war ended (Schredl & Piel, 2006). These findings point to the fact that emotionally intense waking-life experiences have a higher chance of being incorporated into dreams. Using a daytime diary with eliciting waking-life events and ratings of their emotional intensity as well as a dream diary, two studies (Malinowski & Horton, 2014a; Schredl, 2006) were able to demonstrate that emotional intensity but not emotional valence increases the probability of dreaming about a waking-life experience. The idea that we dream preferentially of negative life events was not supported. From a methodological viewpoint, it seems very important to use a prospective design to study this factor, as retrospective studies – e.g., Vallat et al. (2017) – asked the participants after they dreamed of the waking-life event about its emotional intensity and valence. It seems plausible that this might bias the results, as a person might think: "I dreamed about it; thus, it might be more important than I previously thought."

Hartmann (2000) showed that we dream relatively rarely about focused cognitive activities like reading, writing, or doing math, even though a considerable amount of time during the day is spent on these activities. These findings were confirmed by subsequent studies (Schredl & Erlacher, 2008; Schredl & Hofmann, 2003) and emphasized that the type of waking-life activity affects its chance of being incorporated into dreams. Hartmann (2000) speculated that the brain, in REM sleep, is not as capable of performing these cognitive activities, compared to the waking brain. Based on the personal experience of the author with his own dreams and dreams of others, there are some everyday topics that very rarely show up in dreams – e.g., riding a train for several hours, waiting a long time in the consulting room of a physician, and so on. Thus, there seems to be preferences for what waking-life experiences show up in dreams. Another finding of Schredl and Hofmann (2003) was that the participants dreamed relatively often about spending time with friends in relation to the time spent with friends in the waking state. This finding was replicated by studies (Tuominen et al., 2021; Tuominen, Stenberg, et al., 2019) investigating the Social Simulation Theory (SST) and termed this result "sociality bias." As this theory states that dreams provided the opportunity to improve social skills, the finding that social interactions play an important role in dreams and are overrepresented compared to other waking-life activities would fit in very well.

Even though it seems plausible that personality dimensions can moderate the magnitude of continuity between waking and dreaming, research in this area is scarce. For example, persons with thin boundaries (Hartmann, 1991) have fluid boundaries between sleep and waking, different states of consciousness; thus, one might expect that persons with thin boundaries are more likely to incorporate recent events into their dreams than persons with thick boundaries. Some preliminary evidence supporting this idea was provided by Schredl et al. (1996). One might even speculate that other trait factors, or even genetic make-up, might have an effect on the relationship between waking life and dreams. However, research looking into inter-individual differences regarding the continuity between waking and dreaming is still lacking.

To summarize, empirical dream studies have shown that dreams are full of waking-life experiences, especially the salient ones; however, the whole variety of factors that affect this continuity between waking and dreams has to be studied in more detail in the future. Within this context, it is also important to notice that there is a continuity the other way around; that is, dreams can affect the waking state; for example, dream emotions can linger – positive ones (Stocks et al., 2020) as well as negative ones (Köthe & Pietrowsky, 2001). One study (Schredl & Reinhard, 2009–2010) could even show a second-order continuity; that is, dreams that were affected by the previous day are more likely to affect the day after waking up from this dream. This might reflect a continuous stream of consciousness processing information night and day (Bakan, 1978). The overlapping phenomenology and underlying brain physiology (default mode network) between dreaming and daydream respective mind-wandering (Domhoff, 2018b; Fazekas & Nemeth, 2020; Fox, 2018) fits in perfectly with this concept.

1.3 Does dreaming have a function?

The question "Why we dream?" has puzzled many scientists; a large number of theories have been published over the years (see Table 1.3).

A detailed description of the theories and the evidence supporting the claims of the authors is beyond the scope of this chapter. The focus will be on the simple (or maybe not so simple) question how we can empirically test these theories postulating possible functions of dreaming. In order to follow the theoretical considerations and research designs that have been chosen to study possible dream functions more easily, the theories of Table 1.3 can be grouped into four broader categories (see Table 1.4).

The simulation theories, especially the Threat Simulation Theory (TST) and the SST, emphasize the idea that the dreamer is training her or his skills in dealing with threats or her or his social skills to be better prepared for future, possibly similar, situations. Bulkeley (2019) proposed an interesting

TABLE 1.3 Theories on possible functions of dreaming

Theories	Authors
• Guardian of sleep	Freud (1900/1991))
• Compensation	Jung (1979)
• Iterative programming	Jouvet (1999)
• Reverse-learning hypothesis	Crick and Mitchison (1983)
• Mastery hypothesis	Wright and Koulack (1987)
• Systematic desensitization	Perlis and Nielsen (1993)
• Threat Simulation Theory	Revonsuo (2000b)
• Selective mood regulation theory	Kramer (2007)
• Protoconsciousness theory	Hobson (2009)
• Sleep-dependent memory consolidation	Wamsley et al. (2010)
• Social Simulation Theory	Revonsuo et al. (2015)
• Dreaming as imaginative play	Bulkeley (2019)
• Empathy theory of dreaming	Blagrove et al. (2019)
• Overfitted brain hypothesis	Hoel (2021)
• Network exploration to understand possibilities (NEXTUP)	Zadra and Stickgold (2021)
• Constructive episodic simulation hypothesis	Wamsley (2022)

TABLE 1.4 Categorizing theories on dream functions

Simulation theories	Within dreams, we practice skills to prepare for future events.
Memory theories	Dreaming is involved in sleep-dependent memory consolidation.
Emotion regulation theories	Dreams help us to regulate (negative) emotions.
Creativity theories	Dreaming stimulates waking-life creativity.

analogy between dreaming and children's play. Interestingly, already, Maeder (1912) emphasized this analogy; that is, comparing dreams with children's play. Even though playing has no specific goal or learning objective, the child is training his or her skills in many ways while playing – e.g., motor skills but often also social skills. The analogy would be that the subjective experiences during sleep – i.e., dreaming – prepare us for coping with upcoming issues in waking-life more effectively.

The memory theories assume that dreaming plays a role in sleep-dependent memory consolidation. A vast body of research shows that sleep is, indeed, beneficial for memory consolidation (Berres & Erdfelder, 2021; Diekelmann et al., 2009). Although a strong and statistically significant association between task-related dreaming and memory performance was reported in a meta-analysis (Hudachek & Wamsley, 2023), the question whether dreaming just reflects the workings of the brain or whether dreams play a crucial and active role for memory consolidation is still open for debate (Wamsley, 2018). If the latter (just reflecting), dreaming would not have an extra function in addition to the function of sleep.

Sigmund Freud's theory of dreams as guardians of sleep can be grouped into the emotion regulation theories, as the dream process fulfills an unconscious wish that, otherwise, would have caused awakening. In modern theories of mood regulation (Kramer, 2007), nightmares (dreams from which the dreamer wakes up) can be seen as a failure of the mood regulation function; thus, the emotion was too strong to be processed and "softened" during sleep – indicative of the mood-regulating function of dreaming. Interestingly, Walker and van der Helm (2009) postulated a similar theory for the function of REM sleep; that is, on a physiological level (possibly without involvement of dreams or maybe dreams just reflect this neuronal processes in some form), a decoupling between content of the experience and its emotions takes place. The idea that dreaming is comparable to systematic desensitization (a frequently used cognitive-behavioral technique) was based on the idea that muscle tone is very low in REM sleep (Perlis & Nielsen, 1993); but the problem is that, in waking life, low muscle tone is typically associated with anxiety-free, relaxed states of mind; this is not the case in dreams, especially in nightmares. So, the idea that dreams can be helpful in reducing fears might not be valid.

The literature is full of anecdotes that dreams stimulated waking-life creativity (Barrett, 2001; Schredl & Erlacher, 2007); for example, Paul McCartney dreamed the melody of "Yesterday" (Webb, 2017). In many models of problem solving, one step is called "brainstorming" (Isaksen & Gaulin, 2005) – i.e., producing ideas or possible solutions without evaluating whether this can actually be realized for the given problem. Given the creative nature of dreaming, in which we make new and unexpected connections (Hartmann, 2007), several authors speculated about dreams being helpful in solving problems (Wright & Koulack, 1987; Zadra & Stickgold, 2021).

Even though all theories presented in Table 1.3 with their categorization in Table 1.4 seem very plausible – dreams help to work through emotional issues and prepare us for the future – the question remains: "Can we test any of these theories empirically; that is, whether dreaming has an important function for humans (or mammals and birds)?" The opposite view might also be plausible; subjective experiencing during the waking state has been important (and still is), especially for humans; for example, for accumulating knowledge, beneficial cooperation in hunting, and finding a mate to produce offspring; but nature didn't bother to "turn off" these subjective experiences during sleep. In this view, dreaming would have no function at all, at the best reflecting what is going on in the mind of the sleeper while the brain is doing its crucial work on a neuronal level (conceptualized in the different functions of sleep).

Prior to discussing possible empirical designs to study possible dream functions, a few theoretical topics that are important in this context will be introduced (see Table 1.5).

The term "function" can be used in different ways; for example, something has a function within a system; for example, it is important for the wellbeing of the person to have mood-regulation mechanisms. On the other hand, an evolutionary function encompasses that the phenomenon (in our case, dreaming) has been selected for by natural selection; that is, humans without dreaming (if they have ever existed, as mammals might also have some kind of subjective experiences during sleep, especially REM sleep) would have had much lower chances of reproducing than humans who dream. As mentioned earlier, this sounds relatively simple at first; that is, dreaming is present in every human because dreaming has helped our ancestors to survive and reproduce. However, if taking a closer look, the picture gets more complicated. First, the unanswered question of whether animals dream (have some kind of subjective experience during sleep) raises the question of whether natural selection might have worked on mammals long before human species showed up on Earth. Second, as dreaming is a complex phenomenon linked to a lot of other complex phenomena like thinking and mind-wandering in the waking state, it might be difficult to differentiate whether dreaming is a specific function or is just some kind of "byproduct" of these other characteristics that might have been selected for.

Zadra and Stickgold (2021) explicitly emphasized that dreaming fulfills its function (exploring possibilities to facilitate coping with future challenges), even if not remembered. This accounts for the fact that even prodigious dream recallers can remember only a small portion of all dreamed dreams,

TABLE 1.5 Theoretical topics regarding dream functions

Topic	Content
• What do we mean by "function"?	Function within the psyche – e.g., mood regulation – vs. evolutionary function.
• Dreamed dream vs. remembered dream	Does dreaming – even if not recalled – have a function or are only recalled dreams beneficial?
• Possible dream functions differ from functions of waking consciousness	Possible functions between dreaming and daydreaming might overlap (default mode network).
• Subjective level (dream consciousness) vs. physiological level (brain)	Are changes in neural networks related to dreaming?

let alone the less prodigious dream recallers, recalling one dream per month or even reporting never having recalled a dream for years. The question is, how can something have a vital function if it shows up so rarely (remembered dreams). On the other hand, waking-life creativity was always stimulated by remembered dreams (Klepel et al., 2019); otherwise, it would not be possible to link a new idea to a dream (as it might have come up in the waking state). However, testing the function of unremembered dreams – that is, whether they are beneficial for waking life – seems (or is) impossible to do (see the following).

Given the overlap between dreaming and mind-wandering (daydreaming) regarding their phenomenology (Kunzendorf et al., 1997) and neuronal underpinning (Domhoff, 2018b; Fazekas & Nemeth, 2020; Fox, 2018), the question arises whether daydreaming and dreaming may have similar functions. However, this question is still unanswered. One can easily imagine that this might be the case for creative input – ideas stemming from dreams have been reported – but also, ideas can pop up during mind-wandering (the creative periods of artists). The last point presented in Table 1.5 refers to the distinction between the physiological level – e.g., neuronal activity – and the psychological level (subjective experiences). One can easily imagine that a lot of physiological processes are happening in the sleeping brain; for example, sleep-dependent memory consolidation by strengthening connectivity between neurons or pruning (disconnecting neurons); however, these processes are very likely not reflected in dreams. This is not specific for sleep; also, in the waking state, the brain is processing a lot of information – for example, regulating breathing – without any subjective awareness. That is, even though research has shown that sleep has a lot of vitally important functions (Krone & Vyazovskiy, 2019), this does not automatically imply that dreaming also has a function or even plays a role in the functions postulated for sleep.

After presenting some of the theories and theoretical issues that are related to possible dream functions, the question is, what approaches researchers have selected to test whether dreaming has any function in a sense that it played a pivotal role in evolution by providing an edge in the process of natural selection. So far, four paradigms have been used in empirical dream research (see Table 1.6).

TABLE 1.6 Paradigms to study possible dream functions

- "Dream deprivation"
- Effects of specific dream content on waking life
- Sleep-dependent memory consolidation
- Lucid dreaming

The simplest way to test whether dreaming is beneficial for subsequent waking life is to experimentally manipulate the occurrence of dreaming. An even simpler way would be to compare persons who dream with persons who do not dream, but this is not possible, as researchers agree that dreaming is present during every night in every person, even if the person does not remember any dreams (Schredl, 2018b). The first study aiming at manipulating the amount of dreaming was titled "The effect of dream deprivation" and was carried out and published by Dement (1960). In those days, the concept that dreaming was almost exclusively present in REM sleep prevailed. Foulkes (1962) was the first to show that this concept was not correct, indicating that NREM dreams, especially in the second part of the night, can be as elaborated as REM dreams, even though most of the NREM dreams are shorter. In his study, Dement (1960) woke up eight young, male volunteers as soon as they entered REM sleep for 3 to 7 consecutive nights. He achieved a reduction of REM sleep of 65% to 75% but had to perform up to 30 awakenings per night because the brain tried to make up for the lost REM sleep – a phenomenon called REM rebound (which was also present in the recovery nights after REM sleep deprivation). After the REM sleep deprivation nights, the participants reported increased anxiety and irritability as well as difficulties in concentrating and an increase in appetite. These negative effects were not so strong in the control condition; the participants underwent a second set of nights with NREM awakenings with a similar number of awakenings per night (in this condition, the percentage of REM sleep was not reduced). Luckily, all these negative effects of the REM sleep deprivation vanished after a recovery night with sufficient REM sleep. There are two major problems with the study of Dement (1960). First, the findings did not allow for the differentiation between physiological and psychological levels, as the effects might be explained by the REM sleep deprivation and the dramatically altered sleep pattern (up to 30 awakenings per night). Thus, the title "Dream deprivation" was misleading. In addition, this type of experiment would have to differentiate between functions of dreaming during REM sleep and dreaming during NREM sleep, as NREM sleep and, therefore, NREM dreaming was not different between the two conditions (never outlined by the authors). Secondly, the NREM awakenings always happened after the REM awakening block; this was necessary to match the number of awakenings per night. One can easily imagine that the participants got more used to the stressful protocol the second time around and, thus, the negative effects were not as strong as during the first block. Subsequent research (Ellman et al., 1991), indeed, showed that REM sleep deprivation was not interfering with mental health in a special way, indicating that the stress of being awakened 30 times a night was the main factor in explaining the negative effects. As some theorists (Noble, 1950) linked schizophrenia with dreams – that is, that symptoms of schizophrenia are dreams breaking through into waking consciousness – one hypothesis was that dream deprivation might trigger schizophrenia. This was not the case (Ellman et al., 1991). For patients with depression, it was even the other way around; for a substantial number of patients (about 60%), REM sleep deprivation had positive effects on their mood of the next day (Vogel et al., 1975). As total sleep deprivation is as effective as REM sleep deprivation and much easier to carry out, today, sleep deprivation is used as therapeutic tool in the treatment of mood disorder (Geoffroy & Palagini, 2021). But, for the purpose of studying possible functions of dreaming, the REM deprivation paradigm is not adequate.

The second approach is illustrated by the study of Cartwright et al. (1984). They studied dreams obtained in two nights with REM awakenings in the sleep lab from N = 10 non-depressed divorcees (females, age mean = 37 yrs) and N = 19 depressed divorcees (females, age mean = 37 yrs) and found that dream roles like "wife," separated, or "ex-wife" and "alone" were more prominent in the non-depressed group compared to the depressed group. Their conclusion was that these dreams related to the divorce, and the changing life circumstances had helped the divorcees to work through the difficult transition period. One argument against this interpretation is that dreams just reflect processes that occurred during waking – i.e., the waking consciousness has achieved the adaptation and the dream consciousness is just re-iterating these changes. A second argument is that changes in waking life could be attributed to the dream processed in the waking state. That is, I dreamed about my ex-husband; thus, I should think about this and increase my efforts to cope with this. In this line of thinking, the beneficial effect of dreams is only present if the dream is recalled and stimulates the waking consciousness to solve this problem. Even more obvious is this in the case of creative dreams, as only the remembered dream provides the creative input. If the person would not have recalled a dream and had an inspiration in the morning, you can never be sure whether this was part of an unremembered dream or simply an inspiration that occurred during the waking state. Thus, looking closer at the paradigm of studying effects of specific dream contents on subsequent life indicates that this approach also does not allow us to study the function of dreaming (including all the unremembered dreams) directly.

The third approach combined the paradigms applied in studying sleep-dependent memory consolidation and in dream research. Wamsley et al. (2010) studied N = 50 healthy students, presenting them a learning task (maze task on the computer with different routes to find), allowed them to sleep (an afternoon nap in the sleep laboratory), and retested their performance after five hours. Four participants reported a dream related to the maze task; however, the definition of incorporation was very broad – e.g., hearing the music played while doing the task was one dream classified as task-related. These four participants increased their pre-nap to post-nap performance much more than the participants with no dream reports. However, the performance levels of the both groups were similar in the post-nap test; the "dreamers" started much worse compared to the others. So, one critical question might be: "Did they dream about the maze because they worried about their bad performance?" Even though Wamsley and Stickgold (2019) could replicate this finding (interestingly, the "maze dreamers" also started with worse pre-sleep testing scores than the rest group), the meta-analysis carried out by Hudachek and Wamsley (2023) showed that REM dreams that were task-related were not associated with performance increases after sleep – only task-related NREM dreams. But, regarding the task at hand – namely, testing whether dreams has any function – this research paradigm is also not helpful, as the authors (Hudachek & Wamsley, 2023) indicate that task-related dreams might reflect processes that are involved in sleep-dependent memory consolidation but are not responsible for the improvement. In order to really test a possible dream function, it would be necessary to manipulate dream content without the knowledge of the dreamer, as was done in the movie "Inception" (Fleming, 2012). So far, this is not possible in the real, non-cinematic world.

This experimental manipulation of dream content is possible in a specific form of dreaming: the so-called lucid dreams. Sophisticated, lucid dreamers can carry out tasks the experimenter suggested to them prior to sleep onset (Dresler et al., 2022). In one study (Erlacher & Schredl, 2010), participants were instructed to train a coin-tossing task (trying to toss a coin into a cup from a distance of two meters) in the evening and – if they became lucid in their dream – to train the same task in their dream. The basic principle is analog to the mental training athletes carried out in the waking state and which has been shown to improve performance (Vealey, 2007). And, indeed, the successful lucid dreamers (N = 7) were able to improve their performance more than the unsuccessful lucid dreams (N = 13) and the control group (N = 10) (Erlacher & Schredl, 2010). In a subsequent study using darts throwing as a task (Schädlich et al., 2017), it could be demonstrated that only the participants (N = 4) who were able to practice in a systematic way during the lucid dream improved their performance, whereas the other lucid dreamers who had problems with the training in the dream (distractions, darts deforming, etc.) did not improve. This is interesting in the context of the studies looking at memory consolidation and dreaming, as the task-related dreams – even if they coincide with performance increases in the post-sleep test – are not really practicing dreams – i.e., the dreamer is practicing actively the task but just a more or less distant association with the task (see the Wamsley study, earlier). Although not systematically studied, it is the impression of the author that normal (non-lucid) dreaming very rarely (if at all) depicts training sessions in a sense that the dreamer is practicing a skill in a formalized way for several minutes (as had been done in the lucid dream studies). Thus, the lucid dream research – even though it shows that lucid dream training can improve waking performance – seems unhelpful in answering the question of whether normal dreams have a function in the sense that skills are trained while dreaming (see simulation theories).

To summarize the brief review about studying possible functions of dreams empirically (see Table 1.6): the honest answer to the question "Does dreaming have a function?" is "We don't know, yet." As direct approaches like experimentally manipulating dream content or decoding dreams using imagining techniques without having to rely on the dream report to test whether dreams have been or are beneficial for survival as a species are currently not available, the question is whether there might be indirect clues to possible dream functions; for example, the findings regarding the sociality bias (we dream proportionately more about social interactions compared to cognitive activities) might point at a function of dreaming being to improve social skills (Tuominen, Revonsuo, et al., 2019). In Chapter 11, the author will discuss whether the extensive analysis of the long dream series presented in this book might provide any clues about possible dream functions.

Lastly, it is important to emphasize that working with remembered dreams in waking is beneficial (Edwards et al., 2015; Hill & Goates, 2004), even though dreaming itself might have no function at all.

2

HISTORY OF LONGITUDINAL RESEARCH WITH DREAM SERIES

Several early dream researchers (Calkins, 1893; Köhler, 1912; Kraepelin, 1906; Maury, 1861; Saint-Denys, 1982; Van Eeden, 1913) recorded their own dreams in order to have material for doing statistics – e.g., sensory perception in dreams (Calkins, 1893), increase in frequency of lucid dreams (French original published in 1867; Saint-Denys, 1982), or unusual usage of language in dreams (Kraepelin, 1906). Also, Sigmund Freud kept a dream diary and included some of his own dreams – e.g., dream of "Irma's injection" as illustrative examples in his publications (Freud, 1900/1991). Even more impressive are Carl Gustav Jung's dreams in his autobiography (Jung & Jaffé, 1967) and *The Red Book* (Harris, 2010).

In addition to dream researchers, dream diaries were kept by a number prominent persons whose dream journals have been published: authors like Franz Kafka, Graham Greene, Jack Kerouac, and William S. Burroughs (Sturzenacker & Pearson, 2012) or writers Heiner Kipphardt (Kipphardt, 1986) and Arthur Schnitzler (Schnitzler, 2012), physicist Wolfgang Pauli (Lindorff, 1995), Gerolane Cardano (1501 to 1576) (Fierz, 1987), scientist Macfarlane Smith (Sladen & Frings, 1990), and an actress (Bender & Mischo, 1960). For example, Bender and Mischo (1961) used the diary approach (the actress was sending the researchers the dreams on a regular basis) to study pre-cognition; that is, the dreamer should state after recording the dream whether it is precognitive dream or not (typically, precognitive dreams are remembered and recorded after the premonition has occurred). Using their prospective approach, they did not find any support for the idea that dreams can predict future events (Bender & Mischo, 1961). In addition to those "celebrities," there are also many persons keeping dream diaries because they are interested in their dreams and are willing to put in the work to write them

DOI: 10.4324/9781003300373-2

down regularly (Brush, 1993; Garfield, 1973; Hoss, 2020; Matthews, 2016; Paquette, 2018; Schmidt, 1999; Sturzenacker & Pearson, 2012); for example, Paquette (2018) recorded 12,224 dreams over a period of 27 years; he was interested in the spiritual content of dreams. In modern times, dreamers post their dreams online; McNamara et al. (2016) analyzed data from 82 dreamers who posted dreams with numbers ranging from six to 262. Published dreams – at least, those published during the lifetime of the dreamer – might have the disadvantage of being selected (e.g., the dreams of Sigmund Freud, in his book *The Interpretation of Dreams*, or dreams that are posted online are likely to be especially bizarre, funny, or intense or related to the dream theory of the author) or edited (this might be the case for writers who fine-tune their dream texts prior to publication).

Another area in which long dream series were collected and analyzed are psychoanalytic treatments (Deserno & Kächele, 2013; Kramer & Glucksman, 2006; Oberlerchner, 2006). For example, Kramer and Glucksman (2006) analyzed the first and the last dream of 24 patients undergoing long-term psychotherapy and found – among other findings – that the percentage of dreams with negative emotions decreased from 53.3% to 19.2%, reflecting the improvement of waking-life symptoms. However, these dream series have to be viewed with caution, as they have been almost exclusively recorded by the therapist and not by the dreamer himself/herself. In their study, Whitman et al. (1963) were able to show marked differences between topics of dreams recorded by the dreamer and the topics of dreams reported in psychotherapy; their explanation is that the dreamer might select (more or less consciously) specific dreams that fit into the context of the ongoing therapeutic process. This would represent a major bias if compared to all dreams the patient could have recorded if s/he had kept a dream diary. Thus, dream series of patients undergoing long-term psychotherapy recorded by the therapist might produce findings that are helpful to understand the therapeutic process but might not provide a valid picture of how the waking life of the dreamer is reflected in dreams.

In this chapter, a selected number of studies will be presented that focused on the longitudinal aspect of dream series; thus, not only collecting sufficient material for cross-sectional analysis but also analyzing changes over time or trying to find temporal patterns within the dream series (see Table 2.1).

One of the first larger longitudinal analyses of a dream series was carried out by Nelson (1888b). He collected 2,490 dreams over a period of 30 months – on average, more than three dreams per night. The author mentioned in his paper how exhausting the process of recording every dream detail is. The mean word count of those dreams was about 100 words. However, the idea that increased blood flow to the brain due to a 28-day cycle is reflected in more intense dreaming are not really supported by the data

TABLE 2.1 Studies with longitudinal analysis based on diary dream series

Author(s)	Number of dreams	Time interval	Topic(s)
Nelson (1888b)	2,490	30 months	Dream recall and a 28-day cycle in a male
Hall (1948)	200	2 years	Stability of themes, settings, characters
Junger (1955)	> 3,650	10 years	Time references to previous dreams, periodicity
Smith and Hall (1964)	649	50 years	Time references to waking, topics like mother and food
Merei (1965)	480	4 years	Effect of imprisonment on social dream content
Kirtley and Hall (1975)	307	10 years	Effect of going blind on dreams
Garfield (1976)	2 x 50	27 years	Changes in self-concept
Corriere et al. (1977)	754	5 ½ years	Changes due to self-development
Jouvet (1979a)	2,525	8 years	Time references of dream elements
Gerne (1987)	9,856	48 years	Frequency of deceased close persons
Sausgruber (1989)	3,638	14 years	Frequency of partner dreams, mother dreams over time
Uslar (2003)	6,100	53 years	Qualitative analyses, topic like churches, philosophers, horses
Domhoff (2003)	3,116	39 years	Family members, friends, ex-husband
Belicki et al. (2003)	106	16 years	Dreams about deceased wife
Hartmann and Brezler (2008)	44 x 20	Up to 22 wks.	Effect of the 9/11/2001 attacks on dreams
Gackenbach, Sample, et al. (2011)	800	9 years	Effect of medication on dreams
Bulkeley (2018)	6,000	30 years	Frequency of religious topic after a period of intense cult activities
Schredl and Neuhäusler (2019)	132	4 years	Changes in partner dreams after separation

(Continued)

TABLE 2.1 (Continued)

Author(s)	Number of dreams	Time interval	Topic(s)
Schredl (2021e, 2022)	2,025	30 years	Decrease of mother dreams over time, effect of health issues on singing
Schredl and Jacob (1998) **and** Schredl (2021d)	200 to 12,476	31 years	Family members, animals, lucid dreams, partner dreams, pain, clocks, etc.

presented in the article's figures; there are no statistics whatsoever, showing that the relatively small fluctuations in dream recall are associated with the postulated 28-day cycle. It is even difficult to understand how the author defined his "cycle" – being a man, a simple parallel to the menstrual cycle of women seems difficult. Interestingly, the graph depicting the number of dreams over the year showed higher dream recall in the winter months (October to February) compared to the summer months. This might be plausible if the author slept longer in the winter compared to the summer. Although the Nelson (1888b) study represents the first systematic attempt to link dream parameters (amount of recalled dream material) with outside parameters by collecting a large number of dreams, the results are non-conclusive – which is to be expected, as blood flow to the brain (the underlying theory) is not associated with any dream parameters.

Hall (1948) analyzed a dream series reported by a male dreamer over two years. His main focus was to look at the occurrence of specific themes, settings, and characters in the first year (N = 100) and compare those frequencies obtained for the second part of the series. Unfortunately, he did not provide exact figures in the abstract but stated "The incidence of the various types of themes, settings, and characters is practically identical for the two halves of the series in most instances" (p. 274; Hall, 1948). Even though the author is convinced that these data support the notion that dreams reflect the stability of personality dynamics, one has to keep in mind that he didn't provide any statistics, and words like "practically" and "in most instances" point also at differences between the dreams of the two subsequent years.

The author of the paper (Junger, 1955) recorded his dreams every morning for ten years; however, he did not provide the exact number of dreams, as he analyzed the occurrence of 600 themes that have occurred in his dreams, an overall occurrence of 100,000 data points. The finding that 42% dream elements re-occurred within one to five days, whereas only 4% re-occur 41 to 50 days makes sense, as specific topics show up in dreams quite often. However,

TABLE 2.2 Data of a single, female dreamer (Smith & Hall, 1964)

Years	Number of dreams	Mother dreams
25–46	100	11%
46–68	100	11%
67–71	100	9%
71–73	100	9%
73–75	100	10%
75–76	100	12%

the author was also looking for longer periodicities – e.g., cycles of one year – and provided the example that he had dreams about cars on August 17, 1943, on August 22, 1944, on August 25, 1945, and August 28, 1946. Given the large number of data points and the wide range of the one-year interval, one might speculate that searching long enough for periodicities in this data set will provide some results. As no statistics have been applied, these findings might be explained by chance.

Madorah Elizabeth Smith (1887 to 1965) recorded 649 dreams, the first one when she was 25 years old, the last ones when she was 75 years old. As she studied and taught psychology, she was the first author of the paper based on the collaboration with Calvin S. Hall (Smith & Hall, 1964). Whereas the findings regarding possible time references of dream elements occurring in waking life were inconclusive, interestingly, dreams about her mother occurred relatively frequently, between 9% to 12% (see Table 2.2), a figure that is comparable with other dream series (Schredl, 2013b). Even though the mother died when the dreamer was 61 yrs old, the percentage of mother dreams remained stable, clearly indicating that the mother was a very important and dear to the dreamer. Unfortunately, little is known about the dream material itself – e.g., dream length – and statistical analysis are also lacking. On the other hand, it was possible to compare dreams reported at very different phases of the dreamer's life.

A very unique dream study was published by Ferenc Mérei, first in his native language – Hungarian (Merei, 1965) – and later in English (Merei, 1994). The psychology professor was imprisoned for political reasons for four years. Each year, he recorded his dreams for about a month; after he was released, he recorded his dreams for a month and started again recording for another six months after being released. Overall, he recorded in these six months 480 dreams. Needless to say, that this was an unpleasant experience – and something that cannot be done within a research study. His core family consisted of five persons, and 25 persons were his close friends. Even though family members and friends show up in the prison dreams (see Table 2.3), the

TABLE 2.3 Data of a single, male dreamer (Merei, 1994)

Years	Family	Friends	Fellow inmates and prison guards
Prison (Year 1)	13%	11%	29%
Prison (Year 2)	15%	9%	33%
Prison (Year 3)	13%	11%	40%
Prison (Year 4)	13%	10%	42%
Directly after release	21%	23%	40%
Six months after release	16%	20%	22%

frequency increased when he was released and able to meet them in person. On the other hand, the frequency of dreams with inmates or prison guards (overall, 189 different persons) was very high during his imprisonment but significantly decreased after he was released, as seen in the dreams recorded six months after imprisonment. As the frequency is still high (22%), one might speculate whether the dreamer kept contact with some of his fellow inmates (via mail), but no information was given in the article. Although the changes are impressive, statistical tests were not provided, which is especially critical, as the author did not specify how many dreams there were in each of the six recording periods.

Kirtley and Hall (1975) had the opportunity to analyze 206 dreams of a young man (out of his longer dream series) who become fully blind at the age of 12 yrs. The dreams included less physical aggression than the norm (Hall & Van de Castle, 1966), but also included less friendliness and happy emotions (more apprehensive feelings) in his dreams. Therefore, the dreams indicate that the loss of his eyesight (one eyesight due to an accident, the other due to a disease) was a negative life-event for the dreamer, with long-lasting consequences reflected in his dreams.

Patricia Garfield (1934 to 2021) published many groundbreaking books on dream work, starting with her first bestseller, *Creative Dreaming* (Garfield, 1974), and kept a dream diary from the age of 14 yrs (with more than 20,000 dreams). In one analysis (Garfield, 1976), she compared 50 dreams she recorded when she was 14 with 50 dreams she recorded when she was 41. Whereas some dream characteristics remained stable – e.g., male/female percent of dream characters, number of aggressive and friendly interactions – the sexual interactions increased (Garfield, 1976). Moreover, emotions like fear, worry, and loneliness decreased, whereas anger, annoyance, and hatred increased; this is also reflected in the lower percentage of being a victim of aggressive interactions. Thus, this analysis clearly parallels the development from a teenager to a middle-aged and successful woman.

The authors (Corriere et al., 1977) had the opportunity to study a dreams series (N = 754) of a 28-year old man who underwent three years of "Feeling Therapy." As he had kept the dream diary already two years prior to therapy, it was possible to demonstrate that the clarity and the freedom in expressing emotions in dreams increased during the therapeutic process.

The renowned sleep researcher Michel Jouvet, whose work contributed a lot to the understanding of REM sleep physiology, recorded his dreams from December 1970 till August 1978 (N = 2,525 dreams). He was mainly interested in the time reference of dream elements, so he found that the most frequent reference of an element was to something that happened the day before – the so-called "day residue" effect (Jouvet, 1979a). In addition, he also found that, during his travels, the new surroundings showed up only after about eight days he arrived at the new location and also stayed with him in his dreams a few days after the end of the journey back home (for a German translation, see Jouvet, 1994).

Very long and extensive dream series were recorded by "Alice," who kept a dream diary from 1937 to 1985. The researcher (Gerne, 1987) selected dreams before and after the death of four persons who were close to the dreamer (husband, mother, close female friend, close male friend). The series were quite long, as Gerne (1987) selected 200 dreams recorded prior to the respective death and all dreams recorded after the death within one year (168 to 322 dreams). Interestingly, the overall frequency of the respective deceased person did not decline after his/her death within the dream series, but the person was more often dying or dead in the dreams; thus, the loss in waking life is reflected in the dreams of the mourning person (Gerne, 1987).

The Austrian psychiatrist and psychotherapist Herwig H. Sausgruber recorded his dreams from the age 21 to the age of 34 yrs – 3,638 dreams in total. In one of his papers (Sausgruber, 1988), he suggested how to deal with such an amount of material, using tags like "father" and "mother" on punch cards (the early days of digitalization). In one analysis, he found a decrease in the frequency of mother dreams, starting with about 30% at the beginning of the series to about 12% at the end. His romantic partner, with whom he had a relationship from age 18 to age 25, showed up in about 11% to 20% during the relationship period (in some phases, more frequently than his mother), but after the break-up, the frequency rapidly decreased, with about less than 3% at the end of the recorded dream series (Sausgruber, 1989). Unfortunately, the depiction of the longitudinal findings in graphs is not very precise, and again, analysis showing that these changes are statistically meaningful are missing.

A very special dream series was published by Detlev von Uslar (1926 to 2022), a German philosopher and psychologist who taught, for 20 years, theoretical aspects of psychology at the University of Zurich, Switzerland. In his book (Uslar, 2003), he not only presented analyses regarding his dreams but also included a CD with a database containing the original dreams and associations related to the dream – overall, 6,100 dreams. He also made these dreams available online, within the website "Dreambank.net," created by Domhoff and Schneider (2008b). Most of the book deals with qualitative analyses – e.g., all dreams related to an intense dream with two churches, loud noises, the feeling of being paralyzed; the author related about 5% of all dreams to the thematic issues that came up in this intense dream. He only presented a few longitudinal analyses; for example, the frequency of churches in dreams – the percentage varied from 1.4% (Dreams 4001 to 5000) to 3.2% (Dreams 1001 to 2000) – thus remained relatively stable. An interesting theme is the occurrence of philosophers in his dreams (in person, in writing, in conversations): Martin Heidegger (1.9%), Hans Georg Gadamer (0.9%), Nicolai Hartmann (0.8%), and Helmuth Plessner (0.4%). The dreamer had personal contact with them and stated that Heidegger was very influential for his own work (Uslar, 2003). The frequency of the dreams with the four different philosophers varied over the years – e.g., Nicolai Hartmann and Helmuth Plessner occurred most often in the first thousand dreams, whereas Hans Georg Gadamer was more prominent in the second half of the dream series, as, at this point, the dreamer came into contact with him and his work. Given the fact that the dreams are available, Schredl (2011a) was able to extract that the dreamer's wife, Emme, showed up in 20.4% – a figure that was paralleled by other studies looking at the frequency of partners within dreams (Schredl, Cadiñanos Echevarria, et al., 2020; Schredl & Wood, 2021; Selterman et al., 2014). Interestingly, the author was not interested in analyzing why this dream character occurred frequently.

In an extensive researched dream series analyzed by Domhoff (2003), the pseudonym of the dreamer is "Barb Sanders." Her dreams can be found online (dreambank.net) – the first analyses included 3,116 dreams – but "Barb Sanders" provided a sequel of additional 1,138 dream reports she recorded after contacting the researcher. The major advantage of these series is that Domhoff (2003) has collected a lot of data about the dreamer's waking life. In addition, she agreed to answer questions from other researchers regarding her waking life. For example, Han and Schweickert (2016) analyzed, in all 4,354 dreams, co-occurrences of dream characters in one dream as a measure of the dream social network and were able to obtain emotional closeness ratings from Barb Sanders (via Bill Domhoff). As expected, persons of Barb Sanders' social network who are close to her and/or know each other in waking life tend to co-occur more often in dreams than unrelated persons of her social network. Interestingly, systematic longitudinal analyses have not been conducted using the dream series. Domhoff (2003) took a closer look at dreams about Barb Sanders' ex-husband (N = 164 dreams out of the 3,116 dreams); the marriage and divorce were very stressful, so the dreams (divided into four time periods) showed more aggressive interactions between the dreamer and her ex-husband (see Table 2.4) than friendly ones;

TABLE 2.4 Data of a single, female dreamer over 25 years after the divorce (Domhoff, 2003)

Period	Aggression/friendliness percentage (ex-husband)
Segment 1	57%
Segment 2	59%
Segment 3	61%
Segment 4	34%

for example, with the ex-husband asking for sexual activity she did not want. Only after a very long time, the dream interactions with her ex-husband became friendlier (see Table 2.4).

A widower recorded every dream in which his deceased wife occurred (N = 106) for 16 years. Belicki et al. (2003) tried to find a typology of the course of grieving processes in the dreams – e.g., numbness, disorganization, and reorganization. The findings did not show a clear progression along these phases, even though the frequency of dreams in which the deceased wife is alive again decreased over the years.

A very unique approach was carried out by Hartmann and Brezler (2008); their aim was to study the effects of the 9/11/2001 attacks on the twin towers in New York on dreaming. They contacted the national sleep societies (SRS, AASM) and the International Association of the Study of Dreams (IASD) in order to search for persons who have kept a dream diary (at least for two years) prior and after the terrorists' attack. From these dream journalists, they requested the last ten dreams recorded before 9/11 and the first ten dreams recorded afterwards – unedited, of course. Interestingly, they found no direct reference to the actual attacks – e.g., planes hitting the buildings – but attacks in general – e.g., encounters with frightening people or animals – were more frequent in the dreams after the attack (Hartmann & Brezler, 2008). Overall, the emotional intensity of the central image increased. One has to keep in mind that these dream journalists were not directly affected by the attacks (they were not survivors or somehow related to victims who died in the attack); they were US citizens who were exposed to the intense media coverage of this event, the gruesome violence of these attacks unknown to that point. This study highlights the unique potential long-term dream journalists have for empirical dream research. One might imagine similar studies for other events like the global COVID-19 pandemic.

A high-end video gamer who suffered from obsessive-compulsive disorder blogged his dreams (more than 800) regularly over about nine yrs. Gackenbach, Sample, et al. (2011) analyzed, for example, the years when he took medication for his disorder (fluoxetine). Although, the dreamer underwent major changes from adolescence (medication intake from the age 14 to 17) to young adulthood (18 to 23 yrs), the finding that aggression occurred less often in the drug-period dreams than later is astonishing clear, especially the percentage of the dreamer himself being the aggressor in the dreams (0% in the drug dreams, compared to 44% of the later dreams). Unfortunately, the topic of good fortune in dreams was also rarer in the drug dreams (0% vs. 12%) (Gackenbach, Sample, et al., 2011).

Bulkeley (2018) analyzed 940 dreams of the series, encompassing 6,000 dreams, because these dreams have already been transcribed by the dreamer (average word count was about 54 words per dream). The dreamer was intensely involved in the Hare Krishna group in Los Angeles, practiced regularly, and was also – being a writer – responsible for the public relations of this group, but she had left behind the practice by 2006. This religious engagement is clearly reflected in her dreams (see Table 2.5), as the frequency of dreams with religious content dropped drastically in 2006. As the frequency of reading/writing dreams of a control sample of the author (Bulkeley, 2018) was 6%, the dreams also reflect clearly that the dreamer was concerned with writing, especially in 1996. Bulkeley (2018) formulated a total of 26 inferences about the dreamer's waking life based on the dream findings (change over time and the comparison to a control sample with N = 3,095 dreams); for example, the dreamer is not interested very much in sports, as she reported about 1% sports dreams, compared to the control sample who reported 4% sports dreams. On the other hand, Bulkeley (2018) predicted that the dreamer is less concerned with family, as only 12% to 26% of the dreams included family members (compared to 40% of the control sample). Although, the dreamer confirmed 23 of the 26 predictions, it is difficult to determine the statistical significance of the findings, as other persons might have also agreed, at least to some of the predictions.

Although being a relatively small dream series (Schredl & Neuhäusler, 2019), the analysis of partner dreams clearly reflected the waking-life experience of a painful separation; there was a significant shift from friendly to aggressive interaction with the partner/ex-partner in the dreams, and negative dream emotions also increased.

A Benedict nun recorded her dreams, starting at the age of 38 yrs, for more than 30 years (Schredl, 2021a). In one analysis (Schredl, 2021e), it showed

TABLE 2.5 Data of a single, female dreamer over 30 years (Bulkeley, 2018)

Years	Dreams	Religion as topic	Reading/writing
1986	253	25%	13%
1996	253	16%	27%
2006	247	6%	11%
2016	187	4%	10%

that the frequency of mother dreams decreased from middle age to older age (from about 10% to 5% of all remembered dreams), and after the death of the mother, the frequency continued to decline (2.45%). Due to health problems, the dreamer was not able to sing for some time (several years), even though she very much liked this activity (Schredl, 2022). The dreams reflected this change: the percentage of dreams that include singing dropped from about 20% of all music dreams she recorded to about 7% in the period with the health problems (Schredl, 2022).

The first analysis based on the dream series presented in this book was published by Schredl and Jacob (1998). They took 100 dreams while the dreamer was studying electrical engineering and 100 dreams while the dreamer was studying psychology. As most of the fellow students in engineering were male (more than 90%) and most of the follow psychology students were female (about 70%), it was expected that the ratio of male and female dream characters would change. Indeed, the male percent dropped from 63% to 51% (Schredl & Jacob, 1998). Whereas the first figure is close to the percentage of male students, the second value is close to the percentage of female students (Hall & Van de Castle, 1966). That is, the findings from the dream series indicate that the male/female percentage is not inherent to the person – e.g., explained by the Oedipus complex – as suggested by Hall (1984) but mainly reflect the pattern of social interactions during waking. This was supported by additional studies (Paul & Schredl, 2012; Schredl, Loßnitzer, et al., 1998) directly correlating the amount of time spent with males and females during waking with the male/female percent of dream characters. Other published studies based on this dream series looked at the frequency of family members (Schredl, 2013b), romantic partners (Schredl, 2018a; Schredl & Reinhard, 2012), and schoolmates (Schredl, 2012d) over time. As updated analysis of these – and additional – topics will be presented in this book, a detailed description is not included in this chapter.

As already mentioned in this chapter, there is a rich database with more than 20 long dream series available online: the website, "Dreambank.net," was created by Domhoff and Schneider (2008b). Every researcher can use these dreams and will find information about the dreamers on the website, with the most elaborate information about "Barb Sanders."

Overall, the brief review of research done with dream series so far clearly indicates the potential this type of material has; that is, the analysis of dream diaries provided by long-term dream journalists allows us to ask and answer questions that are not easy or even impossible to tackle by even the most sophisticated research projects. So far, I only know one dream content study (Lortie-Lussier et al., 2000) that was able to collect dreams of 21 women for a second time (on average, 15 years after participating in the first study). Overall, 109 women participants as students in the dream studies; of those, 69 could be located, and the 21 agreed to participate. In order to keep the workload low, dreams were only collected for three days. The findings indicate a decrease in aggressive and negatively toned dreams over the years (Lortie-Lussier et al., 2000). However, compared to the large number of dreams per participant in the "natural" dream series, the research study did not provide much data (only a few dreams per time point). In addition, one might speculate why so many persons refused to participate (48 of 69 = 70%). Shorter longitudinal studies with similar small samples have been carried out in children (Foulkes, 1982) and adolescents (Strauch et al., 1997). The lack of longitudinal studies within larger samples in the field of dream research underlines the importance of using long-term dream journalists as a valuable data source.

From a methodological viewpoint, the overview presented in this chapter also highlights the weaknesses of many of the published dream series studies. It seems important to present the descriptive statistics regarding the dream reports, as it makes a difference whether dream reports are, on average, 54 words long (Bulkeley, 2018) or 184 words ("Barb Sanders" series; Domhoff, 2003). The longer dreams should include everything, on average, more often. Second, the analysis of large data sets without any theoretical background (or even incorrect theoretical background) – for example, looking for a periodicity of 28 days in dream recall (Nelson, 1888b) or for annually recurring dream topics (Junger, 1955) – harbors the danger that the findings are chance findings. With one eye on the next chapter, it seems obvious that the statistical procedures applied to analyze dream series of single persons should be improved in the future, in order to provide estimates whether longitudinal changes in these series might be chance findings or pointing to specific interactions between dreams and the waking life of the dreamer.

3

STUDYING DREAM SERIES – PROS AND CONS

Studying long dream series that are typically collected outside of research settings offers unique advantages but also poses a few challenges in addition to handling the often-abundant material itself – especially if the dream reports are handwritten. The most important pros and cons are summarized in Table 3.1.

Keeping a dream diary and recording all dreams remembered in the morning can be an arduous task, especially for prodigious dream recallers (Garfield, 1973; Nelson, 1888b); for example, Nelson (1888b) recorded more than 1,000 dreams per year. In typical research settings, participants were asked to keep a dream journal for 2 to 6 weeks (Zadra & Robert, 2012), but the motivation to record dreams can decrease even after one week of journal keeping (Schredl, 2002). Thus, material from dream diaries kept over years or even decades can offer unique insights into whether and how dream content changes over time. An illustrative example is the decline of dreams with the former romantic partner over years, showing that, even after nine years, about 3% of the dreams included the dreamer's former partner (Schredl & Reinhard, 2012). Domhoff (2003) studied the interaction quality in dreams featuring the ex-husband, showing that it took many years before the friendly interactions outweigh the aggressive interactions between dreamer and ex-husband in her dreams.

The next topic is related to the nature of live events that can be studied – as a high number of events happening in the "real" world cannot be re-created in an experimental setting. An illustrative example is provided by Hartmann and Brezler (2008). They contacted dream journalists and asked them to provide ten dreams recorded prior to 9/11 and ten dreams recorded afterwards. Overall, 44 dream journalists provided the requested material.

DOI: 10.4324/9781003300373-3

TABLE 3.1 Pros and cons of studying dream series

Topic	Example(s)
Advantages	
Studying long time intervals	Frequency of schoolmates in dreams recorded 20 years after finishing school (Schredl, 2012d)
	Interaction quality with ex-husband in dreams recorded more than 15 years after the divorce (Domhoff, 2003)
Studying the effects of unusual life experiences	Comparing dreams prior and after 9–11, obtained by dream journalists (Hartmann & Brezler, 2008)
	Effects of four years of political imprisonment on social interactions in dreams (Merei, 1994)
Dream material not influenced by demand characteristics	Dreams were recorded prior to the researcher analyzing them (Domhoff, 2022)
High number of dreams per person	Parallel between personality testing and determining typical dream characteristics of the person (Domhoff, 2022; Schredl, 1998)
Disadvantages	
Possible selection bias	
Who is recording dreams?	Personalities of persons who keep dream journals (Schredl & Göritz, 2019b)
Motivation (Which dreams are recorded?)	Only partner dreams (Schredl & Neuhäusler, 2019)
	Dreams of the deceased wife (Domhoff, 2015)
Who is providing his/her dream series for research?	Curiosity of the dreamer about the partner's reason to break-up the relationship (Schredl & Neuhäusler, 2019)
	Being a dream researcher (Schredl, 2013a)
Possible effects of keeping a dream journal on dream content	Regularly keeping a dream journal might be also reflected in subsequent dreams (Schredl, 2015b)
Statistical issues with handling binary time series with gaps	Using h-statistics (Domhoff, 1996)
	Using regression models developed by Klingenberg (2008); see, for example, Schredl (2018a)

The findings indicate that direct references, like tall buildings and airplanes, were not more frequent, but the intensity (predominantly negatively toned) was increased after the 9/11 attacks. Another example is the study of Merei (1994) that was originally published earlier in Hungarian (Merei, 1965). The author, a psychology professor, was imprisoned for four years for political reasons (Hungary). As expected, the percentage of friends and family members in dreams went up after he was released, whereas the percentage of fellow inmates or guards went down. For comparison, a social seclusion experiment with students lasted four days in single rooms on an isolated island; they found no changes regarding the frequency of close persons in the frequency of the dreams during the seclusion period compared to the period afterwards being at home in their usual everyday world (Tuominen et al., 2021).

Another interesting approach is to analyze dreams of "celebrities"; Hall and Domhoff (1968), for example, analyzed the dreams Sigmund Freud (N = 28) and Carl Gustav Jung (N = 31) published; although the authors addressed the possibility that Freud and Jung might have selected specific dreams to illustrate their respective theories, there have been interesting findings; for example, Freud was more sociable in his dreams, compared to Jung. Another interesting comparison was made between Arthur Schnitzler, who recorded a lot of his dreams (Schnitzler, 2012), and Sigmund Freud, as they were acquainted and Freud referred to Schnitzler as his "Doppelganger." In dreams, Schnitzler was, more often than Freud, the befriender – that is, initiating friendly interactions – but also showed more physical aggression in dreams; possibly, Freud selected "tame" dreams to be published, whereas Schnitzler's dreams were published posthumously. Such famous men typically do not participant in academic dream studies; even though the researcher has to rely on their published dream reports (with pros and cons), analyzing such material offers unique insights. Interesting within this context is a publication of a botanist who remained anonymous; in her dream series of 5,000 dreams, about 90 different plant species occurred, reflecting her very unique profession (Woman, 1915).

Domhoff (2022) pointed out another advantage of analyzing dream diaries with dreams that were recorded long before the researcher had a chance to see them; that is, the material is not influenced by demand characteristics. Uga et al. (2006), for example, carried out a diary study in order to analyze the frequency of music-related dreams and recruited for their study advertising with this agenda ("Music and dreams"). In their non-musician sample (psychology students), 18.2% of the dreams included references to music, significantly less often compared to the musician group (40.1%) but also much higher than in a sample of psychology students who recorded their dreams in the course of a study about dream recall that was not at all related to music; the percentage of music dreams in this study was 8.13% (König & Schredl, 2021). The fact that participants knew what the study was about – music in dreams – had a marked effect on the findings, increasing the percentage of music dreams dramatically. Another example was a re-analysis of sleep-dream diaries kept for over 100 days by students (Schredl et al., 2006). Long after the data-collection period, the researchers looked up the moon phases during the study periods (diaries included dates) and correlated dream recall with the occurrence of the full moon. The finding was that dream recall was not affected by the moon in persons who did not know about or focused on moon phases during the diary period. If a research group were to advertise a study called "Possible effects of moon phases on dreams," the results based on sampling with this recruitment strategy might be different.

However, the usage of this archival material also raises some questions that might be labeled as possible disadvantages. The most important questions are (see Table 3.1): Who keeps a dream journal? Are these dream journalists special, different from the general public? As there is growing body of knowledge on this topic, an extra section is dealing with that issue (see Section 3.1). In a nutshell, there are differences in personality; for example, that is, findings based on long dream series should be evaluated carefully whether these differences might have affected the results. For example, dream journalists are more likely to be female.

Another critical question is the selection of dreams that have been recorded; for example, one dreamer recorded only her dreams about her partner and then ex-partner because she wanted to learn more about the reasons why it did not work out (Schredl & Neuhäusler, 2019). Another dreamer – a widower – only recorded the dreams about his late wife in order to cope with the mourning process (Domhoff, 2015). These selection methods are obvious, but one can imagine many other possible biases – e.g., the dreamer only records dreams that are extraordinary, puzzling, or distressing. In this case, findings based on such dream diaries might yield different results compared to dreams of journalists who try to record all or almost all dreams they remember – e.g., Garfield (1973) or Schredl (2013b). In the first case, dreams, in general, might be evaluated as being mainly bizarre and emotionally intense because the mundane dreams have not been recorded and, thus, were not included in the analysis. The selection issue is even more problematic if the dream reports are published during the lifetime of the dreamer; for example, the dreams Sigmund Freud used as illustrations in his book *The Interpretation of Dreams*. As mentioned previously, these dreams did not include physical aggression (Hall & Domhoff, 1968), which is unusual, as many dreams, especially in males, also include physical aggression (Hall & Domhoff, 1963). One might speculate that Freud, being the founder of the psychoanalytic school, did not want to disclose all of his dreams.

The last issue in this section is about the question what dream series can be analyzed by dream researchers; that is, what kind of journalists are willing to hand over their dreams to a researcher who even publishes these dreams on a website (not with the real name of the dreamer and with changed names of the dream characters to ensure anonymity); for example see www.dream bank.net, a website hosted by William G. Domhoff. Sometimes, the dream journalists contact the dream researcher because they read or heard something about his or her dream research in the media. For example, one woman contacted the authors because she wanted others to learn from her positive experiences looking at dreams to better cope with a break-up (Schredl &

Neuhäusler, 2019). Another dreamer shared her dreams because she wanted to see some benefit of her work of recording dreams over three decades (Schredl, 2021e). Another dreamer ("Barb Sanders," a pseudonym) contacted Bill Domhoff and provided 3,116 dreams she had recorded (Domhoff, 2003), and even provided an additional 1,138 dreams after the first contact with the researcher (Domhoff, 2022). This allows for extensive analysis; however, one has to keep in mind that "Barb Sanders" is a unique person; for example, she experienced a bad marriage ending with a divorce, never remarried, has three daughters, and has interests like playing theater. So, her dreams are clearly not representative for all dreams of different persons, but – and this is the basic idea of the continuity hypothesis of dreaming (Schredl, 2003) – allow us to study how the specific live circumstances of this dreamer are reflected in her dreams – e.g., the emotional quality of interactions in dreams with her ex-husband (Domhoff, 2003). The most obvious motive for analyzing dream series is at work if the dreamer himself or herself is a dream researcher; for example, lucid dream researchers like Saint-Denys (1982) or Van Eeden (1913) used their own dreams as major data source to study this – in this period of time very rarely talked about – phenomenon. Other researchers used their own dream to tackle a rare phenomenon like PSI topic in a series of 12,224 dream records (Paquette, 2018). For his master's thesis, Rizzolo (1922) recorded 100 subsequently remembered dreams, and Sausgruber (1989) analyzed 3,638 dreams he recorded over 13 years for his dissertation. Typically, in these cases (like in the present book), dreams are not included (as there is no anonymity) – with the exception of a few illustrative examples, even though one researcher (Uslar, 2003) included a CD in his book with all 6,100 dream texts (published during his lifetime).

To summarize, findings based on dream journals should be evaluated regarding the dreamer's background, his or her motivation about what dreams will end up in the dream journal, and his or her willingness to provide the dream series for research purposes.

The last issue that will be addressed in this chapter is the statistical issues that are related to analyzing long dream series. On the pro side is the high number of dreams per person; this is necessary, as the dream content varies a lot from dream to dream (Kramer & Roth, 1979; Schredl, 1998). Thus, a sample of 100 dreams or more yields quite stable results regarding major dream characteristics – e.g., friendly and aggressive interactions (Domhoff & Schneider, 2008a; Hall, 1947). The method for testing this stability is quite simple: the researcher took a long dream series and compared the dream characteristics – e.g., male/female percentages of different subsamples consisting of 100 dream reports (Domhoff, 1996). And some research questions – e.g., determining the characteristics of the social network in dreams – that is, what dream characters show up in dream together – require a substantial number of dreams (300 and more) (Han et al., 2016; Schredl & Schweickert,

2022). The major disadvantage is, of course, that, typically, only one participant provided the dream series. The first caveat has been discussed earlier: these dream journalists might not be representative of the general population; research has shown that there are marked differences in traits like openness to experience and conscientiousness (see section "Who keeps a dream journal?"). The second methodological issue concerns the statistical methods applied to the data for testing hypotheses; for example, whether the percentage of cat dreams significantly decreased after the dreamer moved away from home (with cats) in an apartment without cats (Schredl, 2013a). Typical statistical methods assume statistical independence between observations that are given if the measurements are stemming from different participants (Bortz, 1999); this is obviously not the case for a dream series. Specific statistical methods – time series analysis – were first developed for variables measured on interval levels – e.g., mood scale ranging from 0 to 10 – and equidistant time lags – e.g., one day or one hour, etc. (Shumway & Stoffer, 2017). These two requirements are often not fulfilled in analyzing dream series, as the dependent variable might be binary (cat in the dream vs. no cat in the dream), and the time lags vary, as there are nights with several dreams or even nights without any dream recall. To the knowledge of the authors, only one publication (Klingenberg, 2008) addressed the topic of analyzing binary time series with gaps. As these methodological, respective, statistical issues are important, further information is given in the section titled "Statistical issues in analyzing dream series" (see the following).

3.1 Who keeps a dream journal?

Even though early dream researchers (Calkins, 1893; Nelson, 1888a; Van Eeden, 1913) kept a dream journal in order to obtain dream material for their research and modern dream researchers (Domhoff, 2003; Schredl, 2018b) value the contributions made by findings based on long dream series, relatively little is known about the frequency of dream journaling in the general population. For example, such simple questions of how many persons are recording dreams at all or even on a regular basis have rarely been studied. Moreover, the question of whether and in what respect these dream journalists differ from those who do not record their dreams has also not been addressed very often.

The database on dream recording frequency in the general public increased dramatically with the introduction of the MADRE (Mannheim Dream Questionnaire), as this questionnaire included an item about dream recording: "How often do you record your dreams?" with eight answering options, ranging from several times a week to about once a year, and never. Most of the studies, depicted in Table 3.2, used this item of the MADRE (Schredl et al., 2014a). Many studies reported a lifetime prevalence (having recorded at least one own dream) between 14.77% and 24.2%, with two exceptions: psychology students (Schredl, 2020b) reported dream recording more often compared to the general population, whereas patients with sleep disorders (Schredl & Schmitt, 2019) reported recording dreams less often (statistically controlled for dream recall frequency and attitude towards dreams; both variables' means were lower in the patient sample). The first difference seems plausible, as psychology students are especially interested in all sorts of inner experiences, including dreams. The second difference might, at least partly, be explained by methodological issues. Most of the MADRE studies shown in Table 3.2 were carried out online and recruited participants who were interested in dreams; for example, dream recall frequency was well above average in the sample of Schredl et al. (2014b) compared to two representative German samples (Schredl, 2008a, 2013c). On the other hand, the patient sample of Schredl and Schmitt (2019) completed the MADRE questionnaire as part of their diagnostic routines and, thus, about 95% of all patients filled in the questionnaire, irrespective of whether they were interested in dreams or not. Therefore, these results were not biased toward a strong interest in dreams. However, it has to be noticed that the sample was older and included more males; both factors – age and gender – are related to dream recording frequency with younger age and female gender associated with higher frequencies (Schredl et al., 2014b). Systematic surveys looking at the frequency of dream recording of representative samples are still lacking.

A small percentage (1% to 5%) of the participants recorded their dreams quite regularly (once per week or more often); these might be dream journalists (see Table 3.2). In a longitudinal study (Schredl & Göritz, 2020) with three measurement points over two yrs, 2.71% of all participants (N = 739) recorded, at each time point, their dreams once a month or more often; that is, they are very likely regular dream journalists. As this study is, again, based on participants with an above-average interest in dreams, one might speculate that the percentage of persons who are keeping a dream journal over extended periods of time is relatively small in the general population.

In order to get an idea of whether a selection bias might be at work, if researchers look at long dream series obtained from regular dream journalists, the question of whether and how persons who record their dreams differ from those who do not has to be studied. The most obvious factor associated with dream recording frequency is, of course, dream recall frequency. If the individual cannot recall any dreams, keeping a dream diary is not possible. Indeed, all studies but one (Settineri et al., 2019) found a substantial correlation between dream recording frequency and dream recall frequency (Ghorayeb et al., 2019; Scapin et al., 2018; Schredl, 2020b, 2021g; Schredl et al., 2014b). As keeping a dream journal can increase dream recall (Schredl, 2002; Zadra & Robert, 2012), the causal relationship is not clear; that is, whether the dream journalist started with high dream recall or improved his or her

TABLE 3.2 Frequency of persons keeping a dream diary

Recording dreams		Sample size	Sample mean age	Sample characteristics	Citation
Lifetime	At least one a week				
16.70%	1.67%	2,929	45.88 ± 14.38 yrs.	Adults	Schredl et al. (2014b)
22.32%	5.52%	357	32.02 ± 14.35 yrs.	Adults	Scapin et al. (2018)
24.2%	4.5%	623	38.26 ± 14.71 yrs.	Adults	Settineri et al. (2019)
18.4%	1.2%	315	38.0 ± 15.6 yrs.	Adults	Ghorayeb et al. (2019)
4.20%	0.72%	1,467	59.56 ± 13.17 yrs.	Patients with sleep-related breathing disorders	Schredl and Schmitt (2019)
46.55%	3.46%	409	22.84 ± 4.03 yrs.	Psychology students	Schredl (2020b)
14.77%		4,849	15.88 ± 11.50 yrs.	Children, adolescents, adults	Schredl (2021g)
19.55%	3.5%	87	25.78 ± 4.50	Young adults	Mediano et al. (2022)

dream recall over the years. One study (Schredl, 2021g) found an additional contribution of nightmare frequency, which is plausible, as some persons use dream recording as a strategy to cope with nightmares, even though it is not very effective (Schredl & Göritz, 2014). The finding (Schredl & Göritz, 2019b) that a more positive attitude is related to dream-recording frequency is also very plausible. This would indicate that dream journalists differ from persons not keeping a dream journal in the same way as high dream recallers and low dream recallers differ. Such trait factors as female gender, openness to experience, and creativity were found in high dream recallers, but it has to be kept in mind that the differences were rather small (Schredl, 2018b).

Even after controlling for dream recall frequency, which is necessary, as, for example, women tend to recall their dreams more often than men (Schredl & Reinhard, 2008), women tend to record their dreams more often than men (Ghorayeb et al., 2019; Scapin et al., 2018; Schredl, 2020b, 2021g; Schredl et al., 2014b). This is also plausible because women are also more interested in dream interpretation (Schredl & Piel, 2008), reading more often books about dreams (Schredl, 2010b) and talking more often about their dreams (Graf et al., 2021). In two studies (Schredl et al., 2014b; Schredl & Schmitt, 2019) analyzing samples with large age ranges, dream recording frequency in older adults was lower compared to young adults, indicating a higher interest in recording dreams in younger adults. In the UK library sample (Schredl, 2021g), adults recorded their dreams slightly more often (17.77%) compared to adolescents (14.49%) and children (14.27%). However, as these are all cross-sectional studies (different cohorts might have different attitudes toward dreams in general and dream recording in particular), the factors that might explain the relationship between age and dream recording frequency are still unidentified. Schredl and Göritz (2019b) reported a small but significant effect of education on dream recording frequency in one analysis, with highly educated persons slightly more prone to record dreams. This fits in with the finding that keeping a diary (for daytime events) is strongly related to recording one's own dreams (Schredl, 2021g). If a person is strongly interested in recording their own experiences, dreams are often included.

Two studies (Schredl, 2021g; Schredl & Göritz, 2019b) so far have looked at the personality factors that might be related to dream recording frequency. The first finding that openness to experience is related to dream recording frequency (even after controlling for dream recall frequency) seems very plausible, as the curiosity found in persons with a high openness to experience might have stimulated them to keep a dream diary. However, the second finding was unexpected; two authors (Garfield, 1973; Nelson, 1888b) strongly emphasized that recording dreams directly upon awakening is an arduous task and, thus, one would expect that self-discipline, which is a facet of the conscientiousness trait, would help. The findings (Schredl, 2021g; Schredl & Göritz, 2019b), however, showed exactly the opposite: low conscientiousness was related to dream recording frequency. Therefore, it might be that other facets of conscientiousness, like being achievement-oriented, orderly, and traditionalistic might be important in this relationship; that is, that dream journalists are more unconventional and less goal-oriented than the average person is. The marked relationships between dream-recording frequency and openness to experience and low conscientiousness also holds for the regular dream journalists in the longitudinal study of Schredl and Göritz (2020).

To summarize, persons who record their dreams regularly differ from persons who do not; they recall their dreams more often, are more interested in their dreams, are more likely to be female, and show high openness to experience and low conscientiousness. These differences have to be kept in mind if one aims at generalizing the findings obtained from long dream series to the population in general.

3.2 Statistical issues in analyzing dream series

Two properties of dream series pose a challenge for statistical analyses: first, there is only one participant; and, second, even if this participant recorded a large number of dreams, these dreams are not statistically independent from each other. For commonly used statistical tests like t-tests, Chi-Square tests, and ANOVAs, this statistical independence is required (Bortz, 1999). Typically, this is the case if each observation was provided by different participants; that is, each participant contributes only one observation – e.g., in this case, a dream report. If – within a sample – participants provide different number of dreams, mixed-model approaches have to be applied – e.g., Schredl and Wood (2021) and Nöltner and Schredl (2023) analyzing interactions between dreamers, partners, and family members in a sample of 1,612 dreams reported by 425 students. However, for time series, still another set of statistical procedures has to be applied: time series analysis (Shumway & Stoffer, 2017). As mentioned previously, most of these procedures and algorithms cannot be applied to dream research, as the dream series shows gaps (nights without dream recall or nights with several dreams); thus, the lags are not equidistant, and the dependent variables – e.g., cat present in the dream or not – are binary and not continuous on an interval level – e.g., a visual analogue scale for mood – ranging from zero (depressed) to 100 (feeling happy). So far, only one statistical paper (Klingenberg, 2008) has tackled this problem. This algorithm can only be used for a very specific question – e.g., is there a significant change of the frequency of a specific dream characteristic from one time interval to another. For example, Schredl (2018a) compared the frequency of partner dreams for different relationships the dreamer had over the years. For P1, the percentage was 16.76%; that is, of all remembered dreams, the partner was present in about 17% of the dreams. For P3, the percentage was 19.20%, which was not significantly different from P1 using the algorithm of Klingenberg (2008). On the other hand, the lower figure for P4 (11.56% partner dreams in this relationship) was significant lower compared to P1 (p = .0073) and significant lower compared to P3 (p < .0001). Thus, the analyses were able to estimate whether the differences are sufficiently large, so it cannot, or to be more precise, can with a very low probability, be explained by chance.

Another approach to describe differences in percentages is using effect sizes (Cohen, 1988). In Appendix D "Statistical Appendix" of his book, Domhoff (1996) provided a table for determining effect sizes "h" from differences between two percentages (Table D.2; Domhoff, 1996). Alternatively, one can also use a formula

h = arcsine (2 x (1 –Percentage 1)-1) – arccos (2 x (1 – Percentage2)-1)

in order to compute the effect size. For illustration, several variables of the comparison of 100 dreams of Arthur Schnitzler with 34 dreams of Sigmund Freud are shown in Table 3.3.

Based on the classification suggested by Cohen (1988) with 0.2 as small, 0.5 as medium, and 0.8 as large effect sizes, one can determine that there are at least small differences between the two men. But the question is: Are these differences statistically significant? In Table D.3, Domhoff (1996) provided cut-offs for effect sizes and sample sizes; for example, for N = 140 sample size, effect sizes larger than 0.24 are statistically significant (p < .05), and for effect sizes larger than 0.31, the probability level that the difference is explained by chance is below p < .01. So, you might argue that the difference regarding sexual dreams is significant; Arthur Schnitzler's series included more dreams with references to sexuality than Sigmund Freud's. However, using the table D.3 (Domhoff, 1996) is problematic, as it assumes independent observations, which is not the case in the previously mentioned study; there were only two participants reporting 134 dreams. Domhoff and Schneider (2015) argued that this simple application might be possible, as the autocorrelations are very small and often non-significant; this was also reported by Schredl (2000). However, this conclusion might be a bit hasty and is, in the end, not statistically sound. Similarly, the argument that dream series do not show repetitive patterns using the Wald-Wolfowitz test (Wald & Wolfowitz, 1940)

TABLE 3.3 Dreams of Arthur Schnitzler and Sigmund Freud (Beuerle & Schredl, 2017)

Category	Schnitzler (N = 100 dreams)	Freud (N = 34 dreams)	Effect size
Friendliness	30%	21%	0.207
Sexuality	7%	3%	0.363
Misfortune	26%	12%	0.187
Success	3%	6%	−0.147

might not be sufficient to justify the assumption of statistical independence between dreams within a dream series.

Two studies (Kramer & Roth, 1979; Schredl, 1998) provided evidence that dream content is very variable; for example, one night, the dreamer experiences a horrifying nightmare and the dream a few days later is about a wonderful holiday in the Fiji islands. A very illustrative study was carried out by Schredl, Ebert, et al. (2015): they selected two dreams from one participant (male, 25 yrs.) and asked external raters to estimate different personality traits of the dreamer based on the dream. Both dreams were rated with positive emotions, but dream 1 (word count: 262 words) did not include any self-rated negative emotions. The dream plot is about a race, which is won by the dreamer, who also has the task of rescuing a woman. After that, he meets with friends and his ex-girlfriend. He is happy to see her, and they connect with each other. He proposes to her and is very happy because she wants to marry him. The second dream (word count: 321 words) included moderate negative emotions. The dreamer does not catch the school bus, and his friends do not wait. He is hurt. Finding another bus, he tries to follow them but driving the bus is difficult. He causes an accident, resulting in a person being severely wounded. The dreamer has compassion with the wounded bus driver. The dream ends with a scene where the dreamer observes sexual activities of two women and three men. Even though he is fascinated, he feels embarrassed, as one of the women points at him.

The 28 external judges who read dream 1 (without negative emotions) estimated much lower values on neuroticism and higher values on ego strength and assertiveness for the dreamer compared to the 32 external judges who based their estimates on dream 2 (with several negative experiences) (Schredl, Ebert, et al., 2015). As the dreams were collected within a dream diary kept over a two-week period, they were remembered in close proximity; that is, the overall life circumstances of the dreamer were unchanged. This study clearly demonstrated that one dream is not enough to make any inferences regarding the dreamer's waking life. From a statistical viewpoint, this implies that the correlation from dream to dream – as computed by Domhoff and Schneider (2015) – is, indeed, very small.

In order to illustrate this issue in a practical way, let us assume a researcher wants to know whether a person is more introverted or more extraverted or something in-between. However, she does not use a personality questionnaire but – this will comparable to dream studies – has, as a data source, randomly selected five min episodes of behavioral observation throughout the day and the night. If the researcher has only one observation period, then it will be very difficult to conclude with the part of the extraversion-introversion dimension the person is, especially if the five-min segment is at night, when the person sleeps. Even if you have a five-min segment of reading or going out with friends, this will also not suffice to make adequate estimates because the introverted person goes out sometimes, and the extraverted person reads now and then. This example illustrates that the researcher needs a lot of observations (5-min segments) to predict the person's introversion or extraversion – let's say, 50 segments – and more segments are even better if you want to know about the fine nuances of how introverted or extraverted the person is. Using this analogy, the statement of using 100 dreams or more in order to obtain quite stable results regarding trait dream characteristics (Domhoff & Schneider, 2008a; Hall, 1947) makes sense. In Figure 3.1, the example is dream aggressiveness. The analogue to the five-min segments to measure extraversion also illustrates that the correlation between different segments or dreams is almost negligible (Domhoff & Schneider, 2015; Schredl, 2000); that is, you cannot predict, by looking at one segment (or dream), what will happen in the next one. However, does this also imply that the observations (five-min segments or dreams) are statistically independent? The answer is no. A quick glance at Figure 3.1 clearly shows that all dreams (or segments, in the analogy) are influenced by the same latent dimension. In the waking-life example, the chance of having a five-minute segment with going out with friends will be higher for an extraverted person (high value in this latent dimension) compared to an introverted person. This clearly implies that using statistics developed for data with statistically independent observations cannot be applied to analyzing dream series, as it has been proposed by Domhoff (1996). See also the previously mentioned example of comparing Sigmund Freud's dreams with the dreams of Arthur Schnitzler.

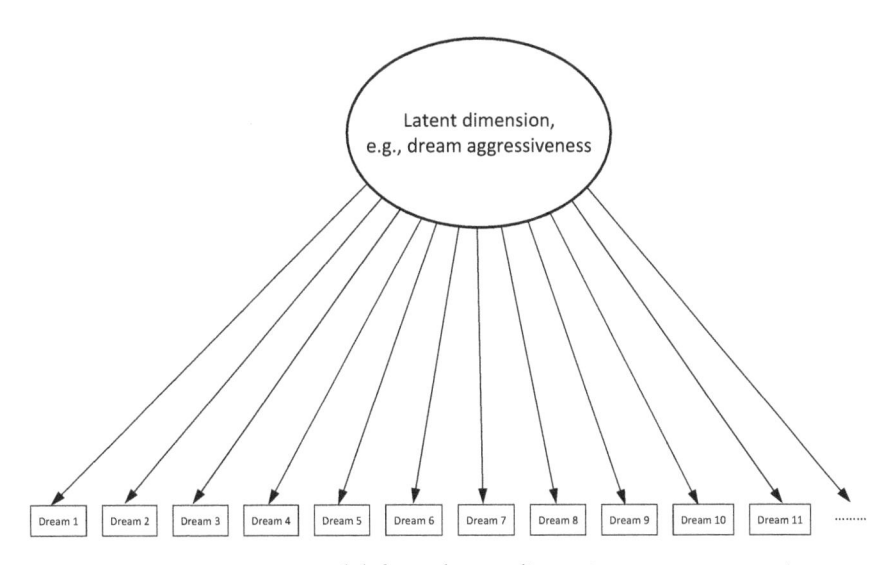

FIGURE 3.1 Measurement model for a latent dimension – e.g., aggression as a trait of the dreamer

To conclude, doing inference statistics for dream series is not an easy task. So far, Klingenberg (2008) has developed a procedure that can test the differences in percentages of two different time periods – e.g., whether the frequency of partner dreams (then ex-partner dreams) drops significantly after the break-up. For other tests – for example, whether cats occur more often in the same time period (let's say one year) – no statistical algorithms can be found in the literature. In order to promote the scientific study of dream series, some advancement regarding the statistical methods is necessary.

4
CURRENT DREAM SERIES – METHOD

Dreamer

The dreamer was born in 1962, the first of three children (younger sister and younger brother), and lived in different small towns in the Heidelberg region. The father of the dreamer worked as a computer specialist in different companies; the mother was a housewife but started later working as a career counselor (state institution). The divorce of the parents was in 1975; after that, the new partner of the mother lived for several years in the family household. After their separation, the mother was a single mother. After finishing school, the dreamer studied electrical engineering in Karlsruhe, Germany (within a distance of 70 km of his home town). During this time, he met his first partner (see section on "Partners in dreams"). Then, he studied psychology in Mannheim, Germany, completed his PhD in dream research – also in Mannheim – and worked as a research assistant, and later, as head of research in the sleep laboratory of the Central Institute of Mental Health in Mannheim (see Table 4.1).

Dream series

The first dream was recorded on the morning of September 5, 1984; the last dream entered into the analysis on December 31, 2016. This encompasses a period of more than 32 years. As the dreamer only recorded 20 dreams in 1984, these dreams were added to the 157 dreams recorded in 1985. The number of dreams per year are shown in Figure 4.1. Even though there were a few years – e.g., 1998 and 2000 – with a relatively small number of dreams, in most years, the dreamer was able to recall a substantial number of dreams – up to 879 in 1992.

DOI: 10.4324/9781003300373-4

TABLE 4.1 Curriculum vitae of the dreamer

Year(s)	Topic
1962	Born in a small town near Heidelberg, Germany
1968–1981	13 yrs education, completed with "Abitur"
1981–1986	Studies in electrical engineering (University of Karlsruhe), completed with "Diplom" (Master)
September 5, 1984	First recorded dream, start of keeping a regular dream diary
1986–1991	Studies in psychology (University of Mannheim), completed with "Diplom" (Master)
1991–1998	Research fellow (Sleep laboratory, Central Institute of Mental Health, Mannheim)
1995–1997	Doctoral fellowship ("Landesgraduiertenförderung")
1998	PhD in sleep and dream research (psychology), University of Mannheim
1998–2001	Research assistant (Sleep laboratory, Central Institute of Mental Health, Mannheim)
Since 2002	Head of the Sleep laboratory (Research), Central Institute of Mental Health, Mannheim
2003	"Habilitation" University of Mannheim
Since 2008	Associate Professor (University of Mannheim)

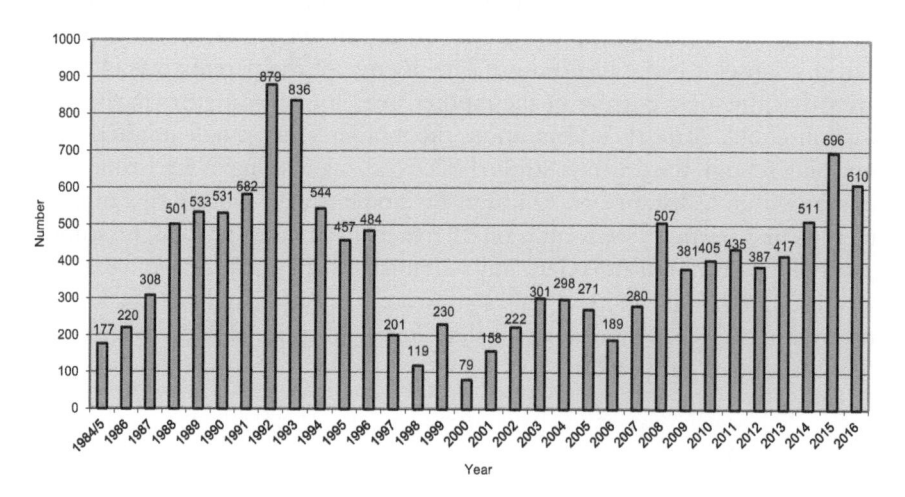

FIGURE 4.1 Number of dreams per year

Most dreams were recorded in the night/morning (N = 11,879); only a small number after a midday nap (N = 51), afternoon nap (N = 666), or a nap in the evening (N = 173). In most cases, one dream per night or nap (midday, afternoon, evening) was recorded. On 3,529 occasions (nights, daytime naps), the dreamer recalled and recorded two or dreams. The number of dreams recalled per sleep period are shown in Figure 4.2. In two nights, 12 dreams were written down, not in one session in the morning, but in several awakening periods in the night and after the final awakening in the morning (during his times being a student, the dreamer had the possibility of sleeping quite a long time).

For all 12,769 dreams, the mean word count was 137.60 ± 85.37, with the shortest dream report consisting of three words ("Sextraum mit P1"/"sex dream with P1") and the longest dream with 760 words. The frequencies of reports with different lengths are shown in Figure 4.3. Most dream reports ranged between 50 and 300 words, but also, shorter dream reports and longer dream reports were recorded.

In Figure 4.4, the mean word counts plus their standard deviations per year are depicted; the mean ranged between about 110 words per dream report (in 1994) to about 180 words per dream report (in 2013). The standard deviations are high in all years, as the report length differed considerably from dream to dream.

Procedure

During his studies in electrical engineering, the dreamer began to develop an interest in psychological topics, reading especially the books of Erich Fromm,

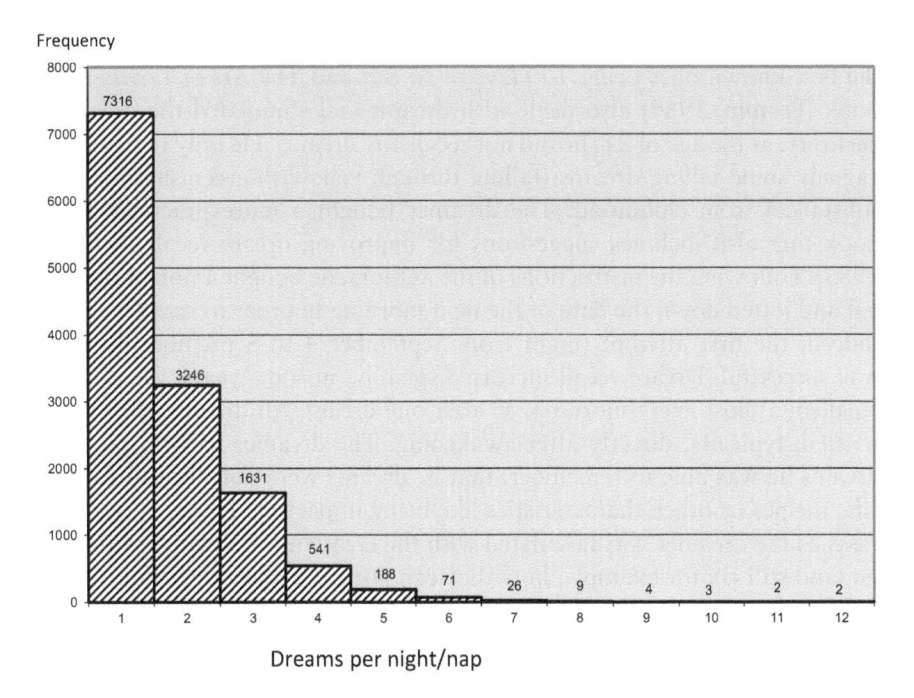

FIGURE 4.2 Dreams per night/nap

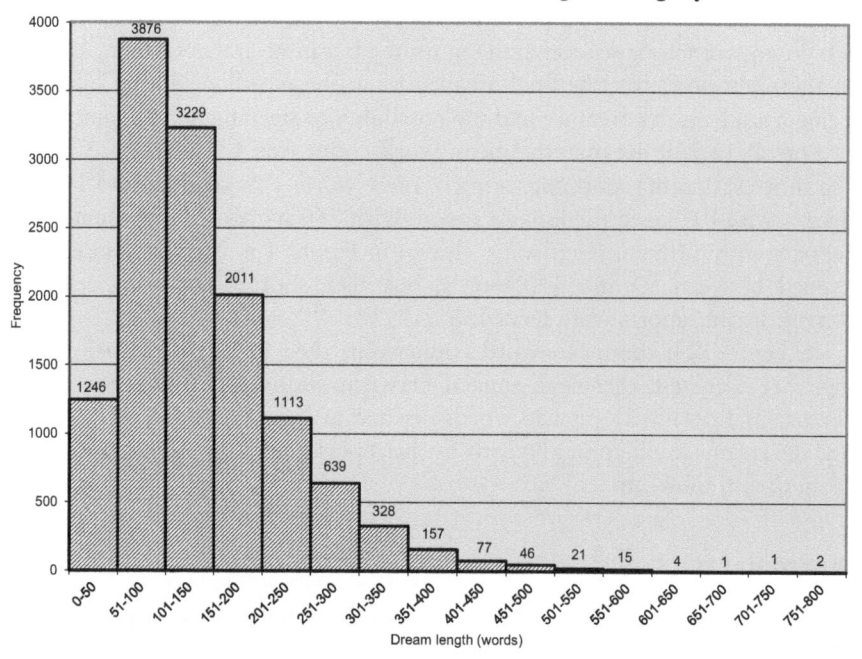

Number of Dreams for each word length category

FIGURE 4.3 Dream length distribution (N = 12,789 dreams)

the best-known ones being *To Have or to Be?* and *The Art of Loving.* One book (Fromm, 1980) also dealt with dreams and stimulated the dreamer's curiosity; at the age of 21, he did not recall any dreams. He only remembered vaguely some falling dreams (falling through yellowish-greenish and sticky substance) from childhood. The dreamer bought a more practical dream book that also includes suggestions for improving dream recall (Faraday, 1985). Following the instructions of the authors, he bought a notebook/journal and jotted down the date of the next morning in order to recall a dream. Indeed, the first attempt (night from September 4 to September 5, 1984) was successful. Dream recall increased steadily; in some years, the dreamer recalled, almost every morning, at least one dream. All dreams were hand-written, typically, directly after awakening. The dreamer tried to recall all dreams he was able to remember; that is, dreams were not selected for specific themes or other characteristics like being impactful. This was relatively easy, as the dreamer was fascinated with the creativity of dreams from early on (and still is); for example, how they can portray the waking-life issues of the dreamer in a very illustrative way.

In 2003, the dreamer started to type his dreams into word documents but switched very quickly to Alchera 3.72 – a dream diary software created

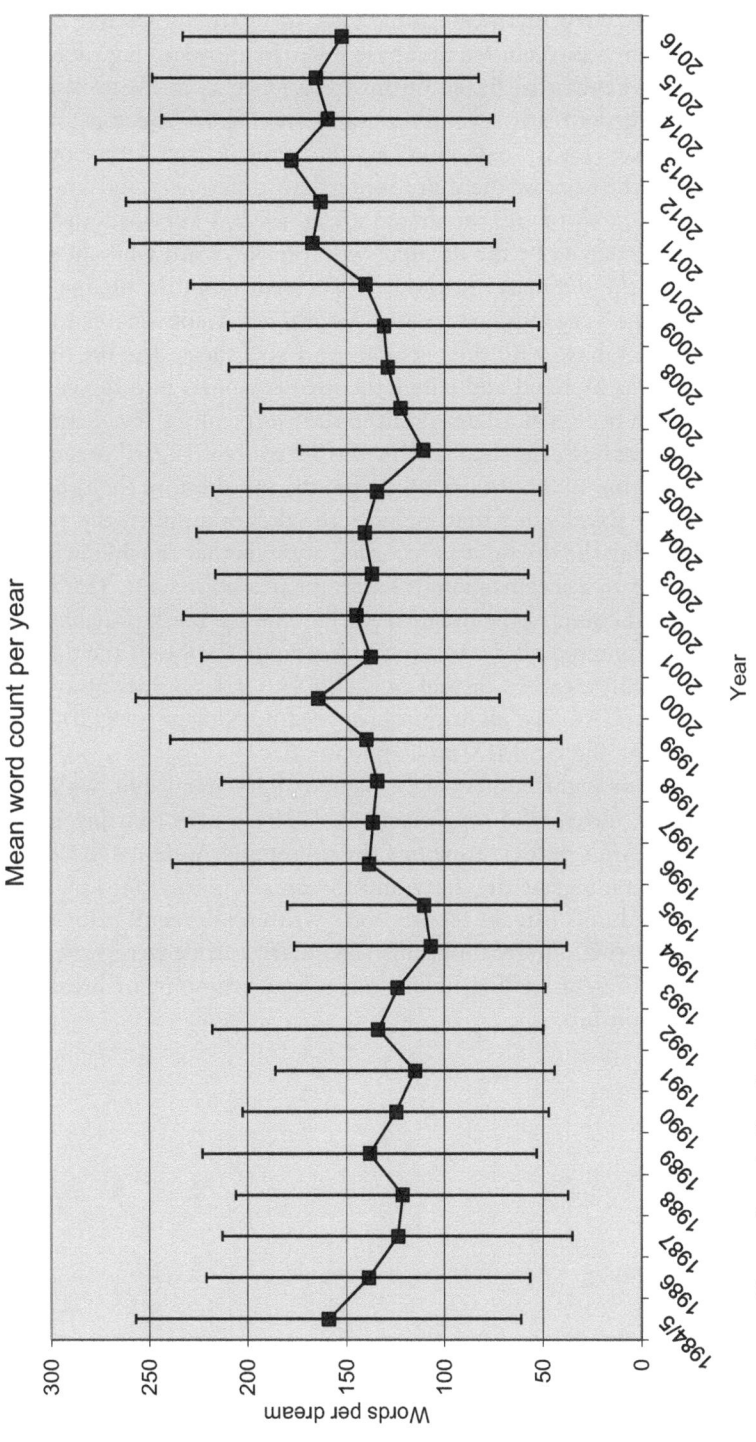

FIGURE 4.4   Dream length distribution per year

by Harry Bosma (www.mythwell.com). This software allows not only for entering the dream reports into a database but also allows to tag each dream with self-defined keywords. Based on his experience as a dream researcher and having recorded already several thousand dreams, the dreamer created a large number of keywords – e.g., father, mother, specific friend, type of sexual activity, colors, etc. – now, there are more than different 1,500 keywords. Within the Alchera software, the dreamer can select a keyword and see all dreams that were tagged by the dreamer with this keyword while he entered the dreams into the database. In order to perform more detailed statistics, Harry Bosma was very supportive and programed a conversion tool that transforms the database with the tags into an Excel sheet. The dreamer still records his dreams by hand and enters the dream reports into the database, and tagging them occurs at a later point in time (typically a few years later). For the present analysis, the data matrix was very large: 12,679 dreams with 1,751 tags, resulting in 22,200,929 data points. In addition, the dreamer is keeping an extra Excel sheet that includes the dream number, the year, the month, and the day the dream was recorded and whether the dream was the first, second, etc., on a specific night (or after an afternoon nap). This file also includes the word count of the dreams. At the time the book project started, the dreamer had entered all dreams until December 2016 into the database. The statistical analyses were carried out with SAS 9.4 (SAS Institute, Cary, North Carolina, USA). The algorithm proposed by Klingenberg (2008) was implemented using the GLIMIX procedure in SAS.

The dreamer also started keeping a regular diary (recording waking-life events, thoughts, ideas, etc.) on December 9, 1986, after starting his psychology studies. After participating in a dream seminar in January 1993, the dreamer began to integrate the diary and the dream journal into one, using differently colored inks (dream reports were written in green); prior to that, the dreamer kept two different journals. The diary entries were very helpful in determining different waking-life aspects – e.g., beginning or break-up of a romantic relationship.

5

DREAM CHARACTERS

5.1 Social dream network (known persons)

Overall, there were 11,088 occurrences of persons known to the dreamer in his waking life in 6,810 dreams (see Table 5.1). That is, 53.33% of the dreams included at least one known person. As unknown persons were not included, this is not comparable to the number of dream characters per dream as it has been determined by the rating systems of Hall and Van de Castle (1966).

Overall, 896 persons or categories were present in the dreams (see Table 5.2). The column with mean occurrence of persons within one category reflects nicely the closeness of these persons to the dreamer in his waking life, with the core family members showing a very high-averaged frequency, followed by romantic partners and friends. Women with whom

TABLE 5.1 Frequency of known persons in dreams

	Frequency	Percent
Nine persons	1	0.01%
Eight persons	0	0.00%
Seven persons	8	0.06%
Six persons	16	0.13%
Five persons	68	0.53%
Four persons	245	1.92%
Three persons	722	5.65%
Two persons	1,691	13.24%
One person	4,059	31.79%
No known person	5,959	46.67%

DOI: 10.4324/9781003300373-5

TABLE 5.2 Frequency of persons grouped into different categories

Category	Number of persons	Occurrences	Dreams with at least one character of this category	Mean number of occurrences of the characters in this category
Family	4	3640	2360	910.00
Kinship/relatives	38	507	418	13.34
Romantic partners	9	1531	1448	170.11
Women (erotic feelings, no partnership)	9	158	157	17.56
Friends	28	726	671	25.93
Colleagues (department of the dreamer)	47	819	666	17.43
Colleagues (Institute)	161	569	499	3.53
Colleagues (others)	97	225	208	2.32
Supervised students	32	140	130	4.38
Engineering studies	30	116	99	5.80
Psychology studies	69	473	421	6.86
School-related persons	101	1012	750	10.02
Known persons – e.g., neighbors, persons involved in the same hobby	161	990	777	6.14
Celebrities	120	180	165	1.50

the dreamer hat brief romantic involvements (without developing into a partnership) occurred not that often in dreams; the same is valid for relatives. Interestingly, the pattern "closeness in waking life and mean number of occurrences in the dream" can also be found in the professional world of the dreamer; that is, colleagues with whom he works (and worked) more closely together (in the same department) occurred, on average, more often than colleagues working in other departments of the institute or in other institutions.

Table 5.3 displays those dream persons with the highest number of occurrences within the dream series. Even though it is to be expected that the core family members occur most often (the dreamer spent very much time with them in waking life during the course of his life), the fact that the brother is slightly more common than the mother is puzzling. One might speculate that

TABLE 5.3 Top 22 dream characters

No.	Code	Frequency	Percent	Description
1	Bruder	1,242	9.73%	Brother
2	Mutter	1,236	9.68%	Mother
3	Schwester	878	6.87%	Sister
4	P3	791	6.19%	Former romantic partner ("true love")
5	P4	416	3.26%	Former romantic partner
6	Vater	285	2.23%	Father
7	G096	153	1.20%	School friend (male)
8	F05	142	1.12%	Close friend (female) during psychology studies
9	G100	116	0.91%	School friend (male)
10	P1	112	0.88%	First romantic partner
11	S24	101	0.79%	Colleague (female), Department
12	V23	88	0.69%	Partner of the mother after divorce (lived in the household)
13	S09	84	0.66%	Colleague and former boss (male), Department
14	N22	75	0.59%	Landlady (sub-tenancy in a family)
15	S35	72	0.57%	Colleague and former boss (male), Department
16	F15	70	0.56%	Friend (male)
17	P5	61	0.48%	Former romantic partner
18	F11	60	0.47%	Friend (male)
19	F06	55	0.43%	Friend and colleague (male)
20	P6	53	0.42%	Former partner
21	G035	53	0.42%	School friend (male)
22	S07	50	0.39%	Colleague (female)

this reflects sibling rivalry, which was quite strong between the brother and the dreamer in their childhood and adolescence and, thus, was personally relevant for the dreamer. The markedly lower frequency of the father can be explained that the dreamer had almost no contact with him after the divorce of the parents (the dreamer was, at that point, 12 years old).

The person with the most frequent occurrences but who is not family was the "true love" of the dreamer, with whom he had three periods of partnership (for more information, see "Partnerships" section). The next most frequent person was the partner with whom the dreamer was about ten yrs together. Three other former romantic partners are among the 22 most frequent dream characters.

5.2 Core family members in dreams

The core family of the dreamer consisted of five persons: the parents, one younger sister, and one younger brother (see Table 5.4). A previous analysis of the dream series, including all dreams recorded until 2007, can be found in Schredl (2013b). Interestingly, the brother occurred slightly more often in the dreams compared to the dreamer's mother. In sample of 1,612 diary dreams reported by male and female students (Nöltner & Schredl, 2023), the mother was the most frequent family member (13.4%), followed by the father (7.6%); siblings occurred less often; that is, sister (7.6%) and brother (5.1%), but these figures are difficult to interpret because the study did not elicit whether the dreamer had siblings or not. Similar findings with the mother the most frequent family member have been reported, for a student sample, by Hall and Van de Castle (1966) and, for two dream series, reported by a female dreamer (Domhoff, 2003; Schredl, 2021e). The frequency of the father dreams is quite low; the dreamer had almost no contact with him for years after the divorce (see Table 5.5). The frequency of the dreamer's sister occurring in dreams is intermediate between father occurrences and brother/mother occurrences.

In order to back up the analysis regarding co-occurrences of family members in dreams, the information given in Table 5.5 is crucial. Until the age of 12, all family members lived together, but after the divorce, the dreamer lived with his mother, his sister, and his brother. During his first studies (electrical engineering), the dreamer had a student flat but was at home every weekend and during the winter and summer breaks. This changed in 1986; then, the dreamer had his own apartment and stayed in contact with his family, with occasional meetings.

The majority of the family dreams only included one family member (see Table 5.6). Overall, at least one family member occurred in 2,360 dreams–18.48% of all dreams. In 881 dreams, there was a co-occurrence of at least two family members. All five family members (including the dreamer) occurred relatively

TABLE 5.4 Core family of the dreamer and their occurrence in dreams

	Born in	*Frequency*	*Percent*
Father	1932	285	2.23%
Mother	1943	1236	9.67%
Dreamer	1962	–	–
Sister	1963	877	6.87%
Brother	1965	1242	9.73%

TABLE 5.5 Timeline of the dreamer living with his core family

Year	
Till 1975	All family members lived together
1975	Divorce (dreamer lived with mother, brother, sister)
1981	Dreamer lived in student apartment but, on weekends, at home (mother and brother; sister had moved out)
Since 1986	Own apartment (dreamer did not live with any family member)

TABLE 5.6 Frequency of core family members in dreams

	Frequency	*Percent*
Four family members	49	0.38%
Three family members	301	2.36%
Two family members	531	4.16%
One family member	1479	11.58%
No family member	10,409	81.52%

rarely in the dreamer (a findings which seems plausible, as the dream recording started long after the divorce and the time period all five core family members lived together).

The time course of the frequency of family dreams is depicted in Figure 5.1. Despite the varying frequencies per year, there is a slight decrease in family dreams over the years ($r = -.284$, $p = .058$, one-tailed). This is expected, as the dreamer spent much more time with his family when he was younger and living at home (see also the years 1984/5 and 1986, when the dreamer was often at home) and this time interval to this period of intense contact is increasing over time.

In Figure 5.2, the time course of the dreams for each member of the core family are depicted. The linear trends for the mother dreams ($r = -.231$, $p = .102$, one-tailed) and father dreams ($r = -.279$, $p = .061$, one-tailed) is parallel the overall decrease of family dreams, whereas the sister dreams

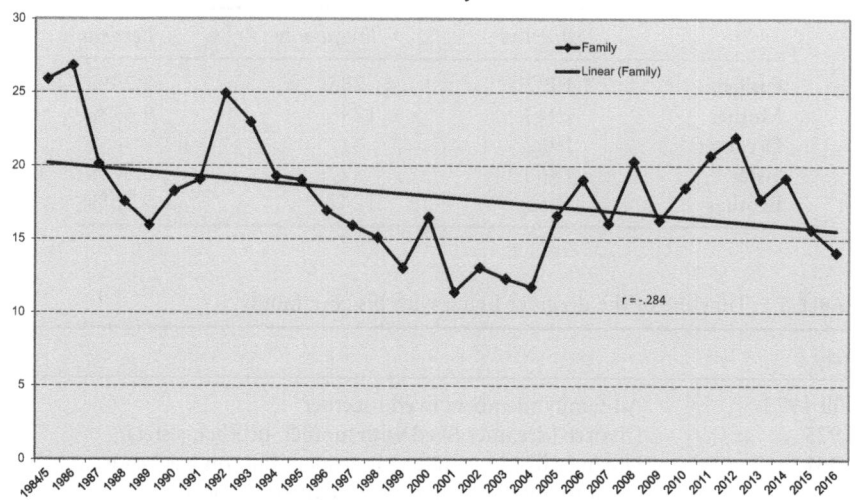

FIGURE 5.1 Time course of dreams with at least one family member

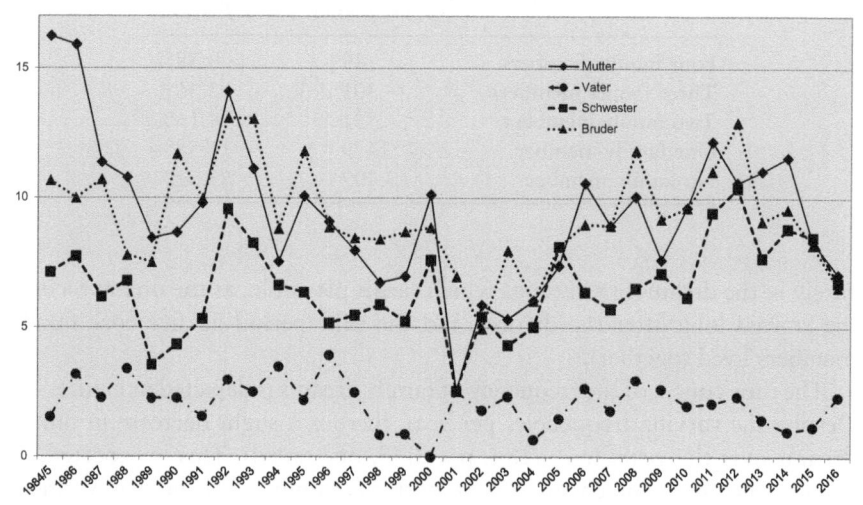

FIGURE 5.2 Time course of dreams with one family member

increased over the years (r = .280, p = .121), leading to comparable frequency of dreams with mother, brother, and sister in 2015 and 2016. The brother dreams also showed a slight decrease (r = -.160, p = .381). One possible explanation for the increase of sister dreams is that she is the only one who

TABLE 5.7 Co-occurrence of core family members in 2,360 dreams with at least one family member

	Frequency	Percent
Father (alone)	107	4.53%
Mother (alone)	274	11.61%
Sister (alone)	571	24.19%
Brother (alone)	527	22.33%
Father – Mother	36	1.53%
Father – Sister	12	0.51%
Father – Brother	26	1.10%
Mother – Sister	112	4.75%
Mother – Brother	199	8.43%
Sister – Brother	146	6.19%
Father – Mother – Sister	6	0.25%
Father – Mother – Brother	17	0.72%
Father – Sister – Brother	32	1.36%
Mother – Sister – Brother	246	10.42%
All four family members	49	2.08%

TABLE 5.8 Percentage of family member occurring alone related to the overall occurrence of this family member

	Frequency	Percent
Father (alone)	107/285	37.54%
Mother (alone)	274/1,236	22.17%
Sister (alone)	571/877	65.11%
Brother (alone)	527/1,242	42.43%

had started a family (three children) and, therefore, played an increasingly important role in the core family.

The family dreams were next grouped according their co-occurrence with other family members (see Table 5.7). Almost two-thirds of the family dreams (62.67%) featured only one family member. Interestingly, the percentage of dreams of occurring as only family member compared to the dreams in which the family member occurred with at least one other family member varies considerably (see Table 5.8). Whereas the mother most often co-occurred with other family members (almost 80%), the sister only co-occurred only in about 35% of the dreams with other family members. Thus, if the dreamer dreamed about his sister, other family members did rarely occur in the dream. Given the family constellations in the dreamer's past (see Table 5.5), this makes sense as the sister was the first sibling who moved out permanently.

Looking at the dreams with at least two family members, the most striking finding is that the number of dreams with all five family members (N =49) is much smaller compared to the number of dreams with the family after the divorce (mother, sister, brother; N = 246 dreams). The second most frequent constellation consisted of the mother and the brother (N = 199), with whom the dreamer also lived together for several years, after the sister moved out.

Death of the dreamer's brother in 2016

The brother of the dreamer died unexpectedly on Aug 31, 2016. The frequency of dreams including the brother in 2016 was 28/418 (6.25%) before his death and 12/192 (6.70%) after his death; that is, no change in frequency. However, dream content was changing after the death. In eight of the 12 dreams recorded after his death, the dreamer had no direct contact with the brother – typically, the dreamer being in the same apartment (family apartment) as the brother, which seems to be a reference to much earlier times. This figure (75%) is lower compared to the percentage of 37% in 100 randomly selected dreams (see Table 5.21).

The following text is the first dream in which the dreamer was aware, in the dream, that his brother was dead.

Dream example (September 27, 2016):

> *I am in an apartment and go into my room, which is out in front. I get a fright, because I see a foot and think that all have flown out, but it is a guest (woman, known). I go back into the hallway, there stands my brother (about 30 yrs. old, slim), he seems quite unconcerned. I am surprised to see him because I know he is dead. He is not fully there, but more like a figure.*

Interestingly, the dreamer's brother was younger and slimmer in the dream than in real life (brother died at 51 yrs and was very obese); that is, a clear mismatch between dream and waking life. The next two dreams, also recorded after the brother's death, involved very dangerous situations, but the dreamer as well as the brother survived unscathed.

Dream example:

> *My brother drives quite fast down the sloping road, I tell him to slow down, but too late. On the right side of the road is sand (several tens of meters), so he cannot brake. The vehicle comes off the road, it goes into the field, but my brother prevents rollover or something similar and comes to a safe stop. We, especially I, breathe a sigh of relief. That could have ended badly – at that speed.*

Dream example:

> *Then we swim in the water, a mountain lake with two outlets (wide) that turn into waterfalls. One person is with me. We get into dangerous water and I want to swim back, but the current is very strong. I misjudge where the current is weaker, but the other person (possibly my brother) is better. I swim forward in the supine position, also doing strong arm pulls, the other person swims in my current shadow. We make fast progress and I am relieved when we are out of the danger zone.*

The last dream with the brother recorded in 2016 included a situation that was not uncommon during adolescence (sibling rivalry between the brother and the dreamer), even though the setting was a current one.

Dream example:

> *I am called in from the next room to help with something on the computer. There are two large rooms (sleep lab) where there are several worksta-tions. I get to the computer, but my brother doesn't release the chair that goes with it, which I think is dumb. I go back.*

In addition to the dreams featuring the brother, the dreamer had five dreams that referred to the death of the brother; the first of these dreams was recorded on October 9, 2016. In this dream, the dreamer tells the institute director about the death of the brother (never done in waking life). Also, the situation in the next dream – seeing some things that belonged to my brother (knowing that he is now dead) – never occurred in waking life (with these types of things). In the third dream, a former school friend is comforting me because of the death of my brother (also never happened). In dream 4, the dreamer sees his father and speculates whether the sadness of the father is related to the loss of his son. The last dream of this kind in 2016 featured the dreamer's mother calling the dreamer's father in order to tell him that the brother (his son) is dead. The dreamer thinks of this is very odd, as the father also attended the funeral and did know that, at that point.

As the present analysis only included dreams five months after the death, future analyses of the dream series could look at the frequency of brother dreams, whether it is declining, and whether brother dreams might reflect the long shared-life history between the dreamer and his brother.

5.3 Romantic partners in dreams

The partnership history of the dreamer is shown in Table 5.9. The first relationship started prior to the start of keeping the dream diary in

TABLE 5.9 Romantic partnerships and frequency of partner dreams during the relationship

Partner	Year	Duration	Dreams	Partner dreams
P1	February 1984 to October 20, 1986	2 yrs, 9 m	370	16.76%
P2	January 17, 1988 to March 16, 1988	2 m	78	6.41%
P3–1	August 6, 1988 to May 2, 1989	9 m	354	16.10%
P3–2	October 1, 1989 to July 31, 1990	10 m	401	22.69%
P4	September 19, 1993 to July 31, 2003	9 yrs, 11 m	2,828	11.56%
P3–3	December 26, 2003 to February 17, 2005	1 yr, 2 m	318	18.24%
P5	November 24, 2005 to December 23, 2007	2 yrs, 1 m	485	8.25%
P6	February 10, 2008 to September 4, 2008	7 m	262	8.02%
P7	July 26, 2009 to September 12, 2009	2 m	28	10.71%
P8	May 25, 2010 to September 1, 2010	3 m	108	7.41%
P9	October 31, 2011 to April 29, 2012	6 m	140	12.86%

February 1984. With one long relationship of about ten years, most of the relationships were rather short. A special case is P3, the dreamer's true love, as they had three different relationship phases, with a brief and a longer gap in-between.

The frequency of partner dreams during the respective relationships varied from about 6% (P2) to about 23% (P3–2) (see Table 5.9); the latter was the most emotionally intense relationship the dreamer has experienced so far. Taking together all three partnership phases with P3 resulted in a frequency of 19.20% partner dreams. The statistical analysis using the algorithm developed by Klingenberg (2008) for binary time series with gaps revealed that P3 occurred significantly more often than P4, P5, P5, P8, and P9 but did not differ from P1 (the number of dreams was too small for comparison to P2 and P7) (Schredl, 2018a). In this dream series, the frequency of partner dreams mainly reflected the emotional intensity of the romantic relationship, as the relationships with low partner-dream frequency were less intense. The exception is the first partnership of the dreamer because it was not very close on an emotional level but, of course, special because everything was new.

In order to analyze whether the frequency of partner dreams changes during a long-lasting relationship, the relationship phase with P4 was divided into ten intervals of almost equal length (about one year). Although the frequency of partner dreams was lower in the last year, and two years in-between, the frequency stayed relatively stable (see Table 5.10). It should be added that the dreamer lived together with P4. The dreams seem not to reflect some form of "cooling" over the course of the partnership. In this context, the findings of Schredl and Wood (2021) are interesting, as their content analysis of 296 partner dreams reported by a large student sample (N = 425) showed that

TABLE 5.10 Partner dreams during the longest relationship

Segments	Start	End	Duration in days	Dreams	Percent
1	19.09.1993	14.09.1994	360	597	12.40%
2	15.09.1994	10.09.1995	360	439	13.44%
3	11.09.1995	05.09.1996	360	475	13.68%
4	06.09.1996	01.09.1997	360	316	6.96%
5	02.09.1997	28.08.1998	360	95	11.58%
6	29.08.1998	24.08.1999	360	231	11.69%
7	25.08.1999	19.08.2000	360	121	8.26%
8	20.08.2000	15.08.2001	360	72	12.50%
9	16.08.2001	11.08.2002	360	199	13.57%
10	12.08.2002	31.07.2003	353	283	8.48%

partner dreams often involved shared activities – e.g., driving a car, visiting someone (about 70%) – whereas sexual activities are only a minor motive in partner dreams (about 4%).

For the next graph, the diary-keeping period was divided into segments – into the relationship periods and the periods in which the dreamer was single (see Figure 5.3). If a segment was considerably longer than one year, it was split into segments of about a one-year duration. The frequency of P3 dreams was highest – as expected – during the three relationship periods P3 and the dreamer spent together. Although there is a slight increase in P3 dreams during the periods of being single (between P6 and P7, and P7 and P8), the frequency is relatively constant about one year after the separation; about 5% of the dreams included P3, even years after their last separation in 2005. Notable is that, during the long relationship with P4, the frequency of P3 dreams was the lowest.

In Figure 5.4, the time course of the dreams including one of the partners during and after the relationship (five one-year intervals) is depicted. After one year, the frequency of the partner dreams with brief relationships (P2, P7, P8, P9) was already relatively low, whereas the longer relationships (P1, P4) were followed by more partner dreams (about 5%). The highest percentages were, however, found for the true love of the dreamer (P3), who showed up quite frequently in the dreams in the year after the separation – and even later. After four to five years, ex-partner dreams were very scarce, except for the dreams including P3.

Although the partners of the dreamer never met in person in real life, 77 dreams featured two (N = 71) or three (N = 6) partners. In most of the dreams (N = 71), P3 was involved, with P4 (N = 33 dreams) and P1 (N = 18) also quite often. A direct verbal interaction between the two partners happened in 14 dreams. The first dream included some kind of shock the dreamer experienced while going out with the current partner (dream occurred during the relationship with P4) and seeing the former partner (P3) (see the following). However, this dream is very creative, and, as the two women started talking, the dreamer relaxes.

Dream example with interaction between two partners (June 30, 1994):

> *Street cafe (small) on the sidewalk in front of a bakery. I wait for someone and eat a slice of bread. P3 is sitting at the next table. At first, I think: "Oh, my God" and want to look away. Then P3 asks P4 if she writes poetry. She has heard about it through others. As she speaks, I notice that her voice sounds different from usual, a little thinner. P4 answers in the affirmative and says that writing does her good. I look at her and P3 quite casually.*

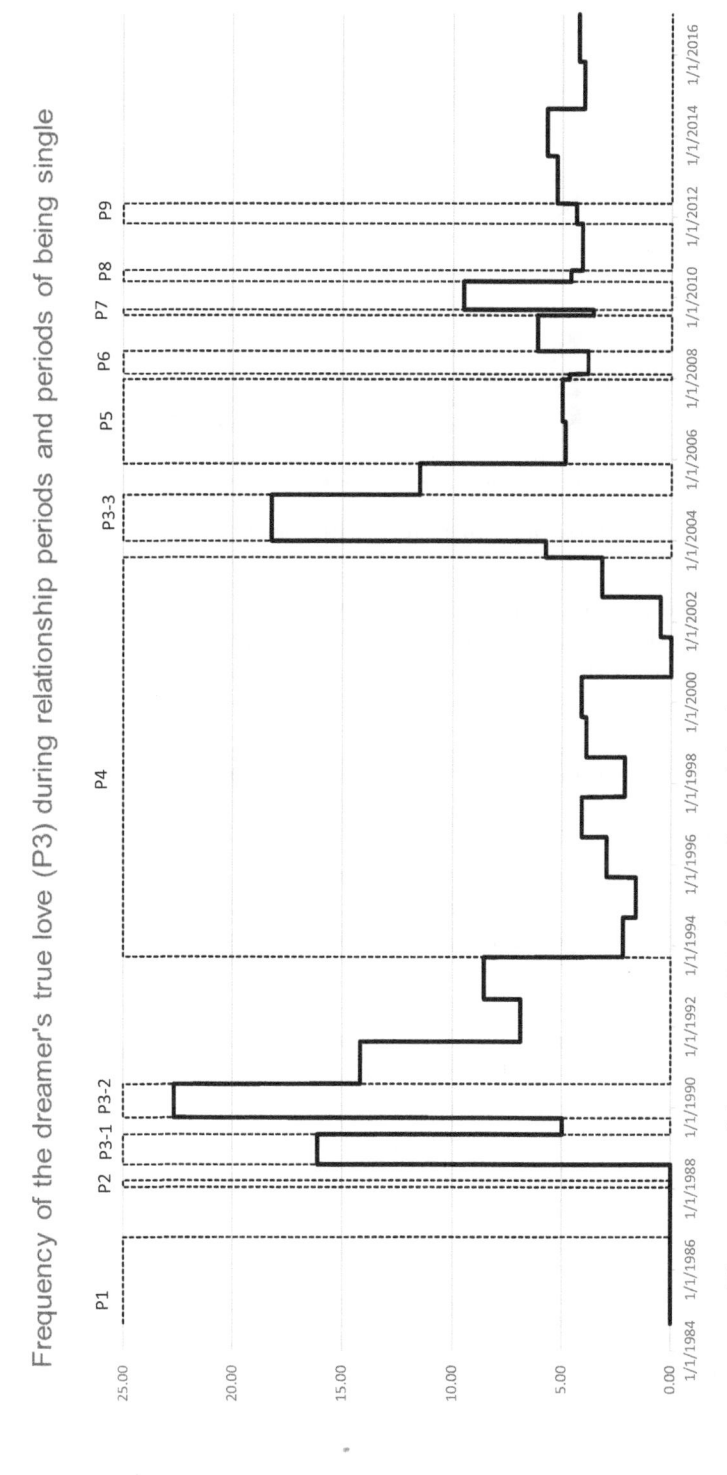

Frequency of the dreamer's true love (P3) during relationship periods and periods of being single

FIGURE 5.3 Time course of dreams with P3, the true love of the dreamer

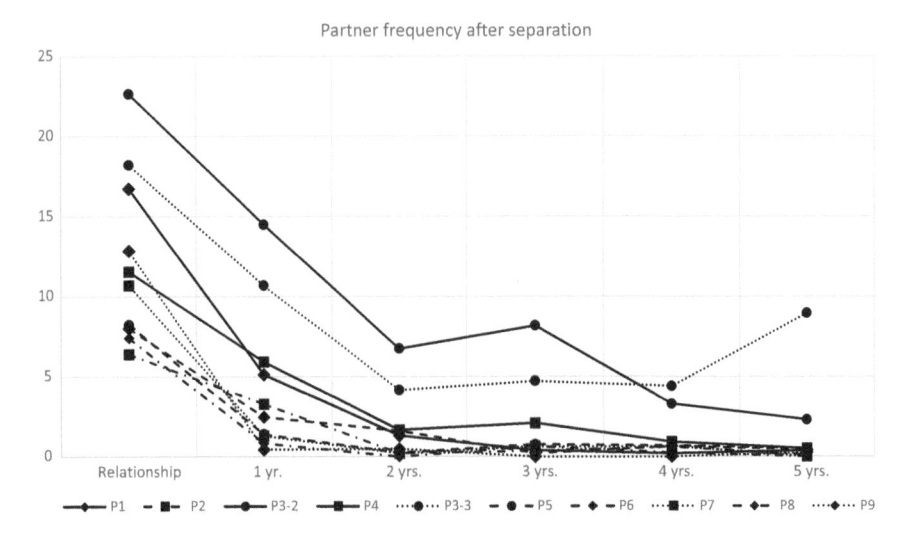

FIGURE 5.4 Time course of partner dreams after separation

In the second dream, the dreamer was frustrated, not feeling close to his current partner (P5). Again, the dream is creative and depict two of his former partners having a close relationship with each other, something the dreamer would like to have with his current partner.

Dream example with interaction between two partners (April 4, 2007):

> *I sit snuggled up close to P5 in a club. I'm not doing so well, being sad. When we leave, P5 pulls me back because I hadn't said anything for a long time, and my desire for closeness is frustrated. Now P4 and P3 are talking. My two former partners develop a better relationship with each other than with me, I think.*

The majority of the dreams with two or more partners were, however, very "dreamy," that is, in 45 dreams, the two partners were blended into one person and/or switching within the dream. The following dream example illustrate this kind of mixing between the current partner (P3) and a former partner (P2) in a sex dream.

Dream example with switching between two partners (November 9, 1988):

> *I sleep with P2. While doing so, I put on a condom. We (now P3) are amazed that it holds so well. It's incredibly horny to penetrate her. I feel the pleasure and move my pelvis. She (?) stands in front of me and soon interrupts, I pull out the penis with condom, it held. In the end, I feel I slept with P2, that it was quite great and that I hurt P3.*

In the next example, a form of merging occurs, that is, the dreamer is doing something with P3 but has the impression that P3 is not only P3 but is mixed with "a little bit" of P4.

Dream example with blending between two partners (October 27, 2009):

> *P3 (perhaps somewhat mixed with P4) and I are in a city on the road. The atmosphere is a bit tense, because P3 still wants to work a bit, while I see it rather casually. We are in the city for vacation. We are in the car and look for the way back to the hotel.*

The next dream occurred when the dreamer was single, not very long after the separation from P7.

Dream example with blending between two partners (November 7, 2002):

> *I come with my partner in a (our) apartment, it is beautiful and spacious. The partner has a lot of P3, something of P4. We then lie in bed, she was previously somewhere else in the apartment. We cuddle, I feel lust, but somehow I also feel confused. We were separated for a while, I do not feel whether I love her, that is, there is closeness and distance at the same time. She is rather reserved, and then walks around the apartment again.*

The last dream example is what Freud would have called a wish fulfillment dream, more exactly a dream with an almost fulfilled wish. The dream occurred when the dreamer was single.

Dream example with blending between two partners (October 11, 2013):

> *I am lying in a large, old-fashioned double bed. On my right is P3, on my left P6. Both are stroking me intensely. I get an erection and think about how it goes to have sex with two women, whether I can do it. P3 embraces my penis, P6 pulls back, so it looks like I will have sex with P3. It feels very nice, but then the alarm clock rings, it's quite early in the morning and without transition P3 gets up. I am frustrated because she is now very cool and wants me to get up too.*

This special feature of dreaming, blending different persons into one, is very interesting. One might think of Sigmund Freud's concept of condensation. In discussing this mechanism, Freud cites several examples of "collective and composite figures" occurring in his own dreams (p. 400; Freud, 1900/1991); for example, he mentioned a dream character whose physical appearance was that of his elder brother, but his manner of speaking and acting were those of Dr. R. For Freud, these condensations were important to fully understand the dream's meaning (Freud, 1900/1991). A modern viewpoint of the same phenomenon was put forward by Ernest Hartmann, who emphasized that dreaming – being a specific state of consciousness – helps the dreamer to make new connections (Hartmann, 2011). He reported that, in his clinical practice, six women had a specific type of blending dreams – e.g. "I was dreaming about my boyfriend 'Jim', and then he turned into my father" (p. 44; Hartmann, 2011). All of these women said that these dreams drew their attention to the fact that there are similarities between their partner and their father that they had not realized before. This new connection can enhance our self-understanding (Hartmann, 2011). A very interesting artistic depiction of this blending phenomenon has been created by Andrew Niccol in his movie "S1M0NE," released in 2002. In the film, the movie director Victor Taransky (actor: Al Pacino) is offered a software that is able to combine the best characteristics of many well-known actresses into one virtual female character (actress: Rachel Roberts). This worked out very well; this virtual actress was exceptional and became famous almost overnight (in the movie).

In the dream series, 142 dreams included the mother of the dreamer and one partner (N = 136), two partners (N = 5) or three partners (N = 1), resulting in 149 occurrences of partners in dreams with the mother (see Table 5.11). The percentage of partner dreams (N = 1,448) that also included the mother of the dreamer was 9.81% – comparable with the percentage of all mother dreams in the dream series (9.67%); that is, there was no hint that the mother was more prominent in partner dreams compared to all other dreams. However, there was a high number of mother/partner dreams with P1 as partner; this might reflect the fact that the first partnership was during a time period when the dreamer still lived partly at home and his partner often visited him there; that is, there was a considerable amount of contact between

TABLE 5.11 Dreams with co-occurrence of partners and the mother of the dreamer

Partner	Partner dreams	Dreams with partner and mother	Percent	Dreams with blending of partner and mother	Dreams with direct interaction between partner and mother
P1	112	26	23.12%	0	2
P2	45	3	6.67%	0	0
P3	791	66	8.35%	3	10
P4	416	36	8.67%	12	1
P5	61	6	9.84%	2	1
P6	55	4	7.55%	0	0
P7	14	1	7.14%	0	0
P8	16	4	25.00%	0	0
P9	23	3	13.04%	0	0

P1 and the dreamer's mother. The high percentages for P8 and P9 should be viewed with caution, as the number of dreams is very small.

A small difference (effect size = 0.046) regarding the frequency of mother dreams was found for dreams recorded during relationship periods (N = 5369) and periods in which the dreamer was single (N = 7400): 8.90% vs. 10.24%. Given the large number of dreams, this small difference might be significant and reflect something along the lines that the mother might be more important to the dreamer in periods without a steady relationship.

The type of interaction between the dreamer's mother and the partner are depicted in Table 5.12. A direct communication between the mother and the partner is relatively rare; more often, both are present in the same dream scene but without having any direct contact. In yet another set of dreams, the partner(s) and the mother had no contact at all, appearing in unrelated scenes in the dream. For example, the dream with the mother and three partners is a dream with P1, P2, and P3 blending into one partner, and this partner occurred in a scene unrelated to the dream scene with the mother. Despite the small sample size, it is interesting that P3 ("true love") was most often involved in direct communication with the dreamer's mother (see Table 5.11), even though P1 and P4 had more frequent contacts with the dreamer's mother in waking life.

The blending of the dreamer's mother and a partner of the dreamer occurred in 17 dreams (see Table 5.12), only with partners with whom the dreamer had a long relationship, especially P4 (longest relationship).

One might speculate whether relationships with partners showing some similar characteristics with the mother – see Ernest Hartmann's reasoning earlier – might have a chance to last longer. On the other hand, one might argue that longer relationships increase the familiarity with the partner's strengths and weaknesses and, thus, a more detailed comparison between the partner and the mother (very high familiarity) can be made. Furthermore, based on Hartmann's ideas, one might speculate whether P4, who had the

TABLE 5.12 Interactions between partners and the mother of the dreamer in dreams where they co-occur (N = 142)

Interaction	Dreams	Percent	Examples
Direct interaction	13	9.15%	Mother is talking to partner; partner is irritated by the mother while having sex with the dreamer.
Being together in a dream scene	65	45.77%	Both are in the same apartment, car, etc., but have no direct contact.
No contact	47	33.10%	Partner and mother occur in different and unrelated dream scenes.
Blending between partner and mother	17	11.97%	See dream examples that follow.

highest number of blending with the mother, is the partner that has the most similarities to the mother. Reviewing the relationship history, there might be something there (personal remark of the author). Interestingly, the percentage of blending dreams including mother and partner related to all dreams in which the mother and one of the dreamer's partner co-occur (N = 142) is much lower (11.97%) compared to the percentage of blending dreams of two or more partners related to the number of dreams with co-occurring partners (N = 77), which is 58.44%. This would imply – again, based on Hartmann's idea – that the partners are more similar to each other than they are to the mother – which makes sense, of course.

Sigmund Freud would have enjoyed the next dream example, with the dreamer, of course, having some knowledge of the Oedipus complex theory.

Dream with blending between partner P4 and the dreamer's mother:

> *P4 wants to go back with others in the car. I want to go by train and run. I make a remark that she should go quietly with her new friends. She decides to change her mind and runs after me. Now it is my mother. She leans against me for a moment, which makes me uncomfortable. I think to myself that I should end this relationship (which is also sexual) with my mother. I am a real Oedipus.*

The following two dream examples also address some kind of confusion related to physical closeness, which is welcomed with the partner but not so with the mother.

Dream example:

> *I cuddle P3, but it is my mother. I kiss her on the toes; she doesn't like that at all because she can't stand the smell. She would smell that if I kissed her on the face. She is annoyed.*

Dream example:

> *Here comes P3, I think at first, into the room, I would like her to lie down with me, which she does. But it's my mother; the physical closeness makes me a little uncomfortable.*

Schredl (2018a) published the frequency of former partner dreams in 2013; the comparison between the years 2013 and 2016 (see Table 5.13) showed that the number of partner dreams decreased significantly (Glimmix procedure: t = 3.1, p < .0012, one-tailed) during this period of the dreamer being single (his last relationship ended in 2012; see Table 5.10). The decrease in

TABLE 5.13 Dreams of former partners in years 2013 and 2016

Partner	2013[1] (N = 417 dreams)		2016 (N = 610 dreams)	
	Partner dreams	Percent	Partner dreams	Percent
P1	2	0.48%	0	0.00%
P2	0	0.00%	0	0.00%
P3	27	6.47%	28	4.59%
P4	10	2.40%	6	0.98%
P5	1	0.24%	0	0.00%
P6	3	0.72%	1	0.16%
P7	2	0.48%	0	0.00%
P8	1	0.24%	0	0.00%
P9	2	0.48%	1	0.16%
Dreams with at least one partner	45	10.79%	35	5.74%

[1]Published in Schredl (2018a).

frequency of former partner dreams has also been shown in a larger population-based sample (Schredl, Cadiñanos Echevarria, et al., 2020). In both
years, the most often occurring former partner was P3, the true love of the
dreamer.

Analyzing the dream content of the former partner dreams indicated
that most of the dreams including P3 were positive and, in almost 50%, the
dreamer had some form of relationship going on (see dream example that
follows). This is in contrast with the analysis of the dream series of "Barb
Sanders" (pseudonym), performed by Domhoff (2003): even a long time after
separation, aggression was prominent in the ex-husband dreams reflecting her
negative experiences in their marriage (ten years) with three children. For this
dreamer, the true love is still imagined as positive, even after three break-ups.

A previous analysis (Schredl, 2011a) indicated that the emotional tone of
the partner dreams with P3 during the three relationship periods was almost
balanced: 44 positively toned dreams, 33 negatively toned dreams, and 150
dreams with no explicitly mentioned emotions toward the partner. Comparing the 2013 and 2016 P3 dreams (see Table 5.14) that occurred long after
the relationship periods ended can lead to the hypothesis that these dreams
idealize P3 (longing for true love) and do not reflect the flipside of the coin;
that is, the problems that had led to the break-ups. Interestingly, more positive emotions in ex-partner dreams compared to current partner dreams were
also found in diary dreams collected from a larger student sample (N = 425)
(Schredl & Wood, 2021). Within the context of a general theory regarding

TABLE 5.14 Former partner dreams during 2016

Dream content	P3 dreams (N = 28 dreams)		Dreams with other partners (N = 8 dreams)	
	Frequency	Percent	Frequency	Percent
Being in relationship with partner in the dream	13	46.43%	2	25.00%
Being separated within the dream	1	3.57%	2	25.00%
Positive emotion of the dreamer toward partner	21	75.00%	2	25.00%
Neutral	7	25.00%	6	75.00%
Negative emotion of the dreamer toward partner	0	0.00%	0	0.00%
Erotic behavior	6	35.71%	5	25.00%

the continuity between waking and dreaming, this might suggest that positive relationship experiences prevail longer in the dreamer's mind than the negative ones. So, this finding might add to the factors that can affect the continuity between waking and dreaming (see Chapter 1.2).

Dream example with being in relationship with P3:

P3 and I are coming back from a trip together. It is morning and we have had a rental car that we still have to return. P3's small car is parked in the parking lot of a small train station. I am busy repacking, among other things I stuff dirty laundry into my small black suitcase . . . but I hug her from behind, at chest level, also feel her breasts. It feels very good to hug her; I am thinking about whether our relationship attempt will work.

Dream example with P4 (not being in relationship):

I am in a room with other people and am talking to P4. She has problems with Xavier, possibly her partner. It is about playing double head, with ambition. I note that it took her quite a long time to play well, in the beginning. She admits that, she says that she dreamed about it at that time. Now she plays very well. She mentions another brother of Xavier, named Peter, who always knows everything better, also speaks English very well. I'm not sure I met him back when I had the relationship with P4.

Erotic dream with P3:

> *I am in P3's apartment, which is on the first floor. Possibly, I live on the 2nd or 3rd floor. The apartment is relatively small, but it goes over two floors. She explains to me that the bedroom is very small because there is a large outside the apartment in the staircase where bundles of newspapers are stacked against the wall. At some point, I tenderly kiss P3, which feels very nice and intense.*

5.4 Schoolmates in dreams

Analyzing a long dream series provides the opportunity to study the frequency of particular dream elements over a long period of time. Even though the dreamer started the dream diary long after finishing school, Schredl (2012d) analyzed the frequency of dreams with schoolmates, teachers, and the school setting itself over a 20-year period (till the end to 2005). The analyses presented in this chapter are an expansion of these earlier findings. The dreamer finished his 13 yrs education in 1981, about three years prior to staring the dream diary. Overall, there were 1,012 occurrences of school-related persons (schoolmates, teachers) in 750 dreams (see Table 5.15). That is, 5.87% of the dreams included at least one school-related person. The percentage of dreams with schoolmates was 5.36%; the percentage for dreams with a teacher was 0.66%.

Overall, 101 persons or categories were present in the dreams (see Table 5.16). Of the 80 schoolmates mentioned, 72 schoolmates finished school with the dreamer. As, overall, 90 persons (including the dreamer) did finish school, 80.90% of these schoolmates showed up in the dreams. The other schoolmates left the particular school prior to finishing (N = 6) or were attending different grades (N = 2). Interestingly, the male percent in the dreams was 78.08% for occurrences of schoolmates and 72.83% for the teachers; that is a clear predominance of males. The gender distribution

TABLE 5.15 Frequency of school-related persons in dreams

	Frequency	Percent
Six persons	3	0.02%
Five persons	2	0.02%
Four persons	19	0.15%
Three persons	35	0.27%
Two persons	112	0.88%
One person	579	4.53%
No school-related person	12,079	94.13%

TABLE 5.16 Frequency of school-related persons in dreams

	Gender	Number of persons	Occurrences
Schoolmates	Male	43	659
	Female	37	185
	Undefined	2	76
Teachers	Male	13	67
	Female	6	25

Note: the two categories of "Schoolmates undefined" are "Schoolmates not specified in the dream" (N = 75) and "Schoolmate in physics" (N = 1).

of the 89 schoolmates that finished school with the dreamer was 46 females and 43 males; thus, almost all male schoolmates showed up in the dreams, but a larger number of female schoolmates were not incorporated into the dreams after finishing school. That is, there is a slight increase in selecting male schoolmates, but the fact that the male schoolmates showed up, on average, more often than the female schoolmates determined the high male/female percentage.

The predominance of male dream characters in regard to female dream characters, in general, was found in male children/adolescents (66.28%; Schredl, Struck, et al., 2019) and young students (67%; Hall & Van de Castle, 1966), even though the dreamer himself dreamed later (2006 to 2015) equally often of men and women (52.94%; Schredl, 2021f). One might speculate whether the high percentage reflects the contact pattern of childhood/adolescents (fitting with the previous findings), whereas later, the balanced male/female ratio is representing a different social network in later adulthood. For example, the male/female ratio in the dreams the dreamer recorded during his engineering studies (predominantly male students) was significant higher compared to the ratio of male/female characters in the dreams he recorded studying psychology (predominantly female students): 63% vs. 51%. The balanced ratio between male and female dream characters is typically found in females (Hall & Van de Castle, 1966; Schredl, Struck, et al., 2019). This indicated that the ratio of male and female dream characters is not gender-specific (being male or being female) (Hall, 1984) but depends on the gender ratio of the waking-life social network (Paul & Schredl, 2012; Schredl, Loßnitzer, et al., 1998).

Table 5.17 displays the seven male and seven female schoolmates who occurred most often within the dream series. All other male schoolmates had frequencies of 23 or below; the frequencies of the other female schoolmates were eight and fewer. The frequencies of the male schoolmates parallel the

TABLE 5.17 Top seven male and seven female schoolmates

	Frequency		Percent	Frequency
James	153	Mary		15
John	116	Patricia		14
Robert	53	Linda		10
David	36	Barbara		10
Richard	27	Elizabeth		9
Charles	27	Dorothy		9
Mark	26	Nancy		9

Note: names were changed.

closeness of the particular schoolmate to the dreamer. James was his best friend in grades one to six. In the last three years of "Gymnasium" (grade 11 to 13), John and Robert were friends of the dreamer. John, David, and the dreamer started together studying electrical engineering, but the contact ceased after a few months, as the dreamer moved away. Richard was a close friend of John, but not particularly close to the dreamer. Richard and Charles were dizygotic twins who attended the physics course (the dreamer's favorite subject in school) with the dreamer in the last two years.

For the female schoolmates, the frequencies are much lower, reflecting the fact that the dreamer had no close relationship (friendship or a relationship of a romantic nature) with a female schoolmate. On a schoolmate (three grades below the dreamer) he had a brief crush on, she occurred, overall, eight times in the dream series.

Former teachers occurred less often than schoolmates; the highest frequency of a teacher was 15. However, the two most frequent male teachers (N = 15 dreams each) and the most frequent female teacher (N = 11 dreams) were the most beloved teachers of the dreamer. With some distance between dreams and school experiences, it seems that the positive impressions teachers gave had a longer-lasting effect than teachers who were not so valued by the dreamer.

The frequencies of schoolmate dreams over the 30 years are depicted in Figure 5.5. The first interesting aspect is that the frequency is not decreasing, as one might expect, as the dreamer rarely had contact with any former schoolmates, aside from occasional reunions and a few meetings with Robert. Whereas the peak in the first year of dream recording (end of 1984 and 1985) can be seen as a recency effect (closest to the actual contacts in waking life), the peak in 2001 might reflect the 20-year reunion, a big party with over 60 persons. Overall, this finding poses some questions regarding the mathematical model of the continuity hypothesis (Schredl, 2003), proposing a decline in frequency with increasing time intervals between waking-life experiences

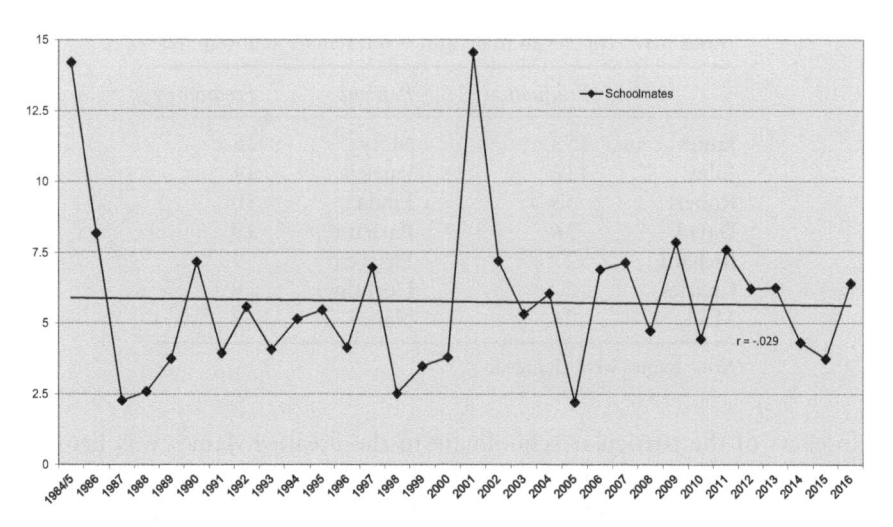

FIGURE 5.5 Dreams with schoolmates per year

and dream. As this relationship was shown for many different topics, like frequency of romantic partners after breakup (Schredl, Cadiñanos Echevarria, et al., 2020), one can only speculate why this is not the case for this particular group of social interactions. One idea might be that the dream occurrences are not solely related to the actual person the dreamer encountered many years ago but to a more general category of person with special traits; that is, the dreamer encountered a person in his current waking life that reminded him of this particular schoolmate. Even though this is not easy to tackle empirically, it seems a promising project for the future to shed light on the facets of continuity between waking and dreaming – as in this case, the continuity is between specific individual traits of waking-life contacts and these traits of dream characters.

The following dream example gives an idea what a dream with several schoolmates looked like. Interestingly, the dream reflects the feeling of being an outsider – a feeling that the dreamer quite often experienced in school.

Dream with several schoolmates:

> *I am in a large lecture hall (university). There is a lot going on. Something is being shown on a large screen for entertainment. The lecture is over. I remember that it is dinner time (about 6:30 p.m.) and join the line to the food counter. Mr. X (senior physician, philosopher) wants something from me, in between he has a resemblance to Robert (schoolmate). It is about the statistics software. He has discovered an error in my software, which is probably due to the fact that not all program parts were installed by me. He starts to explain something complicated. I ask him if he can write it down. Then*

I realize that I forgot my meal tickets and run outside. There Isabell (school-mate), Richard (schoolmate), Jack (schoolmate) and John (schoolmate) are standing on the lawn with their bicycles and are talking. I make a remark that it is nice to see so many persons from my hometown here in Berlin. They take not really notice of me. Isabell leaves quickly. Someone tells her that she has recruited the others for a musical piece they are planning. Paul (school-mate) joins them. I ask if he is doing physics. He says that he does physi-cal chemistry. Me: "I'll never understand the difference between that and chemistry." "It's more applied, industry, etc." He answers in the affirmative. When the others leave, he just goes along without saying anything to me. It's awkward at first. As I walk back into the building alone, I think to myself, they're just like that, and wonder if I'll ever become like that, a person com-municating with other people without goodbyes, attention, etc.

(recorded on December 16, 2002)

The two dream examples with teachers illustrate nicely that the emotional quality of the waking-life experiences with this particular teacher are still continuous with the dream, even though the dream occurred years later.

Dream with teacher (Mr. A.) liked by the dreamer:

I'm going to my High School, I just have something to do there. On my way out, I see Mr. A. standing in front of the door to the music room. I think about it for a moment, then I go up to him. He greets me with a handshake, but doesn't seem to remember me. In addition, the hint of high school graduation in 1981 and the incident in which I got a beer bottle on the head, does not seem to spark his memory. He says that he has grown older. Besides, a teacher's conference is about to start, which he is concen-trating on. Nevertheless, he still asks how I'm doing and what I'm doing. I answer: "Very well," and "graduated in psychology." When he asks further, I tell him about the dream research, about the student and teacher study, which I have not yet evaluated, however. As we talk, I wonder why I have to look up at him. Then the conference starts soon and we say goodbye, again with a handshake. I barely make it out the door, as some teachers, e.g., Mrs. C., are still hurrying to get there on time.

(recorded on August 19, 1995)

Dream with teacher (Mr. Z.) not liked by the dreamer:

Then I settle down in a seat in a classroom. Mr. Z. comes in and starts complaining about the blackboard not being wiped. I hold the next lesson (being also a teacher), but I don't make myself known because I know he is looking for a fight. Someone from the students (all adults) cleans the board, which is difficult because the board is broken. I also make a comment that the blackboard on the right is badly damaged. Mr. Z goes out and gets the principal, Mr. U. I am a little surprised to see him (I know he is retired). However, I see him, the face etc. quite clearly. He manipulates the board going up and down, this works. Then he wants to leave, at our astonishment he says he has to write applications. In terms of mood, he is quite easy-going and relaxed, much nicer than Mr. Z. The two of them walk out.

(recorded on August 14, 2001)

5.5 Studies-related persons in dreams

The dreamer completed two different degree programs: from 1981 to 1986, he studied electrical engineering (MSc), and from 1986 to 1991, he studied psychology (MA). As both of these studies were close to the beginning of the dream series, a longitudinal analysis shows how often persons related to the studies (friends, fellow students, professors) show up in dreams, even years after finishing the degree.

Overall, persons related to the electrical engineering program occurred in 99 dreams (0.78% of all dreams). The 20 persons with overall 116 occurrences were divided into three groups: friends, fellow students, and staff (see Table 5.18). As expected, the friends the dreamer had during the studies occurred more often compared to fellow students without closer contact or staff members. Interestingly, both of the top-occurring staff members were involved in supervising his master's thesis in optical communication techniques; the dreamer especially liked Professor1.

The number of dreams with at least one person that was related to the psychology studies was 673 (5.27% of all dreams). The 76 persons were, again, put into three groups: friends, fellow students, and staff members (see Table 5.19). Similar to the first studies, friends occurred much more often in dreams than fellow students and staff members. In addition, the overall frequency of the persons involved and their occurrences are higher, but one should keep in mind that the dream journaling started in the middle of the engineering studies and, thus, did not reflect the whole picture. The most prominent staff member (Professor1) was a professor the student liked very much and maintained professional contact with after he finished his studies for several years. On the other hand, the dreamer did not like Professor2 and Professor3. For the longitudinal study, the staff members were not included as the dreamer had contact with them long after he finished his studies; for example, during his PhD program, also completed at the same university. In addition, one fellow student was also excluded, as she worked with the dreamer in the same department after several years after graduation. This longitudinal group consisted of 51 persons; they occurred in a total of 499 dreams (3.91% of all dreams).

TABLE 5.18 Frequency of persons related to the engineering studies

Category	Number of persons	Occurrences	Dreams with at least one character of this group	Mean number of occurrences of the characters in this category	Top 3
Friends	4	60	57	15.00	Friend1 (26), Friend2 (13), Friend3 (13)
Fellow students	4	8	8	2.00	Student1 (3), Student2(2), Student3 (2)
Staff	12	48	37	4.00	Professor1 (17), Professor2 (15)
Total	20	116	99	5.80	Friend1 (26), Professor1 (17), Professor2 (15)

TABLE 5.19 Frequency of persons related to the psychology studies

Category	Number of persons	Occurrences	Dreams with at least one character of this group	Mean number of occurrences of the characters in this category	Top 3
Friends	7	319	308	45.57	Friend1 (142), Friend2 (49), Friend3 (48)
Fellow students	45	290	266	6.44	Student1 (35), Student2(30), Student3 (22)
Staff	24	183	164	7.63	Professor1 (31), Professor2 (21), Professor3 (19)
Friends and fellow students (minus student1)	51	574	499	11.25	Friend1 (142), Friend2 (49), Friend3 (48)

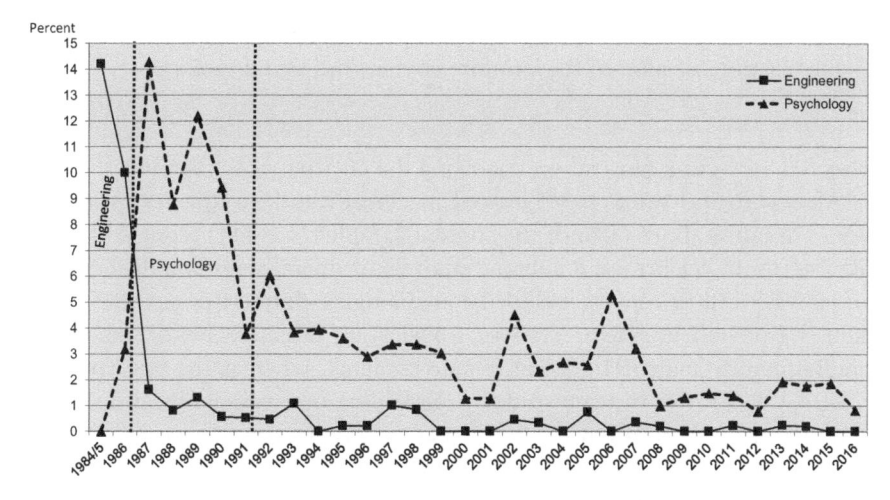

FIGURE 5.6   Dreams with persons related to studying

The time courses of the persons related to the engineering studies and the fellow students related to the psychology studies are depicted in Figure 5.6. Whereas, during the studies, the percentages of persons related to the respective studies are high, their frequencies decline over the years, especially fast for the persons related to the engineering studies. This might reflect the closer bonds with the friends and fellow students the dreamer had had in the psychology program.

5.6 Celebrities in dreams

A large-scaled study in a population-based sample (Moverley et al., 2018) has shown that media consumption affects subsequent dreams, whether this is reading books (Schredl, Samaras, et al., 2018), watching TV (Lambrecht et al., 2013; Stephan et al., 2012), playing video games (Bown & Gackenbach, 2019), or social media (Schredl & Göritz, 2019a). High consumption of violent and sexual media content can affect dreams in a negative way (Van den Bulck, 2004; Van den Bulck et al., 2016). The following dream reported by Gackenbach and Bown (2019) illustrates very nicely that media dreams are not about media consumption itself but the dream scenario that is related to media – in this case, a video game includes the dreamer – that is, the dreamer is not playing the video game in the dream but is "within the game":

I dreamt I was a character in Underworld 2. I was a werewolf character and then I became a 3rd person. I was the two main characters. I was the vampire girl and a hybrid werewolf character, and I was another werewolf character beside them. And, we went into a vampire coven, and we got to the weapons section of the vampire coven. And then I woke up.

(p. 221)

This is a very good illustration regarding the creativity of dreaming.

Alperstein and Vann (1997) looked specifically at the frequency of celebrities in dreams; about 60% of the student sample (N = 241) reported having dreams about celebrities; a content analysis of dream reports indicated that about 8% of those reports included a media figure. Interestingly, these media figures (movie/TV actors/actresses, musicians, athletes, politicians) were predominantly male (91.5%) in female students, whereas the male percent (71.0%) was lower in male students (the difference was significant; that is, male students more often include female media figures – even though the male figures are still more prominent). Moreover, McCutcheon et al. (2021) were able to demonstrate – by using the Celebrity Attitude Scale (CAS) with items like "I am obsessed with details of my favorite celebrity's life" – that persons with a high interest in celebrities in their waking life also dream more often about them – perfectly in line with the continuity hypothesis of dreaming (Schredl, 2018b).

In the present dream series, 165 dreams (1.30%) included 120 different celebrities; their overall number of occurrences was 180 (see Table 5.20). This low frequency of celebrity dreams indicates that the dreamer is not "celebrities-crazy"; see the foregoing McCutcheon et al. (2021) study. The celebrities were grouped into several categories (see Table 5.20), the most frequent ones (actors, actresses, musicians) are also the most frequent categories in the study of Alperstein and Vann (1997). Interestingly, also the gender ratio of the celebrities (of the 120 celebrities, 84.17% were male) for the occurrences (N = 180) was predominantly male: 88.33% (cf. Alperstein & Vann, 1997). For example, in the musician group, there were only two female German singers: Nena and Jule Neigel.

The most frequent celebrity was Thich Nhat Hanh, a Vietnamese Buddhist monk who led a monastery and retreat center in Southern France ("Plum village"). This is plausible, as the dreamer visit his community two times (in 1994 and 1995) and, thus, saw him in person giving talks, but they never communicated directly. Another group of celebrities is related to a hobby of the dreamer, playing chess and watching chess tournaments online (prior to reading about them in chess books and magazines). Magnus Carlsen (current world champion), Garry Kasparow (former world champion), and Robert Hübner (best German player for a very long time) are very important characters in their group. Similarly, in the group of politicians, all three have been chancellors of Germany; that is, the most important person in the German government. As has been reported in the section about music in dreams, the Beatles was one of the favorite bands of the dreamer; thus, the fact that John Lennon is the most frequent musician is not unexpected. George Harrison also occurred three times.

TABLE 5.20 Frequency of celebrities in dreams

Category	Number of persons	Male/Female	Percent	Occurrences	Most often occurring celebrities
Actor	44	44/0	36.67%	63	Bud Spencer (5), Heinz Rühmann (5), Colin Firth (3)
Music	26	24/2	21.67%	43	John Lennon (7), Herbert Grönemeyer (4), Paul McCartney (3)
Actress	16	0/14	13.33%	18	Gwyneth Paltrow (2), Kirsten Dunst (2), Amanda Peet (1)
Baseball	8	8/0	6.67%	9	David Ortiz (2), Andrew McCutcheon (1), Clayton Kershaw (1)
Chess	6	6/0	5.00%	13	Magnus Carlsen (4), Garry Kasparow (3), Robert Hübner (3)
Entertainer	6	6/0	5.00%	6	Eckhart von Hirschhausen (1), Hans Rosenthal (1), Thomas Gottschalk (1)
Sport	5	5/0	4.17%	7	Franz Beckenbauer (3), James Harden (1), Luke Walton (1)
Buddhism	3	2/1	2.50%	14	Thich Nhat Hanh (12), Ayya Khema (1), Dalai Lama (1)
Politician	3	3/0	2.50%	4	Gerhard Schröder (2), Helmut Kohl (1), Helmut Schmidt (1)
Scientist	2	2/0	1.67%	2	Aaron Beck (1), Erich Fromm (1)
Film director	1	1/0	0.83%	1	Alfred Hitchcock (1)
Total	120	101/19	100.00%	180	Thich Nhat Hanh (12), John Lennon (7), Bud Spencer (5), Heinz Rühmann (5)

The next dream example illustrates how media consumption can be integrated into dreams; one half is more about watching and the other half is about being in the dream (being an actor).

Dream example with an actress:

> *I'm in a bedroom and Gwyneth Paltrow takes off her underpants and a piece of sanitary napkin peeks out. She pulls on it and throws it into the toilet. She tells the man who is John Cusack (I am partly him) that she ran out of it. He asks, "Is there more of it." When she gets back into bed, he asks if she needs pads again later. She only has tampons. It's heading toward sex, maybe. With another couple (also actors) there are no problems, I think that here the love of the two is tested and it is not about quick, non-committal sex.*

Whereas the previous example did not refer to a particular movie (there seems no major movie with those two actors), the next example included the actress in her role in the movie *Wimbledon* – a movie the dreamer likes a lot.

Dream example with an actress:

> *I'm playing tennis with a boy against Kirsten Dunst alias Lizzy Bradbury. The big court is in R. (home town of the dreamer), on the left side of the town (seen from W., a town nearby). We make some good shots, although she plays much better. It is fun and familiar.*

In the next dream, Bud Spencer is part of an action scene, but the dreamer participates in the conflict.

Dream example with an actor:

> *Bud Spencer mediates between two warring parties who are in some kind of department store. I see him walk by a woman with a shotgun. She's half asleep and doesn't get it until he's long past. Our leader was impressed with Bud Spencer's courage to go to the other side to negotiate. And he accomplished quite a bit.*

Also in the next dream, the dreamer does not dream about being at a Beatles concert or seeing a film about the Beatles but is amongst them in the dreaming, enjoying it.

Dream example with musicians:

> *I am in a large room, the Beatles' living room. George Harrison is exchanging his electric guitar for a small electric bass, which has only one string (the*

second from the top). When he connects the bass, he sits on a comfortable armchair; there is immediately a great sound with effects. Then he plays on the string, which is groovy and sounds good. Right next to me sits John Lennon, on the right. Also the other Beatles. I think about what such great musicians do all day. Now I know, they make music because they have fun with it. John Lennon goes along with the music. Beautiful atmosphere.

The last dream is a blending dream with a football star and a former teacher; as there is a particular characteristic that both men share in waking life, the dream might have used the blending between the two characters to emphasize this topic of being energetic.

Dream example with an athlete:

I am on the outskirts of a small town, residential area. Around a large table sit about 25 people. There are microphones and speakers, plus a second seating area (also benches) for listening. The weather is nice. It is a public community meeting. It is chaired by a very energetic man (mix between Franz Beckenbauer and Mr. A. (former teacher)). He goes through the agenda items. The atmosphere is relaxed.

Even though the frequency of celebrities in the dream series is relatively low (1.3%) compared to the 8% in a sample of young students, this specific dream topic clearly reflects the waking-life interests of the dreamer. Moreover, these types of dreams nicely illustrate the creative nature of dreaming by putting the celebrities and the dreamer in a shared situation.

5.7 Interactions in dreams

Even though several studies looked at the frequency of family members in dreams (Domhoff, 2003; Hall & Van de Castle, 1966; Nöltner & Schredl, 2023; Schredl, 2013b, 2021e), a systematic study of the emotional quality of the interaction between family member and dreamer has so far only carried out by Nöltner and Schredl (2023). Based on 85 (brother) to 220 (mother) interactions in a diary dream sample reported by students, the results indicate that 70% to 90% of the dreams did not explicitly mention the emotional quality of the interaction. However, if emotions were reported, the negative emotions (ranging from 9.5% to 18.0%) outweighed the positive ones (ranging from 2.5% to 8.0%) (Nöltner & Schredl, 2023). The typical interaction was in shared activities – e.g., driving in a car, sitting on a table (about 50%), direct verbal interaction between the family member and the dreamer (about 25% to 50%) – and no contact in the dream – e.g., being in the same apartment but without any interaction (10 to 30%) (Nöltner & Schredl, 2023).

In Table 5.21, the emotional quality of the interaction between the four core family members and the dreamer is depicted. As the number of dreams were very large for the mother, the brother, and the sister (see previous section), 100 dreams per person were selected randomly. Similar to the findings of Nöltner and Schredl (2023), most interactions were neutral and/or emotions were not mentioned explicitly or could be inferred from the dream description. For the father, the mother, and the brother, the negatively toned interactions outweighed the positive interaction – again, similar to the findings in the student sample (Nöltner & Schredl, 2023). Dream examples for types of negative interactions are presented later – e.g., owing money, uncomfortable handshake (father), not listening in dangerous situations (mother), and rivalry (brother). The highest percentage of negative dream interactions occurred with the father, which reflects waking life, as the father used beatings as a method of education when the dreamer was very small. The rivalry dream with the brother also reflects the rivalry between the brother and the dreamer in waking life, especially during their adolescence. The interactions with the sister were, overall, more often neutral but – if emotions were involved – the positive emotions were more common. The dream following example shows how the sister was helping the dreamer with organizing the moving.

The "stepfather" was the partner of the mother after the divorce who lived in the family's household for several years. The preponderance of positive interactions also reflects the waking relationship, as the dreamer was fond of him and they shared a few hobbies together, like fishing (see the following dream example). The emotional quality of the interactions with the two male friends was balanced, whereas the emotional quality of the interactions with the female friend was very often positive. Even though there were no erotic feelings between the two in waking life (she had a steady boyfriend), 17.79% of the dreams had an erotic component (kissing, making out, sexual) explaining the high percentage of positive interactions. In this context, the dialog between Harry and Sally comes to mind: "You realize of course that we could never be friends. . . . Men and women can't be friends because the sex part always gets in the way" (*When Harry Met Sally* (1989); movie directed by Rob Reiner and written by Nora Ephron). Even though it worked in this friendship during waking, the dreams support Harry's claim. That the sex part can be a burden for cross-sex friendships has also been shown in empirical studies (e.g., Bleske-Rechek et al., 2012). However, the dreams also show an emotional closeness (see dream example) beyond the sex part, reflecting the intense relationship between the female friend and the dreamer. Interestingly, there were also three erotic dreams with the sister not continuous in any way with the waking life, whereas no erotic dreams were found in the dreams with other family members or friends analyzed in Table 5.21. The dream example with the school friend (see the following) reflects a negative interaction, although the dream occurred long after the friendship ended, in

TABLE 5.21 Interaction between family member and friends with the dreamer

		Father (N = 285)	Mother (N = 100)	Sister (N = 100)	Brother (N = 100)	"Stepfather" (N = 88)	School friend (male) (N = 153)	Friend (psychology) (female) (N = 142)	Current best friend (male) (N = 60)
Emotional	Positive	9.82%	3.00%	6.00%	3.00%	18.18%	15.03%	39.44%	13.33%
quality	Neutral	63.16%	83.00%	91.00%	80.00%	76.14%	70.59%	52.11%	75.00%
of the	Negative	27.02%	14.00%	3.00%	17.00%	5.68%	14.38%	8.45%	11.67%
interaction									
Type of	No contact	28.77%	28.00%	31.00%	37.00%	27.27%	11.76%	8.45%	18.33%
activity	Sharing activities	54.74%	40.00%	52.00%	41.00%	55.68%	39.87%	45.77%	48.33%
	Verbal interaction	33.68%	32.00%	19.00%	24.00%	27.27%	54.90%	58.45%	41.67%

Note: N is the number of dreams that were analyzed (all dreams for father, "stepfather," school friend, friend (psychology), and current best friend. For mother, sister, and brother, 100 dream reports were randomly selected.

about 1979 (dream recorded on March 6, 1994). This might be interesting for understanding why this dream with this particular person occurred at that particular point in time. One idea might be that the former school friend is some kind of a placeholder, serving as an illustrative example how the dreamer reacts to this kind of negative interactions (leaving the situation); that is, showing a basic pattern of the dreamer that is not related to specific persons. Lastly, the emotional quality of the interactions between the current best friend and the dreamer was also balanced. The following dream example is indicative of a situation where both enjoy doing something together.

The type of activities between the different dream characters and the dreamer were grouped into three broad categories: no contact (different dream scenes, being around – e.g., within an apartment – just seeing the person in a distance, etc.), sharing activities without direct verbal interaction (being on a trip, eating together, participating together in an event, etc.), and verbal interaction; that is, the dreamer and the specific dream person were communicating with each other. Whereas, for family members and the "step-father," sharing activities was the most prominent type of activity, direct interactions were more common for friends, indicating that friendships are more based on direct interaction – as they have been actively established and maintained by the dreamer and the friend.

Dream example with negative interaction with the father:

> *We, my siblings and I, break into my father's house. He owes us money and we want to get it. I imagined it would be easier. It's the apartment in M. In the living room, we crack a wall safe, it works well, but takes time. There are at most 200 DM in it, much too little, even in the safe in the study there are at most 100 DM in it. We are disappointed. It's dawn and I'm in a hurry, our father could be back soon. I look through the window from above so that we don't run into him. The two others go ahead. He is already there, in the garden and sees us. We shake hands, he holds mine especially long, which makes me very uncomfortable. At first I felt like running away, just away, but now I have decided to tell him about the money issue and confront him.*

Dream example with negative interaction with the mother:

> *My mother, sister, brother and I are driving from Vienna to my father's house to do some business. It's not that cold, but at some point the road is covered in snow. I tell my mother to drive slowly because it is very slippery under the snow. She doesn't listen to me. Then there is a traffic jam. My mother has to brake and sure enough, the wheels lock and we slide along rudderless. We just come to a stop. We think about what to do next.*

Dream example with positive interaction with the sister:

> *I moved in with my sister. She has a bit of a partner. I think that it's nice that she organized helpers, there were no people organized by me. It all went (stuff from both households) in a big truck and the moving went very well yesterday.*

Dream example with negative interaction with the brother:

> *I am in an apartment playing with my brother. We have a small iron ball that we throw to each other. My brother is determined to be better than I am and throws the ball so hard that I can't catch it. That annoys me; I don't feel like playing with him anymore. In my mind, I try to imagine myself throwing hard (like him). Then I go outside.*

Dream with "stepfather (Xavier)":

> *Xavier and I are fishing on a populated beach. He catches several goldfish. We have no landing net and I try to lock a caught fish into a bay. However, the tide drives him out again. One can also see that he is half-dead. He also barely wriggled hanging on the rod. Now we both want to fish differently. Xavier gets a foam board, movable, lays it over the bay, about 5 m and runs on it to the other side. I think about fishing with floater and choose a rod.*

Dream with the female friend:

> *I am in a large hall (old building) and see my friend moving in a queue. It is a study office of the University of Heidelberg. I am very happy to see her. She is happy too. We hug each other intimately, which I notice and like because I feel her body (she is young) very intensely. I ask what she is doing around here. It was about feedback regarding a study she participated in, autonomic parameters were recorded. I make a comment about what they say if they had recorded the peak now. My friend seems to be in a big hurry and runs off, me running behind.*

Dream with male school friend:

> *I am sitting in a lecture in a very large hall and am just talking to someone sitting in front of me in the row. My school friend, who is sitting next to me, interrupts me rather inconsiderately. This annoys me very much, as this is a sensitive point of mine. I pack my stuff, jacket, sweater, bag, and leave. The lecturer comes in, it is about to start.*

Dream with current best friend:

I am in a kind of amusement park, rather small, cozy. On a square, some-one (man) plays children's songs. There are three of us (current best friend, one more person) and we stand next to each other and just do steps and turns, it's fun. I am on the outside (left side) and try to follow the oth-ers. I also say that some people are looking. They probably think we are employees of the park. Then it's more of a space, I think about doing a handstand, on two wooden blocks, but I don't have the strength. My best friend eventually does one against the wall.

6
SENSORY PERCEPTIONS IN DREAMS

Going back to the definition of dreaming as subjective experiences during sleep that can be remembered after waking up (Schredl, 2018b), one has to keep in mind that, in most of these dream experiences, the dreamer thinks s/he is awake; thus, the dream world is experienced as real. A very rare exception are so-called lucid dreams, in which the dreamer is aware of being in a dream state (LaBerge, 1985). This realness of normal dreams led to the conceptualization of dreaming as a simulation of the waking world (Revonsuo et al., 2015). A very interesting aspect is that, in this "real" world, things can happen that are not possible in waking life – like flying, for example. This discontinuous aspect of dreaming is discussed in Hobson and Schredl (2011).

One important element of waking-life experiences are sensory perceptions and, thus, if dreams are experienced as real, perceptions in dreams should be comparable to those experienced in waking life. Several studies (McCarley & Hoffman, 1981; Snyder, 1970; Zadra, Nielsen, & Donderi, 1998) have shown that visual perception is present in every dream (in persons with intact vision) and that auditory perception is also very prominent, occurring in 53% to 76% of dream reports. In contrast, gustatory, olfactory, tactile and pain perceptions are very rare in dreams – i.e., in about 1% or fewer dream reports (Knoth & Schredl, 2011; Schredl, 2011b, 2016; Zadra et al., 1998; Zadra, Nielsen, Germain, et al., 1998). One study (McCarley & Hoffman, 1981) found 8% of dreams include kinesthetic perception (for example in flying dreams) and 3.85% of 104 laboratory dreams include some form of temperature perception.

Strauch and Meier (1996) pointed out that some sensations – for example, touch – might not be explicitly mentioned in the dream report: a female dreamer described that she smoothed a dress that she hung in her closet,

DOI: 10.4324/9781003300373-6

but only after asking additional questions; she added that she clearly felt the texture of the dress. Similar, Plailly et al. (2019) found more dream reports with self-rated perception of olfaction, taste, and touch compared to dream reports with explicitly mentioned sensation – e.g., five dreams included explicit references to olfactory perceptions, whereas the participants reported some form of olfactory perception in 27 dreams. Similar underreporting has been shown for bizarre elements (Schredl & Erlacher, 2003) and dream emotions (Schredl & Doll, 1998; Sikka et al., 2017). This highlights the aspect that dream content analysis done by external judges is restricted to the dream report and the elaborateness of this report; that is, whether the dreamer had described every sensation, thought, emotion etc.

From a theoretical viewpoint, studying sensory perceptions in dreams is very interesting. At the end of the 20th century, Weygandt (1893), working with Wilhelm Wundt, a famous German physiologist, philosopher, and professor, known today as one of the fathers of modern psychology, finished his doctoral thesis on dreams with the sentence: "*Die Träume gehen von Sinneseindrücken aus*" ("Dreams are resulting from sensory impressions"). This viewpoint, also called "*Nervenreizträume*" (peripheral neuronal activity is producing dreams) was very popular at that time, even though some authors also outline the importance of associations based on the dreamer's waking-life experiences (Radestock, 1879). Modern dream research has shown that different stimuli applied during sleep can be incorporated into dreams; for example simple sounds, specific noises, words, light flashes with incorporation rates between 9% to 40% (Schredl, 2018b). Strauch and Meier (1996) pointed out that the external stimuli might be incorporated in a creative way; their example includes a report of a dream in which the dreamer heard sounds that reminded her of odd-screeching doors (the stimulus was a crying baby). Interestingly, several studies (Erlacher et al., 2020; Okabe et al., 2018; Schredl, Atanasova, et al., 2009; Schredl, Hoffmann, et al., 2014) showed that olfactory stimuli are very rarely incorporated into dreams (less than 5%, in two studies: 0%). This is plausible when looking at the information processing of olfactory stimuli in the brain, as the olfactory bulb is more closely related to the limbic system, whereas other sensory modalities are processed within the thalamus and forwarded to the cortex (Gottfried, 2006).

The model (Figure 6.1) includes three possible sources: (1) internal or external stimuli that are present in the body while dreaming; (2) memory sources, waking-life experiences, but also media content, as, for example, it has been shown, for persons with congenital insensitivity to pain, that they can experience "empathic" pain; and (3) "new stuff" – there is form of creativity active while we are dreaming that is able to create completely new experiences the dreamer never has felt, sensed, or experienced before.

In this dream series, different sensory qualities were rated – only if they were explicitly mentioned within the dream. For example, the weather being

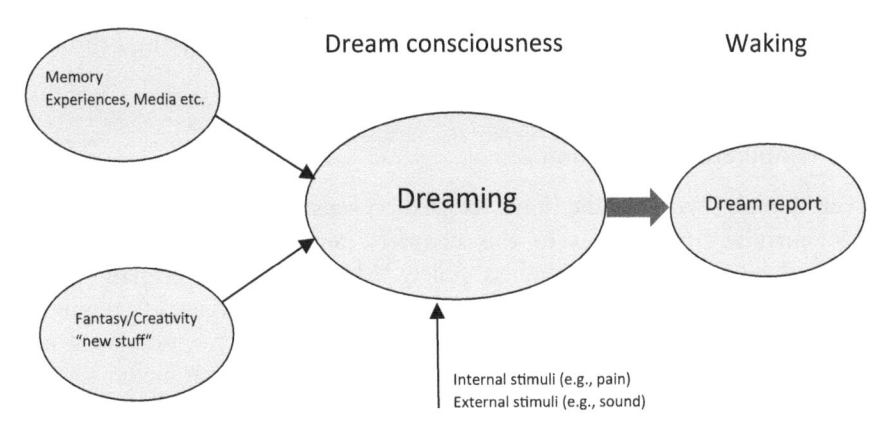

FIGURE 6.1 Model for illustrating possible sources of sensory perceptions in dreams

TABLE 6.1 Dream with explicitly mentioned sensory perceptions in the dream series (N = 12,679 dreams)

Perception	Frequency	Percent
Temperature	131	1.03%
Pain	130	1.02%
Olfactory	60	0.47%
Taste	41	0.32%
Tactile	27	0.21%

nice and warm was not coded, but if the dreamer mentioned that he feels the warmth of the sunbeams on his skin, the presence of a temperature perception was coded. The most frequent perceptions were temperature (hot/cold) and pain, occurring in about 1% of the dreams (see Table 6.1). Olfactory and gustatory perceptions were rarer (see Table 6.1), and the tactile sensations were only reported in 0.21% of the dreams. The low number of tactile sensations underlines the coding rules that were applied, as one can easily image that almost every activity, like walking, grabbing something, kissing, etc., is accompanied by a tactile sensation that would be reported if the person were instructed to focus his or her attention to this type of perception. However, like in waking life, these common perceptions do not enter the mind and/ or are not reported when recalling specific experiences. If you are asked, for example, to recount a recent hiking trip, you would not mention every tactile sensation you experienced when being on the hiking trail; however, if the feet were hurting, it is more likely that the report would include something like

"When I walked on a rough surface, I could feel the underground through my shoes."

6.1 Temperature perception

Even though several studies have focused on sensory perceptions in dreams (see introductory sections to this chapter), temperature (heat/cold) perceptions have rarely been studied. Solely, McCarley and Hoffman (1981) found that 3.85% of 104 laboratory dreams include references to temperature; however, the characteristics of this temperature perception were not specified. One can imagine, for example, a dream report that includes some description that it is sunny and warm outside would not really qualify as an explicit temperature perception, as the dreamer is indoors and does not feel the warmth.

Several illustrative dream examples can be found in the literature. Calkins (1893) reported that only one of her 166 recorded dreams (0.66%) included a clear perception of temperature; the following is an excerpt of this dream: "dream of a sleigh-ride on an intensely cold day . . . was evidently occasioned by a stiff breeze blowing in at the window" (p. 320). Similarly, Weygandt (1893) reported several dreams with temperature perceptions, which he assumed were caused by external stimulation. One poignant example can be found in Schredl (2010c), who reviewed the doctoral thesis of Weygandt. The dream was as follows:

> I was travelling by train up a mountain to a lonely hotel named "Sommerfrische". I felt that it was getting colder and colder. Eventually, there was so much snow that one could not go outside. Snow flurries were hammering at the windows and I was very cold.
>
> *(p. 96)*

He chose this example to support his idea that sensory perceptions in dream were cause by external stimuli and added this comment: "When I woke up, I realized that my bedspread had fallen off of me and a cold breeze had blown into the room." The most detailed study so far was the analysis of Schredl (2016), which included 10,535 dreams – a subsample of the same dream series analyzed in this book. Explicit temperature perception was present in 71 dreams (0.67% of the total dreams). In order to illustrate the point that only explicit temperature perceptions were included, the following dream is presented: "While walking home; I notice a fast driving Porsche that overturns and goes up in flames. Even several hundred meters away, I can feel the warmth clearly" (p. 80; Schredl, 2016). Within this context, it is interesting that, of 90 fever dreams, 10% included a temperature perception – e.g., "The

TABLE 6.2 Temperature perception and the emotional quality of the temperature perception

	Quality of the temperature perception			
Temperature perception	Unpleasant	Neutral/no reference	Pleasant	Total
Cold	23	47	1	71
Cold and warm	2	9	1	12
Warm	3	22	23	48

air is so hot that breathing hurts" (p. 3), whereas only 2.2% of the control dreams included temperature perception (Schredl & Erlacher, 2020). This would support Weygandt's idea that real stimuli present during sleep can affect the dream. However, it should be noted that it is also possible that the temperature perception within the dream is a reflection of feeling hot while awake due to having fever; this would be in line with the continuity hypothesis of dreaming (Schredl, 2003).

Overall, 131 dreams in the dream series (1.03%) included explicit temperature perceptions; with sensations of cold outweighing the sensations of warmth (see Table 6.2). In 12 dreams, both types of temperature perception occurred. The warm/cold perceptions were pleasant in 25 dreams and unpleasant in 28 dreams; in all other dreams (N = 78), no emotional quality associated with the temperature perception was mentioned explicitly. Feeling warm is more often experienced as pleasant than feeling cold (see Table 6.2). In 77 dreams, the temperature perception was related to the weather.

Dream example:

> I'm walking along a raging river that goes in a semicircle within a city. There is also some snow. The city is Montreal and I consider that there are long winters as it is only September (due to all the water in the river) and snow has already fallen. There is quite a lot of spray; I get a little wet, which is very chilly. I am glad that I passed the place with the raging river.

Dream example:

> I'm playing with a small child in a large room, maybe my mother and/or my sister are nearby. I know the child, it's an intense experience, I hold the child, it gets tired (it's night), the closeness, the warmth feels very nice. I want it to sleep because it's time, hold it gently (like one yr. old baby),

it gets tired eventually, closes its eyes. I put it on a small mattress by the window that is open.

Dream example:

P3 and I would like to spend a quiet weekend together and get closer again. We arrive at my mother's and my apartment. She quickly pulls me into the bedroom and wants to cuddle with me. It's nice to feel the closeness and the warmth.

Dream example:

Then we are outside in the open air, under a roof, since it's raining quite a bit. Although the weather is not so nice, cool for local standards here, it is warmer than at home in January. I'm enjoying the milder weather and looking out into the park in the rain.

In 48 dreams, the dreamer directly reacted to the temperature sensation with some form of action. Performing some countermeasure was much more prominent for cold sensations in dreams (N = 33) than for warmth (N = 7). In seven of the eight dreams with both cold and warm perceptions, the action led from a cold perception to a warmth perception – e.g., having cold lips and kissing a woman with warm lips several times or using a heater to battle the cold sensation.

Overall, the most common action (N = 20) was to put on clothes or some textile, bedcover, or flag (see Dream example 1). On very rare occasions (N = 2), the dreamer took something off (see Dream example 2). Other reactions are going away (N = 7) – e.g., going inside – turning up the heating or turning down the air conditioning (N = 6), and closing a window (N = 5). Single occurrences were pulling a hand away from something hot, keeping on moving to get warmer, rubbing the hands on the tights, human warmth (kissing warm lips), and drinking something hot. A very special dream is the third dream example, as the dreamer is deliberately trying to "heat" the water in a lucid dream.

Dream example 1:

I'm in a house and I'm talking to my mother about the heating costs, which are high because the house is poorly insulated (bungalow, reminds me of M.'s apartment). It's morning and I'm walking to the bus stop, which is just outside of town. Since I was cold, I wrapped my bedcover around me, which is nice and warm. While I am waling, I think I'll have to wear the bedcover all day, I could have put on a jacket (although this would be not as warm). It is also expected that it will get (significantly) warmer during the day.

Dream example 2:

> *I arrive with a group of people at a seminar house that is outside in a forest. I have a travel bag with me, which surprises me as I usually travel with a backpack. I'm looking for a pair of shoes that I've temporarily taken off as it's warm.*

Dream example 3:

> *I come to a small indoor pool. I know I'm dreaming. Someone else I know well (male) is there too. The pool is covered with plastic sheeting. The other person (baby) jumps in, but the water is very cold. I try to influence the dream in the direction that the water is getting warmer. Somehow it doesn't work that well, maybe a little bit.*

Unfortunately, it was not systematically recorded whether the dreamer felt warm or cold when waking up from a dream with temperature perception (see the foregoing examples of Calkins and Weygandt). However, as the dreamer is interested in such topics, he would have recorded obvious correspondences. Another counterargument would be that, for example, a dream – e.g., a dream including feeling the warmth of the partner – has not occurred during a night spent with this or a partner together. Another idea to tackle this topic is to study whether temperature perception varies across the seasons, as it is more common to experience warmth sensations during the course of the night in the summer (especially living in an apartment under the roof) compared to the winter months. In order to do this, the temperature perception dreams were divided into two groups: colder months vs. warmer months. The total number of dreams with warmth perception was 60 (for cold perception, 83 dreams), as both perceptions were present in 12 dreams. The number of dreams in each group was almost similar: 66 dreams with temperature perception in the colder months and 65 dreams in the warmer months. Table 6.3 clearly indicates that there is not relationship between outside temperature and "dream temperature" in this dream series;

TABLE 6.3 Temperature perception and seasons (N = 131 dreams)

	Cold perception	Warmth perception
Colder months (November till March)	57.58%	46.97%
Warmer months (April to September)	69.23%	44.62%

cold perceptions were even higher in the warmer months, whereas warmth perceptions were equally distributed.

Studying temperature perception indicated that explicit perception of warmth and cold is rarely described in dreams, but one has to keep in mind that – if the temperature is at a comfortable level – this aspect of the dream world is not particularly salient to the dreamer and, thus, will not be perceived with attention (like in waking life) and, thus, not reported in dreams. This is reflected in Table 6.1 and the previously reported dream examples, as temperature perceptions are cold or warm but not intermediate. It is also plausible that warmth perceptions are more often experienced as pleasant compared to experiences of cold, which often lead to counteractive measure like putting on clothes.

It would be very interesting to study temperature perception in dreams of persons living in different climatic zones, like the Inuit people in the north or peoples living the tropical regions of South America, Africa or the Pacific region – e.g., Indonesia. It would be interesting to find out whether persons living in tropical areas have any dreams with cold perceptions. As far as I know, such studies have not yet been carried out.

6.2 Pain perception

Studying pain perceptions in dreams is a very interesting topic for two reasons. Let's start with an old German saying that "If you pinch yourself and experience pain you cannot dream." Today, one would consider this action a "reality check"; these are – in different forms – part of induction techniques to increase the frequency of lucid dreams (Stumbrys et al., 2012; Tan & Fan, 2022). One research group (Giguere & LaBerge, 1995) was able to demonstrate that dreaming being pinched can produce pain, although the intensity was lower compared to the same pinch self-applied in waking, and about one-third of the participants did not feel pain in the dreams. That is, the old saying is only partly correct. Symons (1993) even argued that it would not make sense – from an evolutionary point of view – to be able to imagine pain, as pain is a bodily warning signal that something is going wrong in the body or there's acute danger to one's health (e.g., putting a finger on hot stove). This line of thinking would imply that pain in dreams would only occur if the person experiences pain during sleep and the dream incorporated the pain into the dream scenario. The following dream that was reported by Weygandt (1893) would support the idea: he dreamed he was carrying a young lady for a while (because the paths were very dirty), not without some trouble, and, after waking up, he experienced the same back pain that he had experienced in the dream. On the other hand, Zadra, Nielsen, Germain, et al. (1998) found that most dreamed pain situations like being stabbed, being shot, being electrocuted, and accidents do not refer to any current or past waking-life pain experience of the dreamer; only one participant who suffered from occasional lower back pain in waking life reported also having dreams in which his back was hurting. In a sample of 28 patients with severe pain due to burn injuries (hospitalized), 39% reported having pain dreams during the study period (five days with interviews about dreaming in the morning), and the dreamed pain was very much the same pain they experienced in the waking state (Raymond et al., 2002). Of 100 patients with chronic lower back pain, 16 were able to recall explicitly a most recent pain dream (Schredl, Kälberer, et al., 2017) compared to 8.5% of the control group. Being asked whether the pain persisted after waking up (see example by Weygandt, reported earlier), eight said "Yes," three "No," and five "Don't know," again supporting the idea that at least some pain dreams might reflect incorporated pain present during sleep. In the control group, the ratio was more balanced: 11 said that the pain persisted in waking life, 12 not, with two participants reporting "Don't know" (Schredl, Kälberer, et al., 2017). This supports the idea that it is possible to dream about pain that is not actual present in the physical body.

The analysis of the pain dreams (N = 130 dreams, 1.02%) has the aim of looking at whether the pain experiences in dreams resemble pain experiences the dreamer had in his waking life; for example, he suffered from chronic tension headaches from 1979 to 1989. Or, whether it is also possible to dream about pain completely unfamiliar to the dreamer (see foregoing model). As the dreamer experienced chronic pain prior to journaling dreams and in the first period of the dream series, the frequency of pain dreams per year were analyzed (see Figure 6.2). There was a small downward trend (r = -.093, p = .692) but it was not significant.

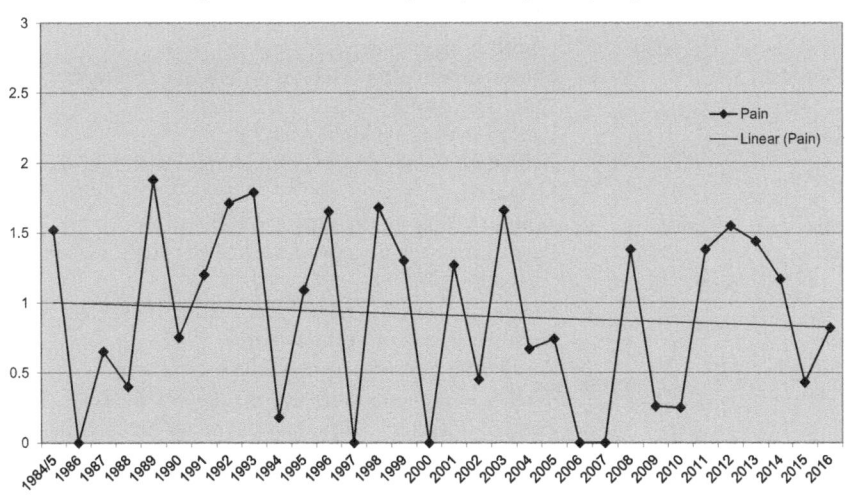

Percentage of dreams with pain perception per year

FIGURE 6.2 Frequency of pain dreams per year

The most frequent part associated with pain was the hand (see Table 6.4). The 12 dreams including pain related to the head were the second most frequent topic; however, only 50% were headaches (illness-related), whereas the other dreams included accidents like being hit by a branch (see Table 6.4). The frequency of the illness-related dream with head pain did not differ in frequency from the time interval the dreamer had chronic headaches (till 1989) and the period after that ($1/1,759 = 0.06\%$ vs. $5/11,010 = 0.05\%$).

In four dreams, two pain locations were mentioned.

TABLE 6.4 Body parts where the pain was experienced (N = 130 dreams)

Body part	Frequency	Example
Hand	22	Ants on a container the dreamer carries bite the dreamer (mildly painful)
Head	12	Branch hits the dreamer while he is flying a kite
Genitals	11	Dreamer plays with a child, who wants to do a somersault (holding hands with the dreamer) and kicks the dreamer unintentionally but quite hard in the balls
Back	9	Flying dream, back is hitting the ceiling of the room
Abdomen	8	Being in a hospital bed, inflammation of the diaphragm, pain in the abdomen
Breast	8	Gun fight, dreamer tries to extract bullets (not life-threating) from chest
Whole body	7	Acupuncture needles all over the body (painful)
Foot	7	Squirrel is bitten by a snake and clings to the foot of the dreamer
Throat	6	Outdoor, camping, cold, sore throat
Arm	5	Mother of the dreamer accidently hurts the dreamer with broken glass (forearm)
Shoulder	4	Shoulder pain after sleeping on the side one night on a hard field bed
Knee	4	Pain in the knee while hiking
Leg	3	Accidently one leg comes into contact with a burning cigarette
Lips	3	A mouse is biting the dreamer in the upper lip
Neck	2	Pain in the neck area because dreamer slept in a sitting position
Ear	2	Consulting an ENT physician because of ear pain
Hip	2	Dreamer gets shot in the hip area
Buttocks	2	Pain in the buttocks from a long bicycle trip
Teeth	2	Teeth and gum are hurting, tongue is swollen
Skin	1	Pointed fingernails of fantasy character hurting the skin
Location not mentioned	14	Dreamer experiences briefly sharp pain, must have had contact with a burning cigarette (no location specified)

The pain intensity within the dreams varies (see Table 6.5). The most extreme pain is typically associated with a situation not experienced by the dreamer in his waking life – e.g., the monsters biting the dreamer.

In Table 6.6, different causes for the pain within the dream are listed. Fighting with others is the most common reason – things not experienced by the dreamer in waking life. The everyday category of feeling pain due to illness – e.g., sore throat or stomach ache – is the second most common cause. Also, the next categories, like hurting oneself while doing something, having an accident, pain inflicted by animals, or pain due to incidentally contact with other persons, can be part of daily life, of course, depending on the kind of pain or, for example, the kind of animal – ants/mosquitos vs. crocodiles. The category of mentally triggered physical pain in dreams is very interesting, as the dreamer experienced this once in his life related to a very intense feeling of jealousy related to P3, his true love. The last category of

TABLE 6.5 Pain intensity (N = 130 dreams)

Intensity	Frequency	Example
Mild	47	Dreamer is soldering cables, slight burning (hand)
Medium	52	Dreamer is stepping on a paper clip, hurts, also while removing it from the sole of the foot
Strong	26	Feeling a bullet in the belly (gunshot wound)
Extreme	5	Many monsters with sharp teeth, the dreamer feels almost unbearable pain in his hand when they bite

TABLE 6.6 Causes of pain (N = 130 dreams)

Causes	Frequency	Example
Fighting with others	25	Enemy chops off the arm of the dreamer (hurts insanely intense)
Illness	21	Person inquires about dreamer's health; he is feeling pain in the stomach
Doing something	20	While cleaning the car interior, dreamer cuts his hand on broken glass
Accident	20	Car accident, neck is hurting
Animals	19	Insect bites the dreamer (left hand)
Incidental contact with others	15	A father is leaning on the dreamer with his elbow, shoulder hurts
Mentally triggered physical pain	6	Seeing partner with two other men, jealous, feeling intense pain in the body
Self-inflicted pain	3	Dreamer cuts his finger while playing a game
Catastrophe	1	Catastrophe including hot ash, but pain diminishes quickly

pain dreams involved a Pompeii-ian dream with hot ashes; this kind of pain experience cannot occur in waking life, as the pain quickly subsided within the dream.

The quality of the pain itself ranges from pain that could, very likely, have occurred in the waking life of the dreamer – e.g., knee pain after a long bicycle trip – to pain that clearly never occurred in his waking life – e.g., pain related to having an artificial bowel outlet (see Table 6.7).

Even though, the pain sensation itself could have occurred in the dreamer's waking life, the situations in which the pain occurred have not been experienced by the dreamer in his waking life, like a situation with pain in the hand inflicted by a lot of small needles or being bitten by a crocodile or being shot (see Table 6.8).

The last section includes a few dream examples to illustrate in what situation what kind of pain can occur. The first dream is directly related to the dreamer's waking life, as he suffered ten years from chronic tension headaches. Within the dream, there is some speculation about the factors that might influence pain intensity; however, in waking life, the dreamer was not able to detect any factors related to pain intensity.

TABLE 6.7 Has the dreamer experienced the pain itself in his waking life (N = 130 dreams)?

Quality	Frequency	Percent	Example
Very likely	41	31.54%	Knee pain, headaches
Probably	32	24.62%	Pain in the ankles
Improbably	20	15.38%	Pain in the knee area and upper body because of being caught between a trailer and a car
Never	37	28.46%	Dreamer is standing in a crowd; someone is pressing against his artificial bowel outlet

TABLE 6.8 Has the dreamer experienced the dreamed pain situation in his waking life (N = 130 dreams)?

Quality	Frequency	Percent	Example
Very likely	8	6.15%	Dreamer's neck is hurting after he slept in a sitting position
Probably	9	6.92%	Ears are aching, thinking about consulting an ENT physician
Improbably	9	6.92%	The dreamer's chest is slightly aching, as the dentist is pressing while he is drilling
Never	104	80.00%	While packing things together, the dreamer gets a lot of small needles in his hand

Dream example (headaches):

> *P3 and I cuddle. It is very nice to feel her. She strokes my head and says that my mother has a bad influence on my headaches. I say that is not only because of my mother, but because of the activities I am doing here. Two weeks before, not in Mannheim, I was fine.*

The next two examples include pain situations that the dreamer never (luckily, you can say) experienced in his waking life. He doesn't even know what it really feels like to be bitten by a crocodile or be shot in the stomach. If one speculates about possible functions of dreaming, the question arises: "Does it make sense to dream about pain one has never had and never will encounter in one's waking life?" Taking a look at the model depicted in Figure 6.1, these dreams clearly support the "creativity" part of dreaming.

Dream example (pain never experienced in waking life):

> *I'm out with P4, we're in the water and we have little boards that we sit on that are propelled. We want to go to a big ship that Gaby came with, which must be around the corner. Area is big lake, rather in the South. Driving through the water is fun, then the scene changes, rather river-like and crocodiles are there. It becomes dangerous because some are quite large. Now we are running, one grabs me by the right foot, I try to shake it off, it is medium sized, it hurts a bit, but it has mainly bitten into the shoe. It seems to be solvable.*

Dream example (pain never experienced in waking life):

> *I go with a woman from a park to a noble building to hear a lecture. While she has her things with her, I have left my backpack on a table near a bench; a notebook lies next to it. She points out to me that it would be better to take the things with me, otherwise they might get stolen. I run back and indeed an older woman has already pocketed the notebook. She hands it back, but there are strange noises when her coat is moving, so I suspect that she has stolen a lot of things. We want to call the police and push her into an indentation so that she cannot run away. I would not act so rigorously or do not want to hold her, but the woman I am with and someone else are very tough. That's when the older woman pulls out a small revolver and starts shooting at me. I feel a bullet in my abdomen.*

The last dream example is linked to the dream reported by Weygandt (1893); even though the dream situation is clearly bizarre and could never have happened in the dreamer's waking life, the pain experience itself – the stabbing pain in the foot – was really there after the dreamer woke up, indicating that some pain dreams are incorporations of internal stimuli (see Figure 6.1). But it also supports the idea that dreams are creative regarding how the pain experience was embedded in the dream – an overall improbable scenario.

Dream example (incorporation):

> *I'm in a large room, walking around, and in the process, I step in a newspaper with leftover lettuce that I want to dispose of. It hurts because there's an office clip in there. It's in the left foot, front, outer part of the heel. I pull on the outer part, it's in very deep, it still hurts. Then I see that there is a worm in the hole, somewhat disgusting and slimy (like an earthworm, but white, about 20 cm long). I pull on it (despite disgust) and get it all the way out. There is still a small piece of entangled flesh that the worm wants to crawl back into (now on the carpet). However, I keep him from doing that. I'm thinking about whether the worm had something to do with the fact that I've had so little strength the last few months. I am also worried that the worm may have offshoots. I'm thinking about killing the worm and taking it to the doctor, so it will become clear what else to look for. When I wake up, slight stabbing pain at the same spot on my left foot.*

Again, the dream pain situation is bizarre, even though the pain experience itself might have occurred during sleep and, thus, persisted after waking up from the dream.

6.3 Olfactory perception

Overall, 60 dreams (0.47%) included an explicit reference to olfactory perception. The olfactory perceptions in the dreams took place in different situations (see Table 6.9). Toilet, feces, etc., and cigarettes associated with unpleasant odors were the most common context. Other contexts were industry-related contexts, perfume, body odor, nature, and a small rest category.

As one can already infer from Table 6.9, the most odor perceptions were negative, with only four dream reports including pleasant smells – e.g., an ointment that belongs to the dreamer's brother (see Table 6.10).

Whereas the reality character of the odor perception itself is something everyone (or the dreamer) might experience in waking reality, hopefully not every day; in the case of the unpleasant smells, a few dreams also featured unusual or even bizarre smells (see Table 6.11). Despite the realistic nature of most smells, the dreamer never experienced, in his waking life, a situation that is comparable to the dream situation (see Table 6.12). The following dream

TABLE 6.9 Context of olfactory perception (N = 60 dreams)

Context	Frequency	Percent	Example
Toilet, feces, etc.	16	46.97%	Dreamer wants to use public urinals that have a strong smell
Cigarettes	11	18.38%	The dreamer smells cigarette smoke in the lobby of the clinic
Industry-related	9	15.00%	A house is burning down, smell of burned things
Perfume	8	13.33%	The perfume of a man smells like pine needles
Body odor	6	10.00%	Dreamer is in a small, closed room with 15 other persons and recognizes the smell
Food	4	6.67%	The dreamer was allowed to smell the poppy-seed cake but did not get a piece
Nature	3	5.00%	A fresh dug pit, the dreamer smells the odor of the earth
Other contexts	3	5.00%	Playing a game in which odors have to be guessed

TABLE 6.10 Quality of olfactory perception (N = 60 dreams)

Quality	Frequency	Percent	Example
Positive	4	6.67%	Ointment that belongs to the brother
Neutral/not mentioned	13	21.67%	I know the perfume (Chanel No.8), but the perception is neutral
Negative	43	71.67%	Dreamer smells the vomit of a woman

TABLE 6.11 Realistic character of the olfactory perception itself (N = 60 dreams)

Quality	Frequency	Percent	Example
Could be experienced in everyday life	55	91.67%	Smelling an incense stick
Unusual for the dreamer	1	1.67%	A complex device for smoking natural substances like tree leaves or drugs, smells good
Bizarre	4	6.67%	Ketchup with a very strong fish smell, feces that don't smell

TABLE 6.12 Occurrence of the situation in which the olfactory perception is in the dreamer's waking life (N = 60 dreams)

Quality	Frequency	Percent	Example
Dreamer has experienced the situation in his waking life	0	0.00%	
Dreamer has experienced something along these lines	1	1.67%	Smelling the feces of animals while being in a zoo
Dreamer never experiences such a situation	59	6.67%	Smell of gas in the cafeteria of his institute

example illustrates this; although the dreamer has smelled pungent cleaning supplies, he was never in a hallway of an Asian snack bar and was almost sprayed with this stuff. Again, this is an indicator of the creativity of dreaming.

Dream example:

In Bergheimer street, I want to go to an Asian snack bar, but only to look at the menu. The way leads into the basement through a pub, a corridor to a counter. Here are Asian customers. One woman's hair looks like food (noodle salad), strange. They are being served right now. I look around briefly; there is no detailed menu on the wall, after looking around, I want to go. But, I don't want to be so conspicuous and go back into the hallway. The woman of the house, small Asian woman, comes towards me, she is snappy and busy. I think that the seats (about 6 to 8 tables) have no light and the ventilation system was certainly not cheap, but was probably already in when they set up the restaurant here in the rented rooms. A man is spraying cleaning supplies on the walls of the hallway. I'm already afraid he's going to spray me. He sprays near me and I make a comment that it is unpleasant, quite pungent smell. I walk through the pub.

6.4 Gustatory perception

Overall, 41 dreams (0.32%) included an explicit reference to gustatory perception. These dream situations were all related to food, with one exception: "the dreamer sucks water out of a mouth piece of a flute (flute could not be played properly), the water having a horrible taste." In contrast to the odor perceptions, the gustatory perceptions were predominantly positive, with 14 dream reports including unpleasant tastes (see Table 6.13).

Similar to the odor perceptions, gustatory perceptions in dreams are typically quite normal in waking life, only a few things – like the taste of a mole head – are somewhat bizarre (see Table 6.14). In most of the situations, the

TABLE 6.13 Quality of gustatory perception (N = 41 dreams)

Quality	Frequency	Percent	Example
Positive	23	56.10%	French roles, tasting delicious
Neutral/not mentioned	4	9.76%	Eating sweet noodles, not explicitly mentioned whether positive or negative
Negative	14	34.15%	Eating a roll that is not fully baked; incidentally biting of the head of a mole (horrible taste)

TABLE 6.14 Realistic character of the gustatory perception itself (N = 41 dreams)

Quality	Frequency	Percent	Example
Could be experienced in everyday life	29	70.73%	Strawberry cake; chocolate
Unusual for the dreamer	3	7.32%	Fruits with an indefinable black sauce
Bizarre	9	21.95%	Bread with cheese and honey

TABLE 6.15 Occurrence of the situation in which the gustatory perception is in the dreamer's waking life (N = 41 dreams)

Quality	Frequency	Percent	Example
Dreamer has experienced the situation in his waking life	1	2.44%	Eating in a restaurant
Dreamer has experienced something along these lines	6	14.63%	Eating sweets that do not taste well
Dreamer never experiences such a situation	34	82.93%	Eating coconut flakes directly from the tree; being served a very delicious dessert (not known to the dreamer)

dreamer tasted something in the dream he never experienced in waking life (see Table 6.15). There are a few occasions with resemblance to waking life situations, but one might speculate that these resemblances are due to the fact that the gustatory experience in the dream is very vague; that is, the dream report did not provide very detailed information about all aspects of the situation – e.g., eating self-made mushrooms. The dream example illustrates a gustatory perception that is very common (coffee with cream) but has not been experienced by the dreamer in his waking life – trying coffee offered by other people and overall, as the dreamer never drinks coffee in waking life.

Dream example: "Then I sit at a large counter in a large, high coffee shop, an old building. A familiar person behind the counter gives two people (a man, a woman) sitting next to me a small cup of coffee to try. The two thankfully decline, as it is quite a strong coffee. I examine the cup more closely, take a mini sip, and put some cream in it, which is first light and then discolored by the coffee, but tastes good. I worry about whether I can sleep, it is evening, about 21:00 to 22:00, especially since I am not used to caffeine at all."

6.5 Tactile perception

Overall, 29 dreams were tagged as including tactile perceptions. However, the dreamer started very late with using this keyword. That is, in the last two years of the series (2015 and 2016), 17/1,306 were coded (1.30%), whereas, in the years before, only 12 of 11,415 dreams were coded (0.10%). This clearly indicates that, for obtaining valid percentages for dreams with sensory perceptions – in this case, tactile sensations – it is necessary to specifically focus on this particular dream topic (see Strauch & Meier, 1996). So, the analysis will mainly focus on a few dream examples illustrating the idea that particularly tactile perceptions might be underreported in dreams.

The emotional tone of the 29 dreams were mostly neutral (N = 19), with one unpleasant dream (strong itching of the leg) and nine pleasant tactile experiences – e.g., petting a cat. The tactile sensations were categorized into four groups: things (N = 11) – e.g., sand, wall; animals (N = 9) – e.g., cat, dog, beaver, sheep; other persons (N = 4); and the feeling one's own body (N = 5) – for example, being outside in fantastic weather and enjoying feeling the whole body.

The tactile experience itself was, in almost all cases, very everyday-like, with one exception: feeling the vibrations of a purring llama. On the other hand, the situational contexts of the tactile perception were almost exclusively never experienced by the dreamer in waking – e.g., when he petted a cat in the dream (which he did in waking life), it was not a cat the dreamer knew, nor in a familiar setting (see the following dream example). The only exception was a dream about washing the hand with curd soap, somewhat similar to something the dreamer used to wash his hands after doing handicrafts in young adulthood.

Dream example:

> In a staircase, I see some cats lying in front of an entrance door (on a blanket). The big red one is very beautiful. I walk over carefully so as not to

frighten her and pet her. She has beautiful soft fur, is a bit critical of me; to her left are three of her kittens, already half-grown, also very cute animals.

The next dream example is related to physical contact with other people; another dream also included the sensation of caressing a female breast.

Dream example:

I am in a large hall (old building) and see old friend (former fellow student, female) moving in a queue. It is a study office of the University of Heidelberg. I am very happy to see her. She is happy, too. We hug each other intimately, which I notice and like because I feel her body (she is young) very intensely. I ask what she is doing around here.

The following dream example is a scenario in which the tactile experience itself plays an important role; in this case, testing for water.

Dream example:

But then comes in not a child, but an older man who tells that they have discovered brown paint in the water on the house outside, which makes them suspect that there may be water in the house. I feel down on the outside wall (below the window), indeed there is a place that is a little damp (although I said before that it is dry in my apartment).

The last dream example is about a bodily perception: feeling the soft forest floor.

Dream example:

I walk up the path, realizing that I am wearing no shoes or socks, but walking barefoot. I feel the soft forest floor; think about whether there could be difficulties on the way. I decide that this will not be the case and run/jog on.

In most of the dream, the tactile perception is not directly in the focus of the overall dream action – e.g., hugging someone is mainly about being happy – but of course, also about the physical contact – feeling the closeness and warmth of the other person. However, one might speculate that untrained dreamers do not report this particular aspect of the experience. Something similar is valid for bodily perceptions – feeling the feet touching the ground is easy to perceive in waking life if the person focuses on that (even though this is rarely done in everyday life), so these perceptions might be present while dreaming but do not get reported. This is different if, for example, the strong itching is unpleasant or the dreamer ties to test whether there is water in his apartment.

6.6 External/internal stimuli affecting dream content

In this section, dreams will be reported from which the dreamer woke up and heard/felt an external or internal stimulus that was also part of the dream (see Table 6.16). These occurrences were rare (12 out of 12,679 dreams = 0.09%). There is an additional example that was not recorded but was remembered even years after occurring: the dreamer sits in in the back of a school bus, looks out of the rear window, and sees a cat running after the bus and meowing loudly. He woke up and a meowing cat was right in front of his face (wanted the dreamer to wake up and to feed it). In most of the dreams, the stimulus was identified correctly – e.g., specific music – and integrated into the dream action in a creative way. Only in dream T11644, the human voice sounding "long, long, long" was phonetically similar but something totally

TABLE 6.16 External/internal stimuli affecting dream content (N = 12 dreams)

Dream No.	Stimulus	Dream
T01821	Radio (sport program including the trainer Biontek and the top tip round [betting])	I'm in a big hall. It's about a coach, Biontek, who has become the national coach (soccer) coming from a small German club. At first, there were difficulties in negotiating, but they wanted him and made him a good offer. I sit in a short skirt in the auditorium-like rows. A woman is doing the top tip round and speaking it on tape. She doesn't quite see the device, though, and occasionally pushes the wrong buttons. At first, I thought the woman was pretty cool because the recording is about to be broadcast on the radio. I feel uncomfortable because I have a naked upper body. I put on my white and blue ringed T-shirt that my partner had on.
T02933	Film music "Diva" was playing	I come into a small gymnastics room. There I am supposed to take over a small group. The previous group leader tells me that one participant is particularly into the Greek dances. Right now, they are dancing to Diva movie music (piano piece 7, actually ran on CD). It's nice and slow and repetitive. There are four, five people. I go to the CD player and want to put in some groovy music. There's nothing there. I could sprint over to my place and get something. But I'm unsure what.

Dream No.	Stimulus	Dream
T03216	Knocking	I am in a small village and want to look around a bit. There is a small cable car with single cabins as a means of transportation. Somehow, I get into it. At first it is nice, but at house roof height, it goes quite roughly around a house. I find out the most comfortable position, but I am afraid that nobody knows that I am sitting in it. It picks up speed and goes out of the village to a slope, first down, then up. I look for the exit button. Difficult, but a small green lever lights up when I flip it. It goes up, but the track gets faster and faster. I get quite scared and was awakened by a (real) knock from my room neighbor.
T03271a	Film music "Hair" is playing	I'm at a seminar and want to go back to the group room, get something, and maybe dance. It's evening and pitch dark in the room, although some are sleeping there. I slowly turn on a dim light. The others don't feel disturbed, it's only 8 pm. Then it looks like a cinema, I sit, almost lie on a cinema chair and look at the screen, a detailed pre-film with good music (in reality "Hair" music is playing). I start rocking to it, some, now there are many people from the seminar, but also strangers, start dancing. The music is great. I get up because I am sitting very cramped. I see a slim, good looking, tall woman, not from the seminar, who I like very much.
T05462	Loud breathing of the bedpartner (having a cold)	Lecture hall. A former professor tells something about a project of his, but it did not work out as he had imagined. My papers, which are discussed within a smaller framework, are good. The professor, who is narrating, breathes loudly. (The stuffy nose of the partner in reality was so loud.)
T05556	Snoring of the partner	I go to a pub. The pub owner snores while standing up. I knock on the table to make him wake up. The first time, he is awake only briefly; the second time, he complains why he can't sleep. I say something about bad impression on possible customers. Later, I am in front of the pub. An older man is trying to make himself comfortable on some kind of rolling board. He also snores. We talk about sleep diagnostics. I ask him if he has ever observed sleep apnea in himself. He denies it. He also doesn't want to know about the whole thing when I say that we have the possibilities to diagnose that, which was not the case before. (Woke up and P4 snored loudly.)

(Continued)

TABLE 6.16 (Continued)

Dream No.	Stimulus	Dream
T07568	Snoring of the partner	Courtyard. A good friend is to sing a song, "Tainted love." He tries hard, sings one line, but then there is a long pause. I hear the loud snoring of an older man. The whole thing takes place in a yard. Then I wake up and my partner is snoring loudly in the supine position.
T08670	Alarm clock	In front of us, a colleague drives her Beetle into one of the last parking spaces. And she has already gotten out and is running toward the building on the left. My former school friend dashes into the space next to it, quite briskly, up to the embankment. There it starts to beep, I think it's some kind of alarm, but it's the alarm clock (real).
T09816	Stabbing pain in the left foot	See dream example in the "pain" section.
T10441	Auditory stimulus "*Ich freue mich*" (I am glad)	I wake up because I hear sentences coming from an MP3 player. First, I want to turn it down, but it is my brother's player. I am annoyed that he does not want to turn it down and walk through the large apartment (Vienna, foreign apartment, visiting, organized). In the room far away, there is a big couch on which I want to sleep, but the sentences do not get quieter. I run back again, determined to find the sound source and turn it off. My brother has gotten up and crept after me to see how I react. I find the MP3 player and already want to break it because I'm so annoyed with my brother. I managed to turn the thing off and sleep in the room with my brother after all. It was a different sentence at the beginning than at the end (the sentence "I'm glad" ran all night).
T10457	Auditory stimulus "*Ich liebe und werde geliebt*" (I love and am being loved)	I am in a kind of group session or seminar. It is about personality. In the room, there are also many books, in shelves and some are on the coffee tables and some still on the floor. I interject that when working with others one can reach a "wall" – i.e., the other person does not want to go on. The leader, older, a bit of a guru type, doesn't really respond to my question, but mentions sentences from two or three books from his spiritual school, there are about ten of them. It's about accepting yourself. I wake up and hear "I love and am loved," which is real going on that night; I don't know if I really woke up

Dream No.	Stimulus	Dream
		or just dreamed about it. I feel quite confident because I know about these questions, even if I'm a bit tense because of the guru, but there is also another leader. With the books, I am a bit worried that it is sectarian or brainwashing to try to answer all the questions with these books.
T11644	Duck quacking	I come into a small cinema. In the front row, my partner has occupied two seats with my leather jacket; she was there earlier and is now out again briefly. It is rather an afternoon performance, not so much going on. In the second row sits a man (thin), I think that he might not see so much if I sit in front of him. I unwrap three cookies, with chocolate or chocolate-like, to eat them. My partner doesn't like that so much because she fears (she says) that, then, in the middle of the film, the bag is rustled, which I, however, do not intend, but only eat the three cookies. We move closer together, snuggle up, which is nice. The last time we went to the movies, we sat farther apart. We hear an announcement or part of a movie; the man says something an English, he repeats himself: "long, long, long . . ." In the awakening process, it goes over into a quacking (loud) from a duck outside (reality).

different from duck quacking. For some nights (about 30 to 50), the dreamer replayed sentences the whole night, a kind of experiment in whether these sentences had a positive effect on the waking life of the dreamer. In two of those nights, the stimulus was incorporated, in one way or another, into the dream. However, without a proper control condition (as the dreamer was, of course, aware what he would hear during the night), one cannot not estimate incorporation rates – as it has been done in experimental sleep lab studies (Schredl, 2018b). In addition, there might be more dreams that have been affected by external or internal stimuli, but if those stimuli have not been present after waking up, the dreamer would never know. Nevertheless, the dream examples clearly demonstrate that the external or internal stimulus are incorporated into the dream scenarios in very creative ways.

Conclusion

In view of the model presented in Figure 6.1, looking at sensory perceptions in dreams offers a very interesting opportunity to study different components the dream consists of, real stimuli from the outside (very rare ingredient), memory fragments (very rarely a full autobiographic memory), and a lot of creativity; the dreamer experiences situations that had not taken place in his waking life in the same way.

6.7 Global warming in dreams

Global warming and climate change with rising mean temperature levels worldwide is a very important and hotly debated topic in politics. In different polls between 1999 and 2017, about 20% to 40% of participants stated that they are worried about the effects of global warming (Bergquist & Warshaw, 2019). In Germany, for example, the number of "ice days" (days with 24 hours of temperatures below zero degrees Celsius [32 degrees Fahrenheit]) decreased from 28 days in 1991 to 19 days in 2019 (Deutsches Klima-Konsortium, 2020).

The question arises – based on the continuity hypothesis of dreaming – whether climate change is reflected in dreams; that is, whether elements like snow, ice, or hail decreased in frequency over the years. In Table 6.17, the overall frequencies of these "cold" elements were presented. For the comparison, the frequency of rain was also included.

Plotting the frequency of dreams with snow/ice/hail over the years show a clear decrease in percentage (see Figure 6.3), with the Spearman Rank correlation of $r = -.251$ ($p = .083$, one-tailed). The correlation is a little bit smaller if the first value (years 1984/5) were excluded: $r = -.176$ ($p = .172$, one-tailed).

In order to control for possible confounders – e.g., the dreamer being outdoors less often over time and, thus, the weather is not that important anymore in dreams – the same analysis was carried out for rain dreams. Rain dreams showed the opposite trend (see Figure 6.4); their frequency increased over the years ($r = .487$, $p = .005$, two-tailed).

Despite the large variability, the decreasing frequency of snow/ice/hail in dreams is indicative for the change in climate in Germany. It would be very

TABLE 6.17 Weather elements in dreams (N = 12,769)

Weather element	Percentage	Examples
Rain	1.47%	Walking home from the supermarket in light rain; waiting at a bus stop; it starts to rain
Snow	1.44%	Walking in a snowy forest; children sledging on a snowy hill
Ice	0.31%	Difficult walking on ice in the mountains; walking along a frozen river
Hail	0.01%	Dreamer experiences brief hail storm outside the house, but got through unscathed

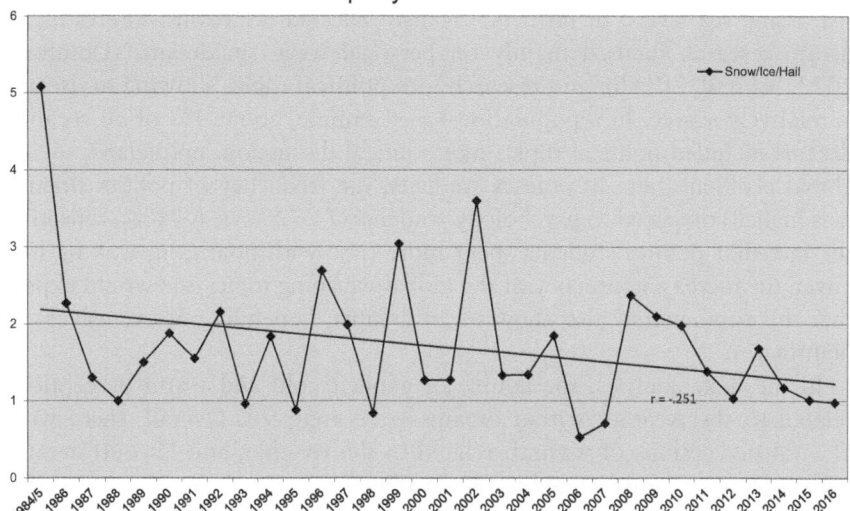

FIGURE 6.3 Dreams with snow/ice/hail from 1984/5 to 2016

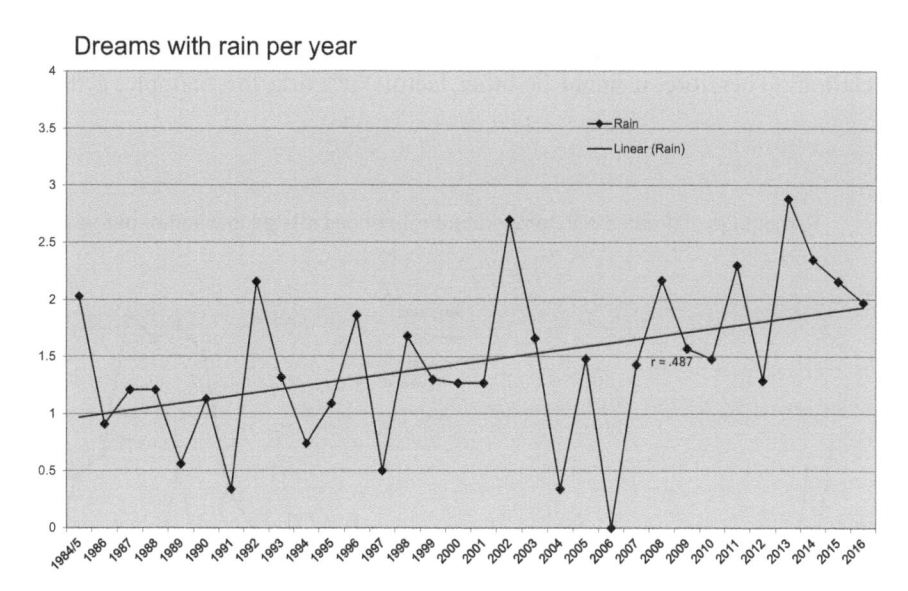

FIGURE 6.4 Dreams with rain from 1984/5 to 2016

interesting to study weather in dreams in people all around the world – e.g., snow and ice dreams in Inuit peoples or flood and storm dreams in individuals living, for example, in New Orleans, USA.

In addition to studying the weather within dreams, it would be also interesting to study whether the current political discussions, demonstrations, and the worries about climate change – for example, inhabitants living near the sea (rising sea levels) or farmers – is also reflected in dreams. Interestingly, dream research focused mainly on personal topics in dreams (Domhoff, 2022; Schredl, 2018b), and research into political topics showing in dreams is relatively scarce. In a population-based sample, about 4% of all recalled dreams included political topics like political discussion, politicians, social/ global problems, etc. In politics students, the frequency of politics dreams was higher compared to psychology students (11.72% vs. 6.71%), reflecting the fact that politics students spent more time with politics in waking life. Given the increasing urgency of the global warming topic, one would expect that this topic would also show up in dreams, hopefully not exclusively as nightmares.

In the next analysis, the course of explicit cold and warm perceptions related to the weather within dreams were analyzed. Overall, there were $N = 24$ perceptions of warmth related to the weather, and $N = 60$ dreams with cold perceptions related to the weather.

Interestingly, the explicit perception of warmth related to weather within dreams increased ($r = .551$, $p = .001$, Spearman Rank correlation) over the years (see Figure 6.5). This would fit in with the global warming during the period the dreams were recorded. However, this increase was also found for perceiving cold weather in the dream ($r = .650$, $p < .001$, Spearman Rank correlation). Therefore, it might be other factors at work; for example, getting

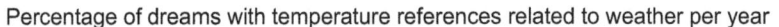

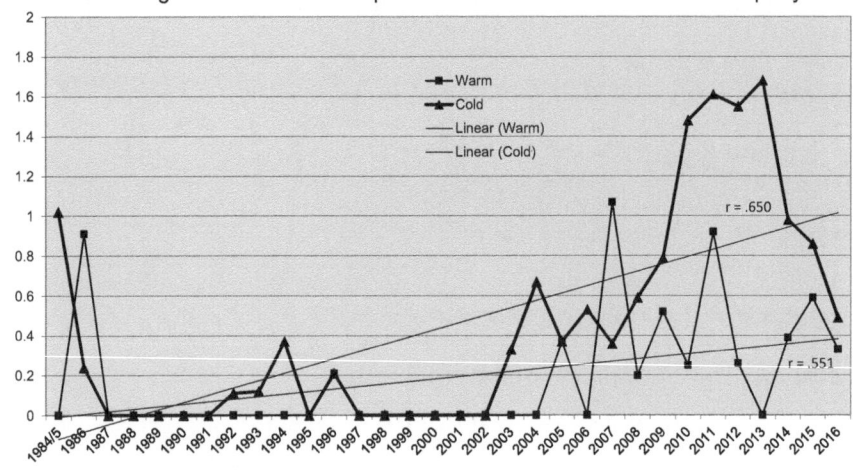

Percentage of dreams with temperature references related to weather per year

FIGURE 6.5 Percentage of dreams with temperature references related to weather from 1984/5 to 2016

older might be accompanied to become more susceptible to warm and cold temperatures.

6.8 Colors in dreams

The interest in the topic of colors in dreams is high because several studies (Bentley, 1915; Husband, 1936; Middleton, 1933), carried out in the first part of the 20th century, reported that a substantial number of participants stated that they see no colors in their dreams – e.g., 40% of the participants in the study of Middleton (1942). Secondly, in spontaneously reported dreams – e.g., recorded in a dream diary – only about 8% (a series of N = 3,638 dreams; Sausgruber, 1989) up to 25% of the reports included a reference to a color (Schredl, 2008d). Moreover, Hoss (2010), analyzing more than 38,000 dream reports, showed that black or white were mentioned most often (18% to 19%), whereas red (15%), blue, green, yellow (each about 10%) did not occur the often. This led to the idea that dreams might be mostly in black and white.

The first idea why people think that their dreams are black and white might be due to recall; indeed, the participants in König et al. (2017) reported that they do not remember colors in over 40% of their recalled dreams. In a sleep laboratory study, the researchers (Rechtschaffen & Buchignani, 1992) asked the participants directly after they were awakened from REM sleep about colors that might have occurred in the dream and found that 80% of the dream reports included some form of color. In a dairy study (Schredl et al., 2008) using the same method – that is, asking participants to list the major dream elements and their colors directly upon awakening and recording the dream – more than 97% of the dreams included colors. These findings strengthen the idea that the impression that dreams might have no colors (are in black and white); it is a memory issue. Looking at another dream element might illustrate this argument: in only about 12% of the dreams are clothes mentioned (Mathes & Schredl, 2013). Does this mean that, in 88% of the dreams, all dream characters are naked, or, much more plausible, is it the case that clothes were not important to the dream action and, therefore, not remembered and/or not reported. That is, is a banana or faces of other people grey (in case of black-and-white dreams); would that be weird and, therefore, remembered? Because it is so normal, in waking life, that bananas are yellow and faces are skin-colored. On the other hand, if the action – e.g., being chased – is so dominant in the dream, the color of the monster is rather unimportant.

The second idea about dream color is related to media; that is, persons might think that dreams are like movies/films. This would explain why the number of participants who dreamed in black and white was high in the first part of the 20th century. Indeed, Schwitzgebel (2003) repeated the Middleton study over 50 years later and found that only 4.4% of the participants (40% in the original study) reported no colors in their dreams. Looking at persons who were born after 1966 – that is, in the area of colored TV – the number of participants who believed that their dreams are all in black and white was even smaller (0.53%) (König et al., 2017). The concept of dreams as being like films had an effect on the evaluation whether there are colors in the dream or not (this can be relevant if the persons do not recall the color explicitly). Interestingly, art students reported colors more often than science and engineering students (Schechter et al., 1965); that is, if color is more important to the person in waking life and probably also in the dream, they are more likely to remember them.

The percentage of dreams with references to color was 9.39% (N = 12,769 dreams). The most common color words were black, white and the three primary colors red, green, and blue (see Table 6.18). This fits nicely with the large study of Hoss (2010). Other colors like brown, silver, or gold were much rarer. Interestingly, there are a number of dreams in which the dreamer saw something colorful but did not specify the color of the dream object. This substantial number of dreams including colors that are not specified support the previously mentioned idea that it might be difficult to remember colors from dreams if they do not play a major role within in the dream

TABLE 6.18 Colors in dreams (N = 12,769)

Color	Frequency
Black	278
Red	252
Green	217
White	203
Colored	146
Blue	128
Brown	85
Yellow	41
Gray	41
Orange	22
Silver colored	21
Blond	20
Purple	17
Pink	17
Golden	8
Copper colored	1
Salmon colored	1

Note: N = 1199 dreams with color(s), multiple different colors per dream possible.

action. If dreams had been mostly black and white, one would, of course, expect a much higher percentage of "gray," as this is the only "color," except for black and white, in black and white experiences. Thus, there are no direct hints of dreams being only black and white (plus gray).

Despite the substantial number of studies on colors in dreams (Schredl, 2012a), so far, no one has investigated the context of color words in dreams – why the dreamer might have used the color word for a particular object – e.g., would someone record something like "I saw a yellow banana"? Or it is more likely that someone would write that I saw a red car on the street. This approach has been applied for 100 dreams of this dream series (see Table 6.19).

The most common context for colors in this dream series was clothing. This makes sense, as color is of importance; for example, for many people, wearing matching colors is important. Using the color is a way of differentiating between clothes – e.g., I am wearing my black shoes (and not the brown ones). In a similar way, color designations are used for nature (blue sky vs. grey sky), cars, everyday objects, architecture, animals, hair color, food (e.g., red wine vs. white wine). In 17 dreams, colors were used in the context of objects belonging to the dreamer; this is also commonly used in waking life to differentiate between objects. Thus, this analysis clearly indicates that color words are used in a similar way to waking life, supporting the idea that the dream experience is similar to waking-life experience regarding its colorfulness.

Interestingly, bizarre colors – that is, objects/characters in dreams displaying colored objects that do not exist in waking life – are rare. In this sample of 100 dreams, only three instances occur: green-yellow-striped lizard, black color of a fresh flesh wound, and intense yellow car tires. You could argue

TABLE 6.19 Colored objects in dreams (N = 113 objects in 100 randomly selected color dreams)

Color	Dreams	Example(s)
Clothing	28	Black shoes, yellow-brown t-shirt
Nature	18	Blue sky, green plants on a veranda
Everyday object	18	Blue office chair, black radio
Car	13	Blue car, black motorcycle
Architecture	9	Red brick wall, white tiles
Toys	9	Blue laser sword, white juggling clubs
Animals	5	Black dog, grey cat
Light	5	Blue light of a police car, brown light seen through lenses
Hair color	5	Blond, reddish hair
Food	3	Red wine, red sauce

that these colored dream objects might exist in principle but they were not part of the dreamer's everyday life. However, these three dreams might be influenced by media – e.g., comics, animated cartoons, etc. – in which sometimes unrealistic coloring is used. For the foregoing examples, the dreamer is not aware of any media-related day-residues. Thus, these examples support the idea that dreams can be creative; that is, it is possible to dream about something that has never been experienced in waking life. Here is another dream passage indicating how creative dreams can be:

(T11462): "A neon (pink, bright) bird flies to a window of a house (similar to a former apartment) and lands on the window sill, rather on the frame. The bird looks like a small kite. I wonder about the bird. My brother says they used to be called partridges. The color comes from the adaptability these animals have. He must have been sitting on an intensive pink surface."

7
DREAM ACTIVITIES

7.1 Relationship issues and erotic topics in dreams

Without doubt, sexuality is a very important topic for humankind and plays a major role in people's waking life (Lehmiller, 2018). Thus, according the continuity hypothesis of dreaming, erotic dreams should be very common. Indeed, the first large-scale studies on human sexual behavior indicated that most of the participants also remembered having sexual dreams (Kinsey, 1953; Kinsey et al., 1948). Several studies (Griffith et al., 1958; Nielsen et al., 2003; Schredl et al., 2004; Yu, 2008) using the typical dream questionnaire ("Have you ever dreamed of?") confirmed that most participants reported having sexual dreams.

The first systematic content analytic study investigating erotic dreams was carried out by Hall and Van de Castle (1966). As they looked at sexuality as a part of social interaction, they devised five categories (S5: dreamer has or attempts sexual intercourse; S4: dreamer has activities related to fore-play, like fondling or petting; S3: necking and non-platonic kissing; S2: sexual overtures, propositions; and S1: sexual thoughts or fantasies). Sexual activities without interaction, like masturbation, were not coded in the Hall and Van de Castle system. About 3.6% of the 500 dream reports of female students included at least one of these five activities, whereas of the male college students' dreams included these themes more often (11.6%). In sub-sequent studies (Domhoff et al., 2005–2006; Geißler & Schredl, 2020; Hall et al., 1982; Maggiolini et al., 2010; Rainville & Rush, 2009; Schredl et al., 2010–2011; Schredl, Sahin, et al., 1998; Zadra & Gervais, 2011), the over-all gender difference was smaller: 7.3% (N = 2,977 male dreams) vs. 6.0%

DOI: 10.4324/9781003300373-7

(N = 6,552 female dreams) but still significant – with an overall effect size of 0.106 (Schredl, Geißler, et al., 2019).

However, studies using retrospective estimates of the percentages of erotic dreams with regard to all remembered dreams reported a much higher percentage of erotic dreams, ranging from 18% to 21% (Schredl, Desch, et al., 2009; Schredl, Geißler, et al., 2019). First, one might speculate that participants might be uncomfortable to record detailed erotic dreams in a diary, knowing that the researcher will read and analyze them. This would result in an underestimation of dreams with erotic content. On the other hand, intensive erotic dreams might be better remembered than mundane dreams long after their occurrence, and thus, retrospective measures of erotic dream frequency might result in too-high estimates. Another methodological issue is related to definition; the study of Schredl, Geißler, et al. (2019) used a broader definition for erotic dreams: "An erotic dream element can be any occurrence of sexually motivated actions such as flirting, kissing, intercourse or masturbation as well as watching sexual actions." This seems important, as erotic dream activities might not always include interactions with other dream characters; for example, masturbation, seeing sexual activities. This might have also contributed to the higher percentages of erotic dreams reported by retrospective studies. The analysis of the present dream series used different definitions; in order to compare frequencies of erotic dreams based on different definitions, the coding rules of different rating systems applied to the dream material.

Interestingly, Selterman et al. (2014) reported that dreams about infidelity were associated with less intimate feelings and more conflict with the dreamers' partners on subsequent days. In accordance, 30% of the participants (married women from Egypt) were reporting that they experienced guilt after having sexual dreams (even though most participants [55%] stated that erotic dreams left behind the feeling pleasure) (Younis et al., 2017). The guilt might be explained by the possibility that the sex partner in the dream was not the husband (see the following). So, this finding poses the question of whether the erotic partner in the dream is the current partner in waking life or another person. In the aforementioned study (Younis et al., 2017), in one-third of the erotic dreams, the husband was the dream character, but in all other dreams, there were celebrities (29%), familiar persons (21%) and unidentified persons (16%). A relatively similar figure of 50% of the erotic dreams featuring the partner was reported by Schredl, Desch, et al. (2009). The most detailed study on this topic was carried out by Vaillancourt-Morel et al. (2021); their results are depicted in Table 7.1. Participants who reported having erotic dreams were then asked to identify the person or persons that are usually featured in these dreams. Whereas the partner was the most frequent "target," there are also others, like acquaintances, strangers, ex-partners, imaginary persons (e.g., gods, goddesses, cat woman), or public figures (see Table 7.1);

TABLE 7.1 Erotic dreams' target in a sample of individuals with partnership (Vaillancourt-Morel et al., 2021)

	Total sample (N = 1,045)
Current partner	52.2%
Ex-partner	23.6%
Acquaintance	44.6%
Public figure	7.7%
Imaginary person	21.6%
Stranger	35.7%

that is, a considerable number of dreams included an infidelity if the same action would be carried out in waking life.

In the present dream series, the dreamer coded many different topics that are related to relationship or erotic topics (see Table 7.2). The most frequent topics are: "Dreamer finds woman attractive" (5.19%), "Talking about sex" (3.02%), "Thinking about sex" (3.00%), "Cuddling" (2.76%), "Feeling close to a woman" (2.22%), "Relationship topics" (2.12%), "Dreamer sees erotic activity" (1.80%), "Feeling lust" (1.79%), "Intercourse" (1.75%), and "Kissing" (1.50%). On the other hand, topics like "Oral sex" (0.02%), "Pregnancy" (0.02%), and "Sexually transmitted disease" (0.02%) were rare. Given that previous studies used different definitions about what to include into the category of erotic dreams, an attempt was made to apply different criteria, with the idea to compare the frequencies of the differently derived indices. The first category (Erotic+) included all topics that were related to erotic topics, thus excluding topics that were relationship-related (see Table 7.2). For example, the "Rape as a theme" was not included, as it contained elements like seeing a man who possibly raped a woman. The category "Erotic (d)" is related to erotic activity the dreamer is actually involved in, thus excluding "Seeing erotic activity," for example. Lastly, the different topics rated by the dreamer were compared to the five categories (S1 to S5) defined by Hall and Van de Castle (1966).

The percentage of dreams related to relationship and/or erotic topics is above 20%, whereas the erotic topics (broad definition as used in Schredl, Geißler, et al., 2019) occurred in about 15% of the dreams (see Table 7.3). This figure is smaller compared to the retrospective estimate of the percentage of erotic dreams (about 22%) provided by men between 31 and 45 (Schredl, Geißler, et al., 2019); thus, one might hypothesize that retrospective estimates might – at least slightly – overestimate the frequency of erotic dreams. On the other hand, the dreamer-related erotic dreams and the erotic dream percentage based on the comparison to the Hall and Van de Castle rating system

TABLE 7.2 Relationship and erotic topics within the dream series

Topic	Freq.	Percent	Erotic +	Erotic (d)	HVC
Woman approaches the dreamer	29	0.23%			
Getting closer to a woman	182	1.43%			
Dreamer approaches a woman	30	0.23%			S2
Dreamer being harassed	29	0.23%			
Dreamer is cheated	9	0.07%			
Dreamer cheats	17	0.13%			
Relationship topics	271	2.12%			
Dating	16	0.13%			
Thinking about sex	383	3.00%	1		S1
Ejaculation	16	0.13%	1	1	
Erection	118	0.92%	1	1	
Erectile problems	17	0.13%	1	1	
Flirting	11	0.09%	1	1	S2
Dreamer finds woman attractive	663	5.19%			
Woman finds dreamer attractive	163	1.28%			
Dreamer is looking for a woman	22	0.17%			
Friendship	3	0.02%			
Woman caresses dreamer	33	0.26%	1	1	S4
Feeling remorse	67	0.52%			
Getting married	5	0.04%			
Homosexuality	87	0.68%	1	1	
Kissing	192	1.50%	1	1	S3
Feeling lust	229	1.79%	1	1	
Dreamer sees naked woman	124	0.97%			
Dreamer is passive	7	0.05%			
Feeling close to a woman	284	2.22%			
Oral sex	3	0.02%	1	1	S4
Orgasm	12	0.09%	1	1	S5
Penis is mentioned	70	0.55%			
Penis is examined	12	0.09%			
Petting	4	0.03%	1	1	S4
Pornography	61	0.48%	1		
Talking about sex	385	3.02%	1		
Pregnancy	2	0.02%			
Dreamer sees erotic activity	230	1.80%	1		
Longing	18	0.14%			
Masturbation	112	0.88%	1	1	
Intercourse	224	1.75%	1	1	S5
Intercourse with problems	81	0.63%	1	1	S5
Dreamer wants sex	96	0.75%	1	1	S5
Sexually transmitted disease	2	0.02%	1	1	
Sexual fantasies	28	0.22%	1	1	S1
Dreamer caresses woman	102	0.80%	1	1	S4
External intrusion stopping sex	16	0.13%	1	1	S5

Topic	Freq.	Percent	Erotic +	Erotic (d)	HVC
Break-up of a relationship	90	0.70%			
Unusual sexual practice	4	0.03%	1	1	S5
Rape as a theme	9	0.07%			
Contraception	75	0.59%			
Falling in love	52	0.41%			
Procreation of children	4	0.03%	1	1	S5
Dreamer rejects woman	71	0.56%			
Women rejects dreamer	127	0.99%			
Cuddling	352	2.76%	1	1	S4

TABLE 7.3 Percentages of dreams with relationship and/or erotic content

	Frequency	Percent
Relationship and/or erotic topics	2,811	22.01%
Erotic topics (broad definition)	1,668	14.63%
Erotic topics (dreamer involved)	1,101	8.62%
Hall & Van de Castle S1	409	3.20%
Hall & Van de Castle S2	41	0.32%
Hall & Van de Castle S3	192	1.50%
Hall & Van de Castle S4	464	3.63%
Hall & Van de Castle S5	389	3.05%
Hall & Van de Castle – At least one S1 to S5	1,158	9.07%

(both about 9%) are slightly higher than the aggregated figure of 7.3% in diary dreams of males. This might suggest that frequencies of erotic dreaming based on content analyses of diary dreams might slightly underestimate the figures, as it might occur that not all participants are frank enough to record every erotic dream. This, of course, would only be valid if the dreamer who had recorded this series has a "normal" frequency of erotic dreams; the fact that the figures are in-between the figures for the retrospective studies and the diary studies would lend support for this assumption.

The direct comparison indicates that the definition – what is included in the category of erotic dreams – is of importance; the difference between the broad definition category is about 6% compared to the other two definitions (see Table 7.3). That is, studies using questionnaires should include some kind of definition – what kind of erotic activities are included; this was not done, for example, in the study of Vaillancourt-Morel et al. (2021).

The frequency of relationship and erotic dreams vary considerably over time, with the lowest value at 11.58% (1994) and the highest value at

33.58% (2005) (see Figure 7.1); however, there was no correlation with year (r = -.078, p = .670). The similar results were obtained when looking at the broadly defined category of erotic dreams (min: 7.90% [1994]; max: 20.66% [2005], r = .011, p = .954).

Thus, the findings of cross-sectional studies (Schredl, Geißler, et al., 2019; Schredl et al., 2010–2011) reporting a decrease of erotic dreams with age were not corroborated. On the one hand, this could be a specific characteristic of this dreamer or the effects found in the retrospective survey (Schredl, Geißler, et al., 2019) and, in the content analytic study of most recent dreams (Schredl et al., 2010–2011), might be interpreted as cohort effects; that is, persons that grew up at different times have different frequencies of erotic dreams. Longitudinal studies in larger samples would be necessary to clarify this issue.

Analyzing the dreamer-involved erotic dreams and dreams with intercourse, the pattern is similar (see Figure 7.2); the range is quite high but there no significant relation to age (r = -.190, p = .297 [dreamer-involved erotic dreams]; r = .157, p = .391 [intercourse]).

The dreams were divided into dreams recorded during one of the relationship periods of the dreamer and into dreams recorded when the dreamer was single (see Table 7.4). Interestingly, relationship and general erotic topics were slightly higher in the single-periods dreams compared to the being-in-partnership dreams, whereas the dreamer-involved erotic dreams and dreams with intercourse occurred equally often in both periods. As the dreamer was considerably less active sexually (with a female partner) in single periods, one

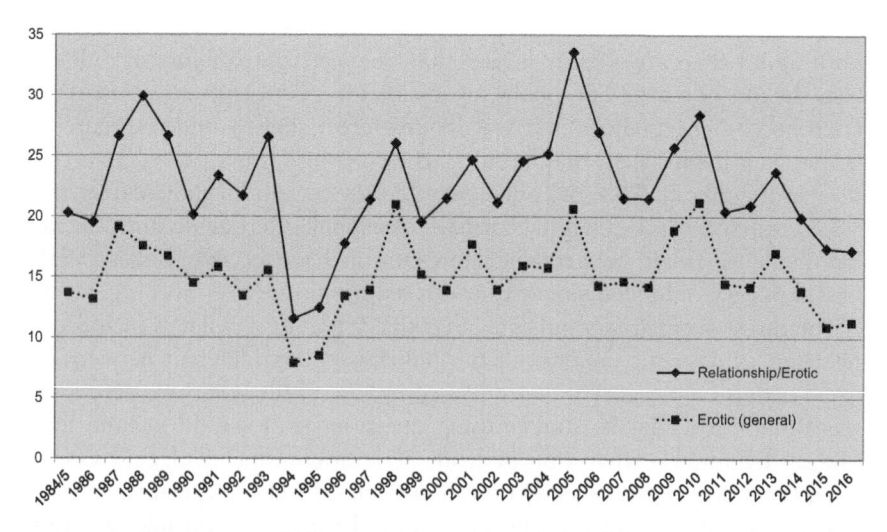

FIGURE 7.1 Percentage of dreams related to relationship and erotic contents per year

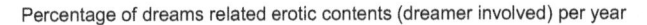
Percentage of dreams related erotic contents (dreamer involved) per year

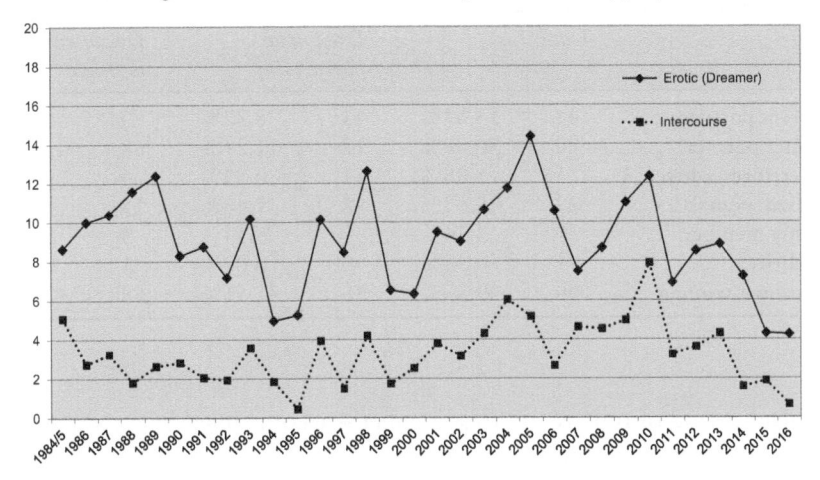

FIGURE 7.2 Percentage of dreams related to erotic contents per year

TABLE 7.4 Percentages of dreams with relationship and/or erotic content in different periods of the dreamer's life

	Dreamer in partnership	*Dreamer is single*	*Dreamer is single (since April 29, 2012)*
Number of dreams	5,369	7,400	2,525
Relationship and/or erotic topics	19.46%	23.86%	19.60%
Erotic topics (broad definition)	13.54%	15.42%	13.15%
Erotic topics (dreamer involved)	8.57%	8.66%	6.30%
Hall & Van de Castle – S1 (intercourse)	3.02%	3.07%	2.14%

might speculate whether the lack of decrease of erotic dreams in single periods (and even more general erotic dreams) might be in line with the finding of Schredl, Desch, et al. (2009), who were able to demonstrate the frequency of erotic dreams was not related to the frequency of sexual behavior (intercourse, masturbation) in waking life but the frequency of sexual fantasies in waking life. After the last separation (2012), the percentage of dreamer-involved erotic topics and intercourse decreased (see Figure 7.2). However, additional data of the following years would be helpful to clarify whether this reduction is stable and continuous with waking life, as being single for

TABLE 7.5 Sexual partners (N = 266) in non-lucid dreams with intercourse

	Total		Dreams in partnership		Dreamer is single	
Current partner	41	15.41%	41	38.32%	0	0.00%
Former partner	80	30.08%	12	11.21%	68	42.77%
Lover/former lover	5	1.88%	1	0.93%	4	2.52%
Known woman	23	8.65%	8	7.48%	15	9.43%
Family member	10	3.76%	7	6.54%	3	1.89%
Celebrity	1	0.38%	0	0.00%	1	0.63%
Unknown woman	106	39.85%	38	35.51%	68	42.77%

a longer period of time is – in this dreamer – accompanied by a reduced frequency of sexual activities.

The last analysis of the section is looking at the 281 dreams with intercourse; more specifically, looking at the women the dreamer had sex with (in three dreams, women belonging to two different categories occurred, resulting in 284 sex partners). As the dreamer was explicitly searching for a woman in order to have sexual interactions in the lucid dream (see chapter on lucid dreams), these 18 lucid dreams with intercourse were not included in Table 7.5.

The largest group of sex partners in intercourse dreams are women the dreamer had sex with in his waking life (partner, former partner, lover/former lover), followed by unknown women. Known persons (acquaintances and family members) and celebrities are quite rare. The intercourse dreams dreamed within a partnership include, in about 40%, the current partner, followed by unknown women. This fits nicely with the findings of Schredl, Desch, et al. (2009) and Vaillancourt-Morel et al. (2021). Former partners and other groups were relatively rare. Here are differences to the Vaillancourt-Morel et al. (2021) study (see Table 7.5), as participants reported more dreams with acquaintances and imaginary persons who did not show up in this dream series. Interestingly, former partners play a major role in dreamed intercourse in periods when the dreamer is single. The most frequent former partner was P3 (N = 61), followed by P1 (N = 7), P4 (N = 4), P2 (N = 3), P6 (N = 2), and P7 (N = 1). For the coding of the former partner, see section about romantic relationships in Chapter 5.

To summarize, analyzing the frequency of erotic dreams in this dream series gave some hints regarding methodology – e.g., how erotic dreams are defined/categorized or how the percentage of erotic dreams was determined (retrospective estimates or content analysis of dream reports). In addition, looking at the partner within the dream revealed that the dreamer of this series (as well as other dreamers) is not always faithful to his or her current partner when having sex in dreams. In this series, for example, dreams with feelings of remorse did occur (N = 67), whereas dreams of explicit cheating or being cheated, thus knowing in the dream the dreamer has a steady partner and nevertheless has sex with another partner, are very rare (see Table 7.2). The research in this area is still in its infancy, as it is not so easy to obtain a significant number of authentically reported erotic dreams, especially those with taboo topics like having sex with a family member.

7.2 Foreign languages in dreams

The use of complex language is unique to modern humans (*Homo sapiens*) and seems to have played a crucial role in the evolutionary history of human-kind – e.g., coordinating hunting activities, sharing knowledge, and passing on knowledge to the next generation (Knight et al., 2000). Given that impor-tance, it is plausible that language is also common in dreams; for example, 63.6% of 500 dreams obtained by the REM awakening technique include verbal activities (Meier, 1993). One of the first authors explicitly addressing language in dreams was Kraepelin (1910), who analyzed 274 dreams with explicit speech occurrences and reported that language usage was, almost every time, appropriate and similar to using the language in waking life.

Studying language in dreams offers, also, a very useful way to study the continuity between waking and dreaming, especially if looking at the usage of foreign languages in the dream. That is, persons who are learning a new language or regularly use a second (or third) language in waking life should also have dreams of this non-native language. For example, the German psy-chiatrist Alfred Hoche collected 900 segments of his own dreams, includ-ing explicit speech; 20% of those used foreign languages like Latin, Greek, French, Italian, English, Hebrew, and Russian – all languages the author spoke in his waking life (Hoche, 1927). He also reported that he more likely dreamed in Italian while he was in Italy. Interestingly, Hacker (1911) – also a German researcher – reported an interesting dream example of using English – "Please, have you these boots smaller" – because, in the dream, he was in an shoe shop in England. As he was not proficient in the English language, he also reported dreams with incorrectly used English expressions. Before sum-marizing the empirical studies looking into the relationship between foreign language used in waking and the occurrence of foreign languages in dreams, it is interesting to note that the study of language in dreams can also shed light on the creative aspects of dreaming; that is, are there dreams including languages the dreamer never heard or spoke in waking life – or even dreamed about a fictive language that does not exist in waking life.

In a sleep laboratory study with REM awakenings to obtain dream reports, De Koninck et al. (1988) found that Anglo-Canadians who incorporated the new language (six weeks of an immersive and intense French course) very early into their dreams did improve their language proficiency faster. However, a re-analysis and expansion of the data (N = 16 participants) showed that this effect (early incorporation of French into dreams predicts French proficiency) was relatively small and not significant; feelings of frustration and anxiety related to the foreign language in dreams were related to lower levels of French; thus, these dreams reflected the struggle of the dreamer learning the new language.

Three studies (Bautista et al., 1992; Garcia, 2000; Sicard & de Bot, 2013) investigated the language used in dreams reported by international students; that is, students who are studying in a country in which another language – not their native language – is spoken. The first study was carried out at San Jose State University in the US (Bautista et al., 1992). For students who learned English before the age of six yrs, the percentage of participants with English dreams only was 77.78% (see Table 7.6); this percentage decreased the later the student had started learning English: 56.81% (6 to 10 yrs), 29.31% (11 to 15 yrs) and 0% (> 15 yrs). On the other hand, the percentage of persons with native language only dreams increased: 6.06% (< 6 yrs), 17.42% (6 to 10 yrs), 32.76% (11 to 15 yrs), and 36.36% (> 15 yrs). These findings clearly indicate the effect of the daytime language on dream language, even though a substantial number of participants still had dreams in their native language after many years living in a new country.

In a similar study, also carried out at the San Jose State University, Garcia (2000) included 122 college students whose native language was not English; the early group (N = 100) started learning English before the age of ten, and the late group were ten years or older when they began to learn English. In the first group, 71.0% of the dreams included English, whereas, in the late group, only 31.6% reported English dreams. Again, the percentage of native language dreams was lower in the early group (23.7%) than in the late group (52.6%); the findings are in line with Bautista et al. (1992).

The third study (Sicard & de Bot, 2013) included international students of different universities of the Netherlands who haven't had Dutch or Frisian as native language. The proficiency of the second (or third and so on)

TABLE 7.6 300 students at San Jose State University (native language other than English)

Dream language(s)	Age of language acquisition			
	< 6 yrs	6 to 10 yrs	11 to 15 yrs	> 15 yrs
English	77	75	17	0
Native language	6	23	19	4
Both	16	34	22	7
Total	99	132	58	11

language was highly correlated with the occurrence of this language in the dream (r = .59, p < .001, N = 165 students with 342 non-native languages). Similarly, the duration spent in the second language environment correlated with the dream occurrence of this second language (r = .395, p < .001). Interestingly, some students (N = 9) dreamed of Dutch, even though they cannot speak it (but might have heard it, as they are studying in the Netherlands).

A different approach was chosen by Gabryś-Barker (2015); this author includes a small sample (N = 22) of native Polish students who studied to become an English teacher. They estimated that these students' days are comprised of about 70% Polish and 30% English and the second language they had to study, typically German or French. Almost all participants (95%) reported that they had multilingual dreams; interestingly, they stated very often that they spoke better English in the dream than they were able to do so in waking life. This is an example: "From my early childhood I have wanted to become an English teacher. It was my dream. Today when I have multilingual dreams, they are all connected with English. In such dreams, I am a perfect teacher who speaks as a native speaker of English" (Gabryś-Barker, 2015, p. 12). This looks like wish fulfillment in dreams; this was also reported by several participants of the qualitative study of Leischner (1965) studying 29 dreams of 21 multilingual persons. This highlights the creativity of dreams when it comes to languages, imagining being proficient in the foreign language.

So far, only one study (Foulkes et al., 1993) used a controlled experimental approach to study the effect of the waking environment on the usage of language in dreams. The authors included eight Germans that lived in Atlanta (USA) and eight native English persons living in Zürich (city in the German part of Switzerland). The participants spent four non-consecutive nights in the sleep lab where they were living. The language spoken in the lab during preparing the polysomnography, awakenings, small talk, and so on, was varied, English or German, using a crossover design. The participants were awakened from REM sleep in order to obtain dream reports. Table 7.7 shows that German dreams increased if the participants heard the person speaking in German (and they were asked to respond in German); the effect for English was prominent for the German participants living it Atlanta but

TABLE 7.7 Dream language in 16 bilinguals

	Lab in Zürich		Lab in Atlanta	
Language spoken in the lab	*English*	*German*	*English*	*German*
Dream language				
German	26%	42%	29%	56%
English	22%	30%	73%	50%

not for the native English persons living in Zürich. Despite the small number of participants, the findings indicate the language spoken prior to sleep onset had affected the dream languages, with the exception of the English natives that heard English in the lab.

Only a few anecdotes support the idea of dreams being creative regarding language – if one excludes the non-realistic increase in second language proficiency; that is, the dreamer spoke that second or their language in the dream much better than in waking life (Gabryś-Barker, 2015; Leischner, 1965). In the study of Sicard and de Bot (2013), 28.8% of the 168 respondents have dreamt at least once in languages they do not know. Leischner (1965) reported a case of a linguist who dreamed something in Chinese, although he had never encountered the language. These examples indicate that dreams can create experiences that have not occurred in waking life.

The current dreamer learned English for eight yrs at school, French for five yrs, and never spoke any other language (except, of course, his native tongue, being German). The school education including the two foreign languages was prior to the beginning of the dream series, which he started at the age of 21. Starting with his studies, he began to read scientific papers in English, and later, being a researcher, started writing papers in English. That is, his proficiency is highest in English, French very low, and in other languages, literally non-existent. This is reflected in his dreams (see Table 7.8). Overall, 212 dreams (1.67%) contained a foreign language (overall 223 incidences). By far, English was the most frequent language, followed by French and other languages. A very small number included languages the dreamer never heard in waking life.

Even clearer is the effect of waking-life proficiency on the dream language, if one takes a look at the context of the language within the dreams (see Table 7.9). Whereas English was spoken in about 50% of the dreams featuring English, the dreamer spoke, in only four dreams, in French and, in two dreams, in another language than English or French (Dutch and Spanish).

TABLE 7.8 Foreign language dreams (N = 12,769 dreams)

Language	Frequency
English	169
French	24
Italian	10
Spanish	5
Turkish	3
Russian	3
Dutch	2
Portuguese	1
Danish	1
Unknown language	4

TABLE 7.9 The context of foreign languages in dreams (N = 12,769 dreams)

Language use in the dream	English (N = 169)	French (N = 24)	Other languages (N = 30)
	49.70%	**16.67%**	**6.67%**
Speaking the language	49.70%	16.67%	6.67%
Listening	23.67%	58.33%	73.33%
Reading/writing	8.88%	12.50%	10.00%
Language as a theme	14.20%	12.50%	10.00%
Thinking in the language	3.55%	0.00%	0.00%
Explicit words of the foreign language	53.85%	8.33%	0.00%

In six dreams, thoughts in English were present; in waking life; thinking in the new language is a sign of intense exposure to the language. The fact that thinking in a foreign language in dreams is so rare in this dream series might reflect the fact that the dreamer never spent longer periods in foreign countries – just for scientific conferences or two- or three-week long vacations.

The next dream example features the dreamer speaking Spanish.

Dream example:

> I get into a noble lobby. I also see myself in a foreign suit. Two fine ladies address me in French, I don't hear anything at first. I respond in Spanish. Then I say in Spanish: "Mein Land pflegt zu kämpfen". That's enough to be accepted into noble society, before that I was almost expelled.

Although the dreamer was sure, within the dream, that he used Spanish, the words recalled were German, and he doesn't know these Spanish words in waking life. There were no unknown language words explicitly mentioned in the dream reports – only English words and two French words (see Table 7.9). The next dream example illustrates the listening aspects to languages the dreamer doesn't know and the clumsy use of French:

Dream example:

> Then someone speaks to me, a young woman, whom I don't understand. It's probably Italian (the host country for this meeting). I try to say "Allemande" so that she knows I speak German and don't understand her. A man from the young clique says something in English.

In contrast, the next dream example included explicit English words, and the dreamer would have been able to translate this in waking life – even though this particular story title never came up in his waking life.

Dream example:

> *I see a typewritten page from my fairy tales. N. has just finished reading the first fairy tale. I encourage her to read on. Then I think of a title for a story: Das seltsame Geräusch (ev. Der seltsame Geruch) der Blume auf der Straße. I translate: "The odd noise of the flower on the street."*

As reported previously (Gabryś-Barker, 2015; Leischner, 1965; Sicard & de Bot, 2013), the percentage of dreaming including the English language is higher if the dreamer has spent the previous day(s) in an English-speaking country (see Table 7.10). Although the difference is statistically significant (using as an approximation a Chi-Square test), the percentage of English dreams in an English environment is still very small: one out of 20 dreams. This is much lower than the figures reported by Foulkes et al. (1993) (see Table 7.7), but these participants spent much longer times in the foreign country (USA or Switzerland) compared to the dreamer. This indicates that dream language is relatively slow in switching to the new waking-life environment.

Dreams including a language not in the least familiar to the dreamer are very rare (N = 4, or 0.03% of all dreams). The following two dream examples illustrate this.

> *A bad teacher is trying to teach us something. She dictates sentences. One sentence contains a strange word that I can't write. She repeats the sentence; it could be Native American. I ask what the point of learning such a word is. She can't answer that. I suspect it could be Hopi, no, it's not. She doesn't even know what language it's from.*

> *"I'm in a small village, walking around. A man is talking on a cell phone. He has a loud, shrill voice and speaks a strange language."*

Even though these dreams are rare, they might be of importance for a possible connection between dream content and sleep-dependent memory-consolidation (Schredl, 2017a); that is, would provide an argument against this line

TABLE 7.10 English dreams dreamed in different locations

Country	All dreams	English dreams
Dreamed in English-speaking countries (US, UK, Ireland, Canada)	208	5.29%
Dreamed at home/in non-English speaking countries	12,561	1.26%

Statistical test: $\chi^2 = 25.5$, p < .0001.

of thinking, as it seems wasted energy to learn something that is completely obsolete. However, the studies of De Koninck et al. (1988) might favor the link between dreaming and memory consolidation, as the incorporation of the new language into the dreams while learning this new language reflects or even facilitates language learning. Thus, studying foreign languages in dreams is a very interesting paradigm to investigate the interplay between waking and dreaming.

7.3 Hobbies

Interestingly, the question of how often the hobbies of a person show up in her or his dreams have been rarely studied, even though a recent survey indicated that about 10% of all remembered dreams included a references to one or another hobby of the dreamer (Schredl, Coors, et al., 2022). And, as predicted by the continuity hypothesis, the frequency of hobby dreams was related to the amount of time spent with hobbies in waking life (Schredl, Coors, et al., 2022). The present dreamer had two hobbies he was very much engaged in as a younger man but almost completely abandoned these leisure-time activities when he grew older. Thus, these topics offer a unique opportunity to study the relationship between waking-life engagement and dreaming about this specific hobby over the course of time.

The first hobby was juggling (balls, clubs, diabolo), riding a unicycle, and fire-breathing. In 1986, he was introduced to juggling by a close friend and started regular but light training. Starting in 1989, the training intensity increased; this period included several public performances as an amateur (alone and in a juggling group), attending juggling conventions, and being a trainer for novice jugglers. Due to other obligations (PhD, professional career), the dreamer has almost completely stopped training and other juggling-related activities since 1995.

Overall, circus art-related activities were found in 418 dreams (see Table 7.11). For comparison, in a student sample of N = 1612 diary dreams, none of these activities occurred (Schredl, 2019a), indicating that it is a rare hobby.

TABLE 7.11 Circus art-related activities in dreams

	Frequency	Percent
Juggling – training	267	2.09%
Juggling – performance	53	0.42%
Unicycle	58	0.45%
Acrobatics	67	0.52%
Fire-breathing	2	0.02%
Total	418	3.27%

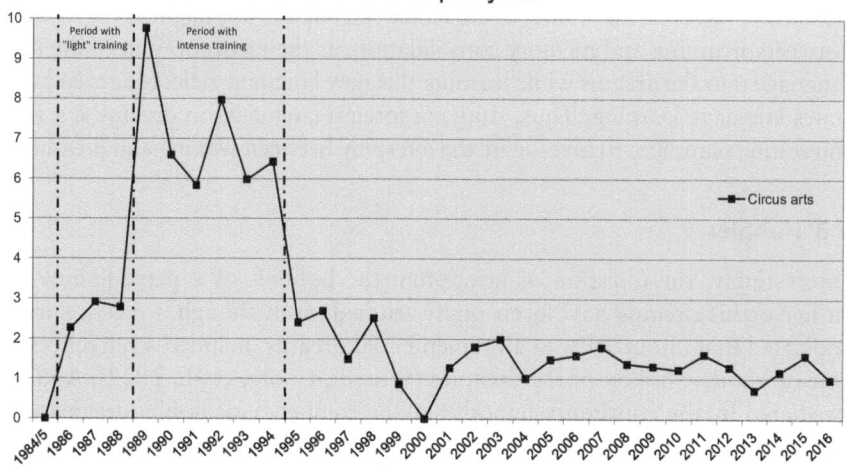

FIGURE 7.3   Dreams with circus art-related activities

The graph (Figure 7.3) is an extension of the analysis presented in Schredl (2019a) and clearly shows the relationship between time spent in waking time with circus art-related activities and the corresponding dreams. Starting with the year 1995, the percentage of dreams with circus art-related activities decreased over time ($r = -.404$, $p = .062$, Spearman Rank correlation), indicating that dreams with those topics refer to waking-life experiences of the more or less distant past.

The second hobby the dreamer was very much engaged in over several years of his life was dancing. In German, it is called "*Freies Tanzen*" (free dancing). This started with weekly events in which a psychologist played music in a small gymnasium and about 50 young persons (including the dreamer) were dancing in every way they wanted to. The dreamer also started to visit discotheques/night clubs for dancing, sometimes up to three nights per week. This stopped in 1993, with moving away from the inner city, focusing on work, and being in a long-term relationship. After that, dancing was only occasionally done (a few times a year). Overall, 252 dreams included dancing as an activity of the dreamer (1.97%). For comparison, dancing as an activity of the dreamer was found in 29 of 1,612 diary dreams reported by 425 psychology students (for more detailed information about this student sampe, see Schredl & Noveski, 2018); that is, 1.80% of the dreams – very similar to the percentage found in the present dream series.

The frequency of dancing dreams per year shows a very large variability from 0% (1998) to about 4% (2004) (see Figure 7.4). Nevertheless, the

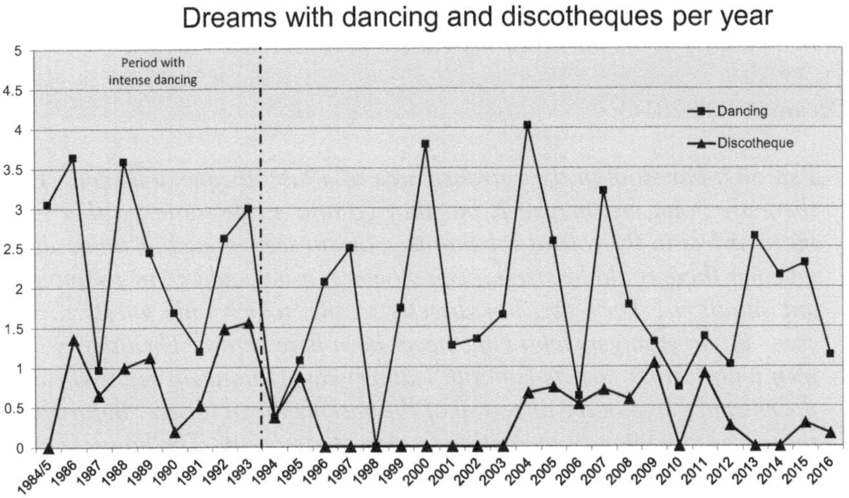

FIGURE 7.4   Dreams with dancing or references to discotheques per year

TABLE 7.12 Dancing dreams and dreams with references to discotheques in two time periods

Time periods	1984/85 to 1993	1994 to 2016	Statistical test
Total Number of dreams	4,587	8,182	
Dancing dreams	2.44%	1.71%	$\chi^2 = 19.1$, p < .0001
Dreams with references to discotheques	1.00%	0.37%	$\chi^2 = 8.1$, p = .0044

percentage during the period of intense dancing was higher compared to the time period after 1993 (see Table 7.12).

The two dreams examples reflect the period long after visiting clubs; the first one seems to be a remembrance of old times, whereas the second dream clearly indicates that the discotheque setting is not part of the dreamer's world anymore.

Dream (27.09.2015):

I am in a small hallway area where dance music is playing; maybe there is a disco in the basement. There are some people dancing, me too. There come 4, 5 young women wearing exactly the same flashy clothes, thin cloth pants, colorful top. They are pretty to look at and dance a bit. In order not to look at them constantly, I dance a little apart, but also see them a little in the mirror of my glasses (like rearview mirror).

Dream (10.08.2016):

I sit on a bar stool in the entrance area of a discotheque, with pub. First there are bouncers, maybe 2, but they go into a side room, so that I am more or less in the role of the bouncer, or am seen as such. I think about whether there could be stress, even violence, if it should come to unpleasant situations. They say, not directly to me, which only guests should come in, no strangers who have never been here before. Then two young men with leather jackets (smooth leather) come and walk safely through the entrance area in the direction of the basement exit (disco). Before that, there was a woman in the entrance area, quite pretty. The bouncers sent her downstairs because she wanted something to eat. I thought about approaching her, but did nothing. After a short while, I think about what I'm doing here, it's not my job, it's risky. I get up and go outside (night). So really I do not know what I want to do.

7.4 Music in dreams

The first evidence for musical instruments (bone flutes) in human history dates back more than 30,000 years (Morley, 2013), and music plays an important role in all cultures around the world (Bohlman, 2013). Especially in adolescents, music is very important; for example, in the study of North et al. (2000), the adolescents spent, on average, about 2 ½ hours listening to music per day. In a population-based sample (N = 1966), only 14% of the participants stated that music doesn't play a role in their lives (König et al., 2018). Based on the continuity hypothesis of dreaming, one would expect that music would also show up in dreams quite often.

In two large-scale and population-based samples, the retrospectively estimated frequency of music dreams ranged from 6% to 7% (König et al., 2018; Schredl et al., 2015). These dreams could include topics like listening to music, playing an instrument, singing, or talking about music-related topics. In an unselected student sample (N = 1612 dreams reported by 425 students), the percentage of dream reports with music topics was 8.14% (König & Schredl, 2021), comparable to the retrospectively collected data. One study (Uga et al., 2006) reported a higher music dream percentage (18.20% in psychology students), but this might be explained by methodological issues, like that the advertising specifically that the study is about music and dream might have biased the sample characteristics and, in addition, they were probed every morning whether music occurred in the dreams and this probing can influence the subsequent dreams elicited with a dream diary. In contrast, the participants of König and Schredl (2021) did not know that the dreams were analyzed for musical content. Overall, the findings indicate that music is a quite common dream topic. As expected, musicians, music students, and choir members reported a marked higher percentage of music dreams (Uga et al., 2006; Vogelsang et al., 2016). Moreover, the time spent actively listening to music and/or playing an instrument/singing was correlated with the frequency of music dreams; thus, music dreams are closely related to musical activity in waking (König et al., 2018).

Listening to self-selected music in waking life is often associated with positive emotions (Liljeström et al., 2013). This is also the case for music in dreams; in two studies, the frequency of music dreams was positively correlated with overall emotional tone of the dreams (Kern et al., 2014; Schredl et al., 2015). Using a within-subject comparison, dream reports with music in them also included often positive and less negative emotions compared to dreams reports without music (König & Schredl, 2021). However, negatively toned music dreams were reported by music students – e.g., "I am supposed to play a concert, but do not know the piece by heart"; or "Sitting in the orchestra, I heard the signal for my entry but did not find my instrument and missed it" (Kern et al., 2014) – i.e., music dreams can also reflect performance anxieties in music students or musicians.

One study (König et al., 2018) also looked at the question of whether the preferred music style in waking – e.g., Classical, Hip-Hop, Rock, Pop, Heavy metal, German folk music, Reggae, Electronic music, and Jazz/Blues/Swing – is also the predominant music style in dreams. The correlation coefficients ranged from r = .380 to r = .603, indicating clearly that a Classical music fan dreams more often about Classical than a person having other preferences, but it might also occur that a non-preferred music style might pop up in dreams now and then. However, a more detailed analysis about music genres in dreams – or even music titles or specific bands that occurred in the dream – has not yet been carried out systematically.

The dreamer started playing acoustic guitar at the age of 17, did some fingerpicking (Folk) and accompany his own singing (at best on an intermediate level). Since 2005 (after taking voice lessons), he started singing in a choir with mixed repertoire (Folk, Swing, Pop, ecclesiastical songs). Training was once per week, with two to four concerts per year. The preferred music genres of the dreamer are Pop, Rock, and Folk. From about 1982 to 1993, he regularly visited clubs (Rock/Pop), with periods up to two to three times per week (free dancing).

Overall, the total frequency of music dreams with any reference to music (listening to music, playing an instrument, singing, talking about music, instrument) was 5.74% (N = 730 music dreams). The percentage of dreams with actual music in them (listening to music, playing an instrument, and singing) was slightly lower: 4.68%. The present findings were contrasted to the diary dream findings of König and Schredl (2021) in Table 7.13. The figures were comparable – the students had more music-related topics without any actual music but, on average, reported somewhat less frequently dreams with playing an instrument.

The fluctuations during the course of the 32 years are quite large, ranging from about 2.5% to 10% (see Figure 7.5). The correlations between year and music percentage were non-significant: $r = .027$ ($p = .883$) for music in dreams and $r = .048$ ($p = .793$) for all musical topics (including instruments and talking about music).

Looking specifically at singing, the time point when the dreamer started singing in a choir clearly marks an increase in singing dreams (see Table 7.14), reflecting the newly practiced leisure-time activity.

TABLE 7.13 Musical activities in dreams

	Present dream series (N = 12,769	Diary dreams of students (N = 1,612
Listening to music	3.87%	4.53%
Music-related topics	0.79%	2.67%
Playing music	0.82%	0.43%
Singing	0.57%	0.62%
Instrument	1.53%	–

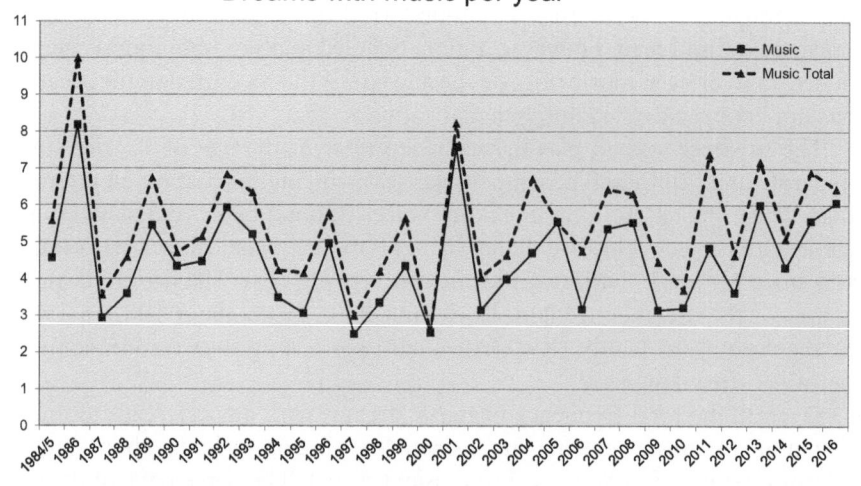

Dreams with music per year

FIGURE 7.5 Dreams with music from 1984/5 to 2016

TABLE 7.14 Singing dreams before and after joining a choir

Time periods	Total Number of dreams	Singing dreams (frequency)	Singing dreams (percent)
1984/85 to 2004	7,680	18	0.23%
2005 to 2016	5,089	55	1.08%

Statistical test: χ^2 = 38.6, p < .0001.

TABLE 7.15 Characteristics of N = 494 dreams including listening to music

	Frequency	Percent	Illustrations
Live music	267	54.05%	Concert, someone is singing, playing the piano
Music not live	227	45.95%	Radio, sound system
Positive emotion	183	37.04%	Enjoying the music
Neutral/Emotions are not mentioned	276	55.87%	
Negative emotion	35	7.09%	Music too loud
Information about genre/ title/artist	152	30.77%	Genre: Jazz, Folk Title: Nirvana – "Smells Like Teen Spirit"
No information about music	342	69.23%	Someone is playing the piano; I am listening to music

In the dreams that included listening to music (N = 494), slightly more dreams included live music – e.g., a band, someone singing or playing an instrument (see Table 7.15). If emotions were mentioned in the dreams that were related to the listening to music, they were much more likely to be positive than negative (see Table 7.15, comparing positive emotions versus negative emotions: Chi^2 = 100.5, p < .0001, N = 218, effect size = 1.850). This is in line with the findings from larger studies (Kern et al., 2014; König & Schredl, 2021; Schredl et al., 2015), indicating that listening to music is most often fun in waking (otherwise you wouldn't do it) and also in dreams. Interestingly, in more than two-thirds of the listening dreams, the music itself was not specified. In about 30%, the music genre or the artist/song title was mentioned (see Table 7.15).

For the 152 dreams with information about the music, only the genre was mentioned in N = 61 dreams – e.g., Rock/Pop (N = 9), Classical music (N = 8), Blues (N = 5), Jazz (N = 5), Disco music (N = 4), Punk (N = 3), Reggae (N = 2), and others. In 91 dreams, the title and/or the artist(s)

were explicitly mentioned in the dreams; the majority of those dreams (N = 63) fell into the Rock/Pop/Disco group – e. g., Beatles (N = 8), Rolling Stones (N = 5), Supertramp (N = 3), Peter Gabriel (N = 3), Van Halen – "Jump" (N = 3). Two references were to the school rock band called "Hitzefrei" with teachers and students of the school the dreamer attended. The dreamer was helping the band now and then when he was a teenager.

The titles that the dreamer heard (see Table 7.16) reflect his waking-life preference – also the time range, as he did not listen much to music after 1994; that is, the list does not include any "modern" songs. This continuity between musical preferences in waking life and dreaming was also found for a large sample of participants (König et al., 2018).

In 105 dreams, the dreamer played a musical instrument. The frequency of these instruments is depicted in Table 7.17. As expected, the instrument the dreamer plays relatively rarely but regularly in waking-life is the most common dream instrument. The instrument learned much later, the didgeridoo, is also found in some dreams. As the dreamer played very rarely very simple tunes on the piano and learned playing the flute for a brief period in childhood, the fact that these instruments also showed up in dreams is plausible. E-Bass and blues harp were instruments the dreamer would have liked to play but never did. In addition, there were also instruments in the dreams the dreamer never played, like organ, saxophone, cello, or accordion.

TABLE 7.16 Music titles (examples)

	Illustrations
Rock/Pop/Disco	Helen Schneider – „Rock 'n' Roll Gypsy"
	Guns 'N' Roses – Knocking on Heaven's Door"
	Edie Brickell – "Good Times"
	Cindy Lauper – "Time after Time"
	Midnight Oil – "The Dead Heart"
	Peter Gabriel – "Solisbury Hill"
	Prince – "Cream"
	Rolling Stones – "Sympathy for the Devil"
	EMF – "Unbelievable"
	Beatles – "All You Need is Love"
	Londonbeat – "9 a.m."
	Matt Bianco – "More Than I Can Bear"
	J. J. Cale – "Cocaine"
Folk	Kansas – "Dust in the Wind"
	America – "Horse with No Name"
Classical music	Piano part No. 7 of the movie *Diva*
	Beethoven Suite No. 21 (Sonata)

TABLE 7.17 Instruments played in the 105 dreams (in one dream, the dreamer played two instruments)

	Frequency	Percent
Guitar	50	47.65%
Piano	11	10.48%
Drums	7	6.67%
Didgeridoo	6	5.71%
Flute	6	5.71%
E-Bass	5	4.78%
Blues harp	4	3.81%

Note: Occurred in one dream: accordion, wind instrument (not specified), Cajon, cello, electric guitar, wooden boards, instrument (not specified), keyboard, clarinet, spoons, mandolin, melodica, organ, percussion, saxophone, plucked string instrument, with two dreams in which the instrument was not specified.

Dream example cello:

I walk with my backpack across a stage that is quite narrow. However, a young musician lets me pass. Then I try out a cello. "Don't worry, I can't play." I adjust the height with the pencil and stroke a bit, the lowest string sounds good. Then I try to add the second string. However, I don't know where to reach. That's about how I get it. We talk about sound volume. I say that the concert guitar doesn't have as good a volume as the cello, for example. He thinks the guitar is good anyway, because it is very good for trills.

Dream example saxophone:

I am in a large music studio practicing playing the saxophone. A man with a flute comes into the room and asks if we'll play together. Another woman also wants to join in. I play beginner level, but it's fun. I clean the big saxophone; there is a lot of white stuff in it, possibly dried spit (rental instrument). I empty everything into a cup.

In both dreams, the dreamer is a beginner, even though the saxophone dream is well beyond the real performance level of the dreamer in waking life, as the dreamer never blew into a saxophone.

Overall, playing an instrument in the dream is more likely to be associated with positive emotions than negative emotions (see Table 7.18); comparing positive emotions versus negative emotions: $\text{Chi}^2 = 27.6$, $p < .0001$, $N = 61$, effect size = 1.818. But, the two dream examples that follow indicate that

TABLE 7.18 Characteristics of N = 105 dreams including playing an instrument

	Frequency	Percent	Illustrations
Positive emotion	51	48.57%	Enjoying the music
Neutral/emotions are not mentioned	44	41.90%	
Negative emotion	10	9.52%	Do not know how to play, instrument is not working properly
Information about genre/title/artist	26	24.76%	Genre: Blues Title: "House of the Rising Sun," "Stairway to Heaven," "Bourrée" (Bach)

negative emotions can occur, not knowing what to play or the instrument is not working well (or not at all). This is comparable with the negatively toned music dreams in music students (Kern et al., 2014). Only about 25% of the dreams include information about the specific genre or title of the music played in the dream. The titles that were mentioned (see Table 7.18) are pieces the dreamer also practiced in waking life.

Dream example with playing an instrument accompanied with negative emotions:

> There is a didgeridoo in the corner. First I think that it is mine (light wood), but there is a plug on top. I loosen it, it is a jackfruit didgeridoo, a large funnel at the bottom. But the blow hole is quite small (small diameter) and besides I have no strength because I was asleep, muscles are limp. With time, the force increases, I blow hard, think that it might work with over-blowing, but I can't get any sound out, even if I hum my lips. The opening of the didge is just too small.

Dream example with playing an instrument accompanied with negative emotions:

> I play in a music group, rather younger people, maybe five or six. Rock group. I have an acoustic guitar, which I grab as I go on stage. It's pretty tight. I don't really have a plan for what I want to play, even know how to play, because I don't have any sheet music and I don't know anything by heart. I pluck away at it. I want to participate, but at the same time I am also frustrated.

Like the music dreams with listening to music or playing an instrument, the singing dreams are generally positively toned, comparing positive emotions versus negative emotions (see Table 7.19): $Chi^2 = 14.5$, $p < .0001$, N = 43, effect size = 1.427); that is, the dreamer enjoys singing most of the time (see dream example that follows). However, some singing dreams are associated with negative emotions; see dream example that follows. In more than 40%, some information was provided: what has been sung in the dreams. Interestingly, only two of the songs were part of the dreamer's choir activity (Supertramp – "Dreamer" and "Santa Claus is Coming to Town"); almost all other songs were songs the dreamer sang at home (accompanied with the guitar).

Dream example with singing accompanied with negative emotions:

> *"Someone plays the piano, then the guitar, he sings the song 'Horse with No Name' by America, I want to sing along despite my impaired voice, but it is much too high for me."*

Dream example with singing accompanied with positive emotions:

> *After a short changeover break, a new music group comes on, which is pretty groovy. The drums are wooden drums, which the previous band also used. They play a groovy song, something like "Knocking on Heaven's Door" by Guns 'N' Roses. Definitely something to sing along to. I'm surprised because the musicians are quite young. Singing along is great fun.*

Overall, three singing dreams were creative, featuring original songs (see dream example that follows). This is in line with the anecdotes put together by Barrett (2001) and Webb (2017); for example, Paul McCartney is dreaming

TABLE 7.19 Characteristics of N = 73 dreams including singing

	Frequency	*Percent*	*Illustrations*
Positive emotion	34	46.58%	Dreamer enjoys singing
Neutral/emotions are not mentioned	30	41.10%	
Negative emotion	9	12.33%	Voice is not strong, being criticized
Information about genre/title/ artist	32	43.84%	"House of the rising Sun" "Blowing in the wind" "Dust in the wind" "Let it be"m" "Puff the magic dragon" "Always look on the bright side of life"

the melody of "Yesterday." Creative music dreams were also reported within another dream series (Schredl, 2022): a Benedict nun who sang a lot but never composed songs on her own.

Creative music dream:

> *Now a rhythmic music/simple rhythm begins. I say: "Es war einmal", it works amazingly well, after one line I translate into English ("Once upon a time"), which also works well. The story is about playing the guitar, learning it, practicing it, singing to it, and performing. The self-made song goes well and is well received.*

Unfortunately, the dreamer did not remember explicitly any melody lines and/or lyrics – like Paul McCartney remembering the melody of "Yesterday."

Lastly, the instruments that were in the dream but not played were analyzed. Overall, 212 instruments in 196 dreams occurred. As expected, the acoustic guitar was found very often (90 dreams); on four occasions, it was even mentioned that it was the guitar of the dreamer. The second frequent instrument was the piano (32 dreams), followed by the flute. All other instruments, like electric guitar, electric bass, didgeridoo, and drums, were relatively rare, with frequencies below 10.

8

MUNDANE WAKING-LIFE ELEMENTS

8.1 Time references in dreams

Time plays a very important role in today's world; for example, using an alarm clock for getting up in the morning, getting to work, to school, to lectures, or being on time for a doctor's appointment. There are train and bus schedules detailed to the minute; if one is late, the train is typically gone. Time is also important for leisure activities like meeting with friends, going to the cinema, concerts, etc.

Based on the continuity hypothesis of dreaming (Schredl, 2018b), one would expect that dreams also include references to daytime, like morning, evening, or night, or include exact times, like 12.14 hrs of the train departure, or even seasons – summer, winter. Even though research that looked at the question of how time is experienced within dreams disproved early claims that time is sped up in dreams (Erlacher et al., 2014), systematic research into actual time references in dreams is scarce. Schredl (2004), for example, analyzed dreams that were recorded in the winter months and compared them to dreams recorded in the summer months (overall 425 students) and found, as expected, that winter topics (skiing, snow, Christmas) were more prevalent in winter dreams (3.8%) compared to summer dreams (2.0%). However, summer themes (hot weather, swimming, etc.) were also more common in the dreams recorded in the winter (8.2%) than in the summer dreams (5.5%), thus only partly supporting the idea that the current season is directly affecting the dreams. However, one might hypothesize that, during cold winter months, individuals might think about summer holiday, even planning summer activities; this was not elicited in the study. In addition, this study did not look for explicit references to seasons but included

DOI: 10.4324/9781003300373-8

a broad spectrum of activities that are typically related to summer or winter (in Germany). Analyzing the same dream sample of N = 1,612 dreams, Schredl and Knoth (2012) found that, in 57 dream reports, the action was set at night, whereas, in 104 dream reports, other references to daytime (morning, midday, evening) were mentioned. Interestingly, the emotional quality of the nighttime dream scenarios was less positive and more negative than dream scenarios that happened at other times of the day; that is, the daytime (or in this case, nighttime) in the dream had a specific function; that is, affecting the emotional tone of the dream. This is continuous with waking life, as most people experience more anxiety if it's dark at night. The results presented in this section are an expansion of the figures reported by Schredl (2015c), who analyzed 10,148 dreams. Clocks, which are important in this context, showed up in 0.7% of the dreams in a student sample (Hall & Van de Castle, 1966), in 1.06% of 4254 dreams reported by a female dreamer ("Barb Sanders", Domhoff, 2003), and in 0.74% of the dreams of the present dreamer (Schredl, 2021d). However, the analysis of Schredl (2021d) indicated that in only 60% of the clock dreams time was relevant – that is, in about 40% of the dreams – the clock was simply an object without providing a time reference to the dreamer. This would result in about 0.43% of dreams with clock(s) and time references. However, one has to keep in mind that time references without clocks might also occur in dreams (see analyses that follow).

In 1,660 dreams, at least one reference to daytime, exact times, days of the week, seasons, and specific dates were present (see Table 8.1). The most references concerned daytime (morning, midday, afternoon, evening, night), whereas dreams with exact dates were very rare within this series.

The most common time references in both dream samples were references to morning and to evening, whereas references to late morning, midday, and afternoon were not a frequent (see Figure 8.1). Interestingly, the student sample showed a very high frequency of nighttime references (30.98%), whereas the percentage of nighttime references of the dreamer was much lower (14.08%).

TABLE 8.1 Time references in the dream series

Category	Dreams	Percent
At least one daytime reference	1,481	11.60%
At least one exact reference to time	515	4.03%
At least one reference to day of the week	274	2.15%
At least one reference to seasons	134	1.05%
At least one reference to a specific date	11	0.09%
At least one time reference (total)	1,660	13.00%

As the dreamer was at the beginning of keeping a dream journal a student, the dream series was divided into three parts (dreamer being a student, dreamer being a PhD student and working part-time, dreamer working as a researcher). The nighttime references were the lowest in the period the dreamer was working and the highest during his PhD period (see Figure 8.2). The figure of nighttime references during his studies (16.28%), however, did not reach the level of the student sample (see Figure 8.1).

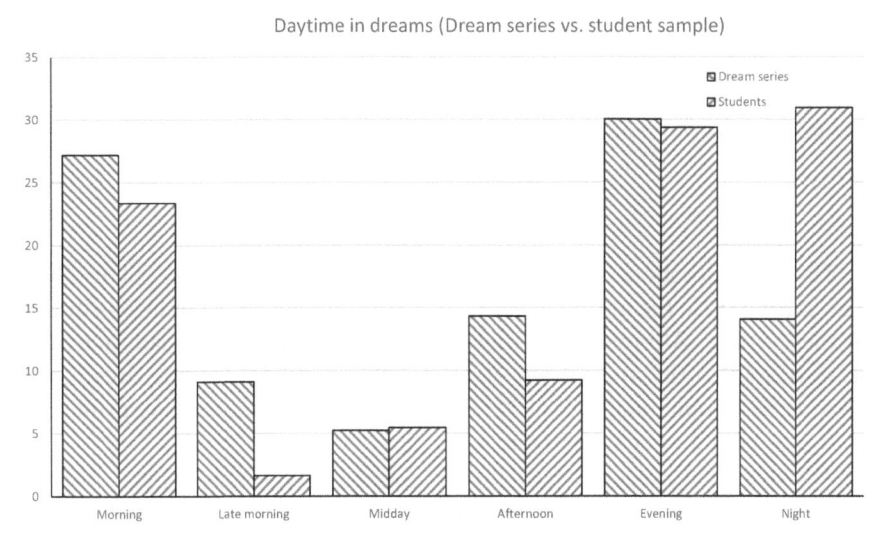

FIGURE 8.1   Daytime references (dreams series vs. student sample (Schredl & Knoth, 2012))

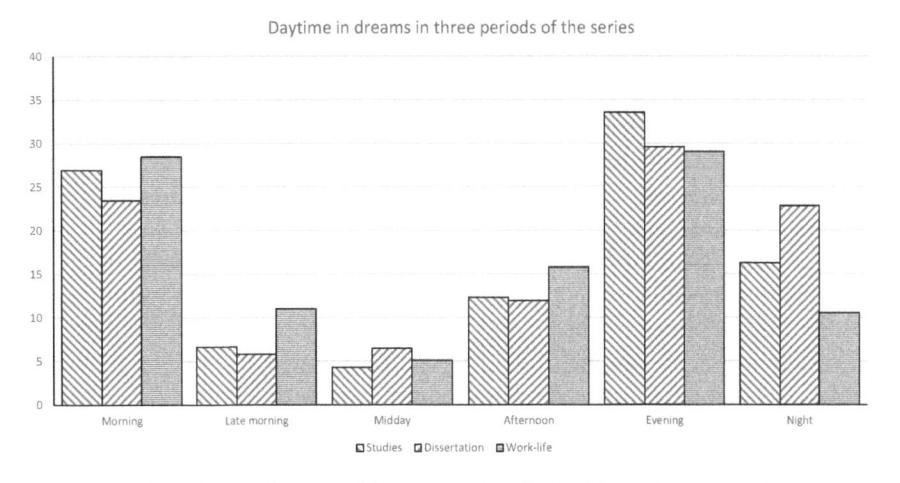

FIGURE 8.2   Daytime references (dreams series divided into three parts)

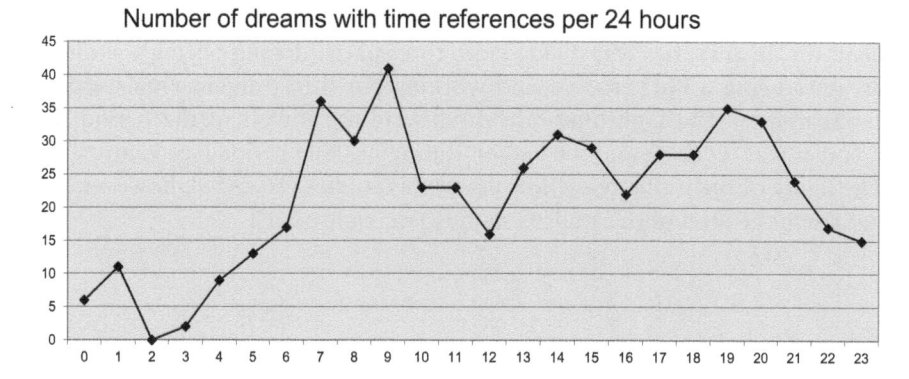

FIGURE 8.3 Distribution of times in the dream over the 24-hour cycle

The next question is whether the daytime references were plausible – e.g., getting up in the morning, eating lunch at midday, or attending a concert in the evening. Although not analyzed systematically, the dream activities were related to the appropriate daytimes. For example, in one dream, the dreamer is complaining that he cannot sleep at night. Another nighttime reference is related to being in a bar.

The next analysis addressed the N = 515 dreams with explicit times – e.g., 13:40. These often refer to times getting up, business appointments, traveling (bus, train, airplane), meeting with friends, concerts, etc. For the graph, the times were categorized into one-hour intervals, starting with 0:00 to 0:59, 1:00 to 1:59, and so on. The distribution over the 24-hour cycle almost resembles an actigraphy (measuring movements with a wrist-worn device), high activity in the morning and in the evening, less activity around midday, and very little activity at the night hours (see Figure 8.3). No dream featured a time between 2 and 3 am. As the dreamer is more of a morning type (referring to the chronotype), reflected in the high number of morning references in the distribution, it would be very interesting to do similar analysis with evening types who often carry out many of their activities late in the evening into the night.

In 274 dreams, 280 references to days of the week occurred; that is, in six dreams, two weekdays were mentioned, most often Saturday/Sunday (four times), Friday/Saturday (once), and Tuesday/Friday (once). Interestingly, the days of the week are not distributed evenly (see Figure 8.4). A Chi-Square test clearly indicated that the weekdays are not equally distributed (X^2 = 166.5, p < .0001, N = 280). Only looking at the working days indicated that even the working days of the week (Monday to Friday) are not equally distributed (X^2 = 17.5, p < .0016, N = 109). The dreams clearly show a preference

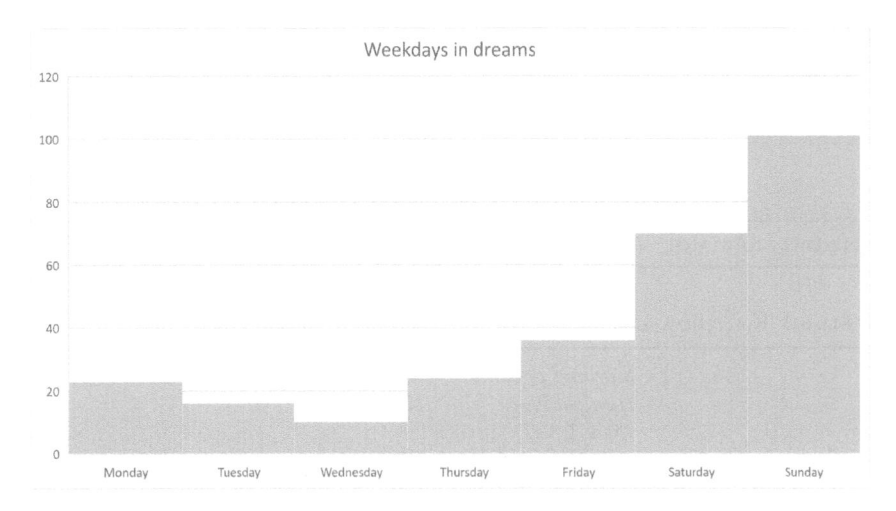

FIGURE 8.4   Weekdays in dreams

for non-working days; that is, the weekend. Even during the week, the later weekday, like Thursday and Friday, are more common that the earlier ones. It, however, would require a thorough analysis why this shift in dreams occur. In the simplest form of the continuity hypotheses, assuming that all waking-life experiences have the equal chance to re-occur in some form or another in dreams, the days of the week should be equally distributed. Several studies (Malinowski & Horton, 2014a; Schredl, 2006) indicate that emotional intensity of the waking-life event increases the probability it will be incorporated into subsequent dreams. Based on this, one might speculate that weekend events are more salient to the dreamer than the average workday event.

Specific reference to seasons were relatively scarce; the 134 dreams included N = 35 references to summer, N = 4 to autumn, and N = 98 winter, with no explicit reference to spring. Similar to the study of Schredl (2004), it was analyzed whether dreams recorded in winter included more references to winter than summer dreams, whereas summer dreams were expected to include more references to summer compared to winter dreams (see Tables 8.2 and 8.3). First, the lower percentages of winter/summer references in the present analysis compared to the Schredl (2004) study can be explained by methodological issues, as Schredl (2004) used a broader definition ("summer-related topics"; for example, outdoor swimming), whereas the present analysis only included direct references to the seasons. Similar to the study in the student sample (Schredl, 2004), references to winter were more frequent in winter dreams compared to dreams recorded in other seasons. This is in line with the continuity hypothesis of dreaming (Schredl, 2018b). On the other hand, again similar to the Schredl (2004) study, references to summer did not differ

TABLE 8.2 References to winter in dreams recorded in the winter

	Winter dreams (Dec/Jan/Feb/Mar) (N = 4,306)		All other months (N = 8,463)		Statistical test
	Dreams	Percent	Dreams	Percent	
References to winter	47	1.09%	51	0.60%	X² = 9.0, p = .0028

TABLE 8.3 References to summer in dreams recorded in the summer

	Summer dreams (Jun/Jul/Aug) (N = 3,307)		All other months (N = 9,462)		Statistical test
	Dreams	Percent	Dreams	Percent	
References to summer	7	0.21%	28	0.30%	X² = 0.6, p = .4251

between summer dreams and dreams recorded during other periods of the year. One explanation might be that the last summer or the upcoming summer is on the mind of the dreamer during the colder months.

Lastly, the references to exact dates are presented in a qualitative way, as there have been only 11 dreams with date information in this dream series (0.09%). This is a much, much lower figure compared to the 515 dreams with exact daytimes. There are some dreams in which the date reference makes sense – e.g., the dates of an upcoming conference (25.2.1987) or a dream in which the dreamer was wondering why his sister already arrived on the 24th (Christmas Eve), as she had planned to come later (dream recorded on December 24, 1986). On the other hand, there are dreams in which the date specifications are out of sync – a date for a juggling training session on December 21 – even though the dream was recorded on January 4, 1993. In one dream, even the day of the week did not match with the time specification; in the dream, January 20, 1987 is a Sunday, whereas the "real" weekday was Tuesday. As for researchers' deadlines – congress dates are important – it is very astonishing that this topic is so rare in this dream series.

The chapter closes with a few dream examples in order to illustrate what role time references can play in dreams.

Dream example (confused about time):

Unknown city, probably Ludwigshafen. I have lost my spatial and temporal orientation. In any case, I have to go back home, first I think that it is Tuesday evening and I have to go to my juggling class, then I see on a church clock that it is 20 to 3 in the afternoon, from this I conclude that it is Thursday, although I lack the memory of Thursday morning. For a short time I walk around completely disoriented, somewhat fatigued, but then I strike a direction. Soon I come to a construction site that looks familiar to me.

Dream example (appointment):

I ride my bike to a village, Walldorf of Rot or so. At 11:00, I have an appointment with a dream group friend, but it is a holiday (Tuesday). It is 10:15 and I meet in front of a large house the others from the dream group. They wonder with me why the group meeting is taking place on a holiday, but also have agreed to this date. Probably she did not know this (that's this date is a holiday) when we made the appointment a few weeks ago.

Dream example (being late):

I wake up at 7:45. That means I am late. Somehow, the alarm clock didn't work. I get up, get dressed quickly to go to the dream group. Somehow, I have some consciousness about being in a dream, but I think I am awake since everything is so real. I talk to some people, maybe family. Everything is delayed; therefore, it takes me over half an hour to get going.

Dream example with two time-references:

It is 20 minutes to 8 o'clock. A friend and I want to go dancing. I run to my apartment, he to his. It's a contortedly part of town, a bit like the old town. I don't find the shortest way, but that doesn't matter. Later there are 2, 3 people (guests) in the apartment (apartment with my family, first it is only my apartment). I ask if they want something to eat, but immediately add that we have nothing to eat in the apartment. It's Saturday, about 12:30. I think about quickly going to the bakery and buy some bread.

Dream example (being aware that the time of the day might not be appropriate):

I call a friend on Saturday morning shortly after 7:00. On the one hand, I think that he is probably on vacation and I talk on the answering machine, but on the other hand, I am worried that I could disturb him. The answering machine comes on, I start to talk on it, but he picks up. It's John Cusack.

Dream example (time pressure):

> *I am skiing at a winter sports resort. It's about 19:00 and at 20:00 they close, so I set out to ski to the valley station to be on time. This won't be so easy, as I'm not that skilled anymore. In-between, I talk to my sister, she tells me that her husband only has to do 10 months of community service (Germany), otherwise it would be more. The family of my sister is also skiing.*

Abbreviated dream example (missing a train):

> *I am at the train station and want go to Berlin. My family is around, but they are doing a lot of other things, are not concentrated on getting the train tickets. Coming to the platform, it is 14:33, the train left at 14:27. I think about other ways to go to Berlin.*

Dream example (time pressure at first):

> *I am in a large bedroom of a large shared apartment (old building). My alarm clock has just beeped, now a second alarm clock beeps in another room for my brother. I get ready to go. It is about 7:45. At first, I think I am way too late, I won't make it to work by 8 o'clock. Then I remember that I am on vacation, there is no time pressure. My mother suggests an activity; we could be in Vienna.*

Dream example (time reference as lucid dream trigger):

> *It's late at night, around 4 o'clock. Since I can't sleep, I'm tidying around in the kitchen. A hanging cupboard is packed full, also on top there is a lot of stuff, e.g. one of my red plates, cake pans, other dishes and household goods. It's not easy as some stuff slides and I have to catch it. I also worry because my mother is sleeping next door. Then I'm outside. I know it's a lucid dream because I am active in the dream but sleeping now.*

Dream example (Daylight Savings Time changeover):

> *I stayed overnight with P3, a large old apartment. We talk to each other, whereby P3 is quite impatient with me, which I do not like, because it creates a lot of emotional distance. I wish for more closeness. It was the first sleepover and I believe that we can get closer. I get up, look at an alarm clock that reads 12:38, possibly, it is 11:38, and the clock is still in the 'old' time (before the Daylight Savings Time changeover). Nevertheless, it indicates that it is late for going to bed.*

Dream example (leisure time activity):

"I am in a pub (cafe style), it is around 7 in the morning. We, a group of about 15 people, have pulled an all-nighter, partying and are now going home."

To summarize, the present analysis clearly indicates that time plays an important role not only in waking life but also in dreams. The dream examples illustrate that the contexts can vary a lot, from time pressure to time confusion to having appointments, having to catch a train, and so on. In most instances, the time references make sense – are not bizarre. But the analysis also supports the assumption that there are factors that affect the continuity between waking and dreaming (Schredl, 2003) – e.g., emotional involvement that might be higher in experiences that are related to weekends and, thus, references to Saturday and Sunday are more frequent than references to working days.

8.2 Money in dreams

Money plays an important role in our waking lives (Davies, 2002), so it would be very interesting to investigate whether money also plays an important role in dreams. This would be expected based on the continuity hypothesis (Schredl, 2018b). However, content analytic studies on the frequency of money in dreams are totally lacking. Only the topic "finding money in dreams" was studied empirically; about 25% to 56% of the participants of different studies (Gahagan, 1936; Griffith et al., 1958; Ward et al., 1961) answered the question "Have you ever dreamed of finding money?" with a "Yes". Based on these figures, one would expect that money – given all the different contexts money can be related to – should occur relatively frequently in dreams.

In the present dream series, 8.92% of the dreams (1,140 dreams) included some kind of reference to money. That is, money plays a significant role in this dream series.

The change of currency in Germany from Deutsche Mark (DM) to Euros offered a unique opportunity to study the direct effect of money on dreams. In Figure 8.5, the money dreams with explicit reference to the currency are depicted for each year. The first year after the introduction of the Euro, the percentage of Deutsche Mark dreams was equal to the percentage of Euro dreams. After that, only a few dreams included references to Deutsche Mark; almost all dreams after 2002 were in the new currency.

In a next step, 200 dreams were randomly selected from the pool of all dreams with references to money. The aim was to evaluate the context in which money in the dream occurred. A look at Table 8.4 indicates that the contexts are "typical" for waking life – e.g., in the context of buying food, tickets, clothing, and so on.

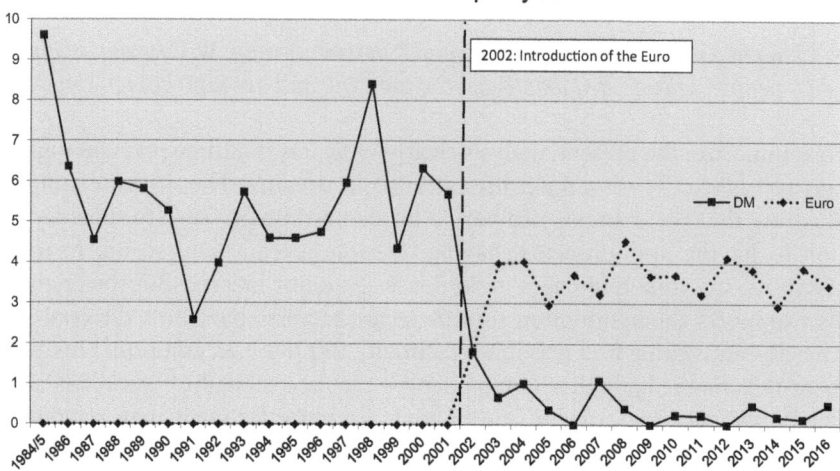

FIGURE 8.5 Dreams with "Deutsche Mark DM" and Euros from 1984/5 to 2016

Interestingly, the situations that involve money are not replays of situations the dreamer has experienced in waking life (see Table 8.5) – e.g., buying an alcoholic beverage for 23.20 DM (see examples in Table 8.4). The dreamer bought drinks in his waking life, but not for this price that is very, very uncommon. Another example is the dream with the stolen purse. This happened once to the dreamer, but the amount of money in the purse was different. Similar, the dreamer never played for money (last example of Table 8.4). This is in line with previous research (Fosse et al., 2003; Malinowski & Horton, 2014b), showing that episodic memories are very rarely replayed in dreams – less than 0.5% in 186 dreams reported by 32 participants (Malinowski & Horton, 2014b). Thus, studying the context of money in dreams provides an excellent opportunity for evaluating how close dreams resemble waking-life.

Even though the dreams did not replay waking-life experiences of the dreamer, most of the situations with a reference to money are realistic; that is, they could have occurred in that manner in waking life (see Table 8.5). Only 14% of the situations involving money were bizarre; see the following examples:

Dream example:

I'm waiting in the clothing section of a department store for my turn. There is only one saleswoman. When it takes quite a long time, I get impatient. I'm looking at socks, there's a pair that costs 64 DM. The tennis socks that hang

TABLE 8.4 Contexts of money in dreams (N = 200 randomly selected dreams)

Context	Dreams	Example
Money without additional context	45	Wallet with 50 DM was stolen
Food	27	Buying an alcoholic beverage for 23.20 DM
Salary-related (other persons)	18	Someone receives 5 DM for babysitting
Restaurant, bar, coffee shop	14	Dreamer pays 2 DM for a glass of table water
Tickets (train, bus, etc.)	13	20 Euros for a train ticket (hometown)
Admission tickets (concert, etc.)	11	5 to 6 DM for outdoor swimming pool
Furniture, potted plants	10	Selling a dresser for 150 DM
Clothing	10	300 DM for a coat, just looking, not buying
Salary-related (dreamer)	9	Dreamer receives 40,000 DM for working 400 hours overtime
Sports accessories	7	Paying 60 DM for Diabolo string
Car/motorcycle (buying gas, etc.)	7	A motorcycle for 4,500 DM
Apartment rent	7	350,- DM rent plus 350,- DM additional costs
Books	7	A teacher gives his student 100 DM for buying books
Jewelry, gold	6	Dreamer looks at gold figurines worth 1,000 DM
Hotel	4	A room for one night is 63 Euros
Research projects (work-related)	2	Planning a research project for 41,000 Euros
Maintenance for a child	1	Dreamer can afford to pay 200 DM per month for a child
Vacation	1	The overall costs for the trip are 1,500 Euros
Playing for money	1	Playing a game with 20 DM stake money

TABLE 8.5 Bizarreness related to the money context and related waking-life experience (N = 200 randomly selected dreams)

Experienced the money-related situation in waking life	Dreams	Bizarreness	Dreams
Experienced in waking life	0	Realistic	171
Unclear	0	Unclear	1
Never	200	Bizarre	28

below are for 10–15 marks. In between, I see patched trousers, red with large black patches. As I take a closer look, I realize it's my old pair of jeans. I show this to the saleswoman, who is now a second-hand dealer, the whole thing is in a large yard. I'm surprised that the trousers cost 500 DM. I would like to take them with me, but would have paid a maximum of 20 DM.

Although there are trousers for 500 DM (roughly $ 250), it is somewhat bizarre to want to sell an old jeans (trousers) for that sum of money.

Dream example:

My family, mother and siblings, get a lot of money. I receive several checks, e.g. one of more than 8 million DM. The checks look quite inconspicuous, handwritten. I say that I can use it to finance my doctoral thesis.

Dream example:

I go to the company where I work to discuss something with my boss; it's about a larger financial sum. I'm in a pretty high position myself. I meet the boss in a large office room, slightly lower than ground level, lots of glass to the outside, 1970s style. He takes a seat in an armchair. I explain to him the profit of a business transaction for which I am responsible. It also turns out to be a considerable sum for me, but the boss turns the pages, a 4-page booklet, large, quite thin paper, there is a long list of numbers that says the profit will be used to pay off my debt. These are around 200 million euros. When I was young, I did something with a friend who is also here now that caused so much massive financial loss. Despite the fact that I'll never be able to earn more than the minimum again, I take it easy, making a comment about the old friend.

Dream example:

I walk to a ticket machine in the train station to top up my card. You have to keep the card on the outside of the machine, and then insert money. I give way to someone who has to get to the train quickly and still needs a ticket. I'm not in a hurry. I put a 20-euro note (it looks different than in reality) straight into the machine, first a little crooked, a very small piece is cut off. It works on the second try.

To summarize, although the dream topic of money might be viewed as very mundane, a closer look revealed that studying this topic elucidates the influence of waking life on dreams in interesting ways – e.g., dreaming of the currently valid currency, dream situations involving money are not a replay of waking-life experience, even though many money dream situations are realistic. It also shows the creativity of dreams; that is, dreams feature highly unlikely and bizarre occurrences of money in dreams.

8.3 Telephone in dreams

The telephone is an important means for communication; in Germany in 1988, 93% of all households had a landline telephone; in 1996, about 10% of the household had also a cell phone; and in 2013, this percentage rose to 92.4%, so that nearly all household had some form of telephone communication (Güll, 2015). Given the importance of telephones in waking life, it is astonishing that empirical research regarding the question how often telephones show up in dreams is lacking.

One of the earliest published telephone dreams is reported in Stekel (1911). The dreamer visits her sister and brother-in-law; their telephone is ringing. She asks about it and is scolded whether she has not read the newspaper; almost everyone in Vienna has a telephone now. The brother-in-law also said that they replaced the unreliable female personnel with highly educated gentlemen, so the system is working better. The dreamer, typically short of money, also wanted a telephone. Her brother-in-low is calling the phone company but the deal does not work out in the dream, as the dreamer would have to invite a disagreeable person working in the company regularly for dinner. Many elements of the dream like telephone operators are not part of the telephone communication system today. However, in her book *The Universal Dream Key*, Patricia Garfield (2001) listed "telephone malfunctioning" (together with machine malfunctioning) among the twelve most common dream themes around the world. This does not include unreliable telephone operators anymore, but topics like dreamer cannot dial the right number, does not know how to operate the telephone, reaches the wrong party, gets disconnected, and so on. In the Hall and Van de Castle (1966) sample of 1,000 students' dreams, collected at the end of the 1940s and early 1950s, 11 references to telephone were coded: telephone (8x), telephone booth (1x), telephone book (1x), and telephone wires (1x), resulting in a percentage of 1.1%. Interestingly, 1,612 student dreams collected in 2000 showed a much higher percentage of telephone dreams (6.89%; unpublished analyses; for more details on the sample see Schredl & Noveski, 2018), very likely reflecting the increase in communication via the telephone over the years. In another study of 442 students' dreams, collected a few years earlier, the figure was slightly lower but in a similar range (4.52%; Schredl & Hofmann, 2003).

Analyzing telephone dreams in the present dream series offers the opportunity to investigate several topics: (1) how frequent are telephone dreams; (2) how often do problems occur with the telephone – as Garfield (2001)

TABLE 8.6 Contexts of telephones in dreams (N = 274)

Context	Dreams	Example(s)
Dreamer is on the phone	161	A colleague is calling the dreamer
Another person is on the phone	77	The dreamer's brother calls the dreamer's sister
Telephone as object/topic	36	Dreamer asks someone for a phone; dreamer sees telephone sets in a department store; a telephone rings as a warning signal

TABLE 8.7 Types of telephones in dreams (N = 274)

Context	Dreams	Example(s)
Landline phone	119	Dreamer is at home, receives a call
Cell phone	56	Other persons are using cell phones
Computer phone (Skype)	1	Neighbor is making a phone call via Skype, very loud
Not specified	98	Dreamer has an intense phone call with a colleague

suggested, there should be a substantial number of dreams; and (3) is the number of references to cell phones increasing from 1984 to 2016 – even though the dreamer himself never owned and very rarely used a cell phone.

Overall, 274 dreams (2.15%) of the dreams included a reference to telephones. In most dreams, the dreamer himself is on the phone (see Table 8.6), but there are also dreams in which the dreamer sees or respectively hears other persons using a telephone and dreams with telephones as objects or topics; that is, not using for direct communication.

In the next step, the telephones in the dream were classified – if possible – into three categories: landline telephones, cell phones, and computer-based telephones (see Table 8.7). Given the time interval of the dream series and the fact that the dreamer didn't own a cell phone, it is plausible that the landline phones in the dreams outweigh the cell phones. Furthermore, it could be identified that, in 40 cases of the 119 landline phone dreams, the phone belonged to the dreamer (33.61%), whereas only 10 dream cell phones out of 56 cell phone dreams belonged to him (17.86%). The second percentage is of interest, as it is discontinuous with waking life, in which he did not own a cell phone.

The percentage of landline phone dreams and cell phone dreams per year are depicted in Figure 8.6. As expected, the frequency of cell phone dreams is increasing; the linear trend is r = .794 (p < .0001; Spearman Rank correlation). On the other hand, there was – in addition to the ups and downs – a slight downward trend for the landline phone dreams (r = -.332, p = .064,

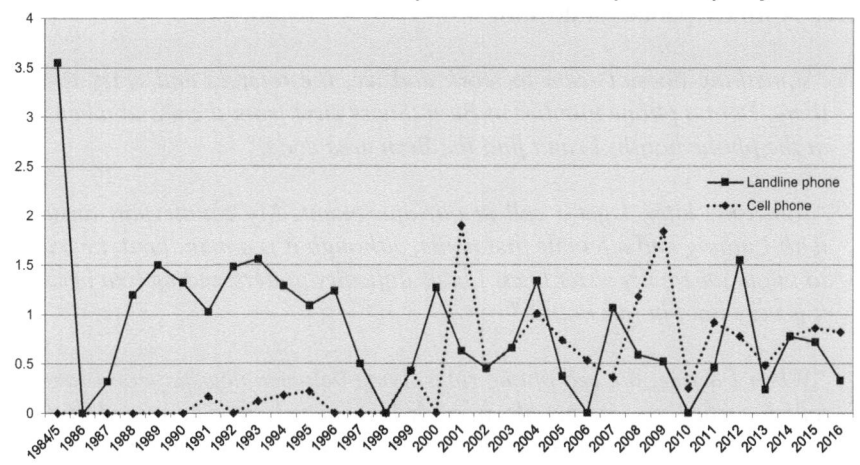

Dreams with landline phones and cell phones per year

FIGURE 8.6 Dreams with landline phones and cell phones per year from 1984/5 to 2016

TABLE 8.8 Problems with telephones in dreams (N = 248)

Context	Dreams	Percent
Dreamer is on the phone	46	28.57%
Another person is on the phone	5	6.49%
All dreams with telephone communication	51	20.56%

Spearman Rank correlation). The increase in cell phone dreams, starting with 2001, clearly reflects the increased use of cell phones in Germany (and the world).

In a next step, it was analyzed whether the dreamer was calling someone or received a call. In 72 dreams, he was the active part, and in 63 dreams, he was on the receiving end of the call (in 26 dreams, it could not be determined who called whom). Overall, in one-fifth of all telephone dreams that included communication (N = 248), problems with the phone occurred (see Table 8.8). Most of these problems occurred when the dreamer himself was on the phone, but in five dreams, the dreamer observed other persons having trouble with the phone. Interestingly, the phone troubles occurred more often for landline phones (30/74 = 40.54%) compared to cell phones (6/26 = 23.08%). On the other hand, the percentage of problematic dreams did not differ whether the dreamer was calling (22/72 = 30.56%) or receiving a call (17/63 = 26.98%).

The following dream examples illustrate some of the problems that might occur with telephones in dreams.

> *"Something doesn't seem to work and we, the referees and I, try to call there. I got a phone number of Bern (Swiss city) from them and when I'm in the phone booth, I can't find the Bern area code."*

> *"Sometime later, I get a call in our apartment. My counterpart answers with Ludwig and a female first name, although it is a man. First, he wants to know where my sister lives. I have difficulty understanding him because it is very loud in our house."*

> *"When I arrive, the cell phone rings, lying between newspapers. I take it, which surprises some people around. However, I am determined, but do not find the button (large screen, some round buttons) to answer, or I press it and it continues to ring. After two or three attempts, it works. It's an acquaintance who wants to take a trip to Ladenburg and asks if we want to come along."*

> *"I lie on my bed (quite large) and talk to my friend on the phone. He has called, it is around 9:30 or so. I look at two clocks, but they show different times, one something like 22:00. I want to find another clock, get up. I cannot hear my friend for a long time. I have an old plastic telephone with a dial and a long cable. I don't like the fact that the connection to my friend is interrupted, I may have to call him again, think of the awkward dialing."*

> *"I am on vacation with my mother. We want to go out for dinner. However, to get to the restaurant, you have to wade through waist-deep water. My mother wants to call my sister at home. She goes to a phone booth and dials the number. At first, she gets a Petra on the phone, because she dialed the wrong number. When she then dials the right number, no one answers."*

To summarize, telephones play a significant role in dreams, even though the percentage of telephone dreams in the present dream series is lower compared to the percentages found in student samples (4.51% to 6.89%; see introduction to this chapter). It would be interesting to investigate whether the amount of time spent with phone calls during the day is related to the percentage of phone dreams. This relationship was reported for using social media; spending more time with social media during the day with a higher involvement was associated with more dreams about social media (Moverley et al., 2018). The increase of cell phone dreams is continuous to waking life, although some of these dreams are not, as the dreamer owned a cell phone in the dream but not in waking life. However, the most astonishing fact regarding telephone dreams is the high percentage of problematic telephone dreams. Even though most people had encountered problems related to phone calls, like not hearing the person, dialing the wrong number, being disconnected, one would assume that does not occur in every fourth dream (28.57% of the dreams with the dreamer on the phone). Following the ideas of Patricia Garfield (2001), this discrepancy between waking life and dreaming might point to a more metaphorical connection of this type of dream to waking life – e.g., the dreamer has problems getting help in waking, with the dream phone not working as the matching metaphor, the relationship to another person in waking life is complicated (phone call in the dream is disconnected), and so on. Even though these metaphorical links between waking life and dreaming are currently highly speculative, it is possible to study them empirically by taking a closer look into the person's waking life – in this case, the social network – and determine whether there are some connections between relationship quality to specific persons and the occurrence of problematic telephone dreams.

8.4 Glasses in dreams

For a severely shortsighted persons, glasses are of the utmost importance. Thus, based on the continuity hypothesis of dreaming (Schredl, 2018b), glasses should also show up in dreams, especially in persons who wear glasses constantly during the day. However, research studying the occurrence of glasses within the dream are almost non-existent. In the diary dream sample (N = 1,000) of Hall and Van de Castle (1966), eye glasses were mentioned in nine dreams (0.9%), but no context was provided; neither the information whether the dreamer actually wore goggles. In a small experimental study that required the participants to wear tunnel vision goggles, 3.45% of the dream reports obtained by REM awakenings (one out of 29 dreams) included a direct reference to wearing goggles (Herman et al., 1979). The first in-depth analysis was carried out by Schredl (2012c) based on the first 7,747 dreams of the present dream series, finding that 0.94% of all dreams included a reference to glasses – very similar to the percentage reported by Hall and Van de Castle (1966). The findings presented in this section are an expansion of the previously reported results (Schredl, 2012c).

The dreamer is severely shortsighted (-6.0 diopters) and has had to wear glasses since his eighth year of life. He has never worn contact lenses. Overall, references to glasses were found in 142 dreams (1.11%). Of those dreams, 18 dreams included references to glasses of other persons; that is, 0.98% of the dreams (N = 124) in this series included a reference to the glasses of the dreamer. As 11 dreams had two different contexts, the total number of different contexts increased to 135 (see Table 8.9). The most common contexts are: "Glasses are dirty, fogged; vision is somehow affected," "Glasses

TABLE 8.9 Contexts in dreams with glasses (N = 135)

Context	Dreams	Example(s)
Glasses are dirty, fogged; vision is somehow affected	38	Glasses are dirty, dreamer cannot clean them
Glasses are broken	31	Dreamer tries to fix his broken glasses
Putting on and taking off glasses	27	Taking of glasses before going to bed
Buying glasses	3	Dreamer wants to buy glasses
Someone gives the dreamer glasses	3	A woman hands the dreamer's glasses to him
Looking for one's glasses, forgetting them somewhere	18	Dreamer has to go back to a room because he forgot his glasses
Glasses do not fit	1	The glasses are too broad, does not fit on the nose
Cleaning classes	3	Dreamer is at work, cleaning his glasses
Packing glasses	10	Dreamer packs to extra glasses for a journey
Being at the ophthalmologist	1	A rough ophthalmologist is examining the dreamer (unpleasant)

are broken," "Putting on and taking off glasses," and "Looking for one's glasses, forgetting them somewhere." On the other hand, buying glasses, simply cleaning glasses, glasses that do not fit, or being at the ophthalmologist are very rare dream topics. Interestingly, only two dreams classified into the "Putting on and taking off glasses" category included the taking off (N = 1) and putting on glasses (N = 1) relation to going to bed or respective leaving the bed.

Most of the contexts in which the glasses occur in the dreams have been experienced by the dreamer in his waking life (82 out of 124) – e.g., fogged glasses, forgetting glasses somewhere, putting on or taking of his glasses. However, other contexts are bizarre (eyeglasses are melting) or have not experienced by the dreamer in his waking life – e.g., another person is breaking his glasses, a new pair of glasses disintegrate into pieces. The overall situations in which glasses occur, however, never took place in the dreamer's waking life. Even the "Putting on and taking off glasses" category does not include a single dream in which the dreamer took of his glasses to lie down in his own bed – an activity that he had done several thousand times in waking life.

Another interesting aspect of the glasses dreams is that only two of them were associated with positive emotions; that is, if emotions are mentioned, they are negative, hampered by blurred vision, sad about the loss of the glasses, etc. (see Table 8.10).

TABLE 8.10 Emotions related to glasses in dreams (N = 124)

Context	Dreams	Percent	Example(s)
Positive emotion	2	1.61%	It is funny to change glasses more often; dreamer is happy because he can read something very well without his glasses
Neutral and/ or no emotion mentioned	87	70.16%	
Negative emotions	35	28.23%	Somebody breaks the dreamer's glasses; glasses are full of sand and break while cleaning

TABLE 8.11 Reading glasses in dreams with references to the dreamer's glasses (N = 124)

Time period	Dreams	Dreams with glasses	Percent of glasses dreams with reading glasses
Period without reading glasses (till September 2002)	6,991	73	0.00%
Period with reading glasses (since October 2002)	5,778	51	23.53%

Lastly, it was analyzed whether reading glasses showed up in the dream series, as the dreamer has had to use them since the age of 40 (see Table 8.11). The first reading glasses dream occurred on December 20, 2004. Prior to wearing reading glasses, the dreamer did not dream about reading glasses. Overall, 13 dreams with reading glasses occurred; in one dream, the dreamer saw reading glasses of another person, whereas reading as an activity was only mentioned in two of the remaining 12 dreams. In one dream, the eye sight of the dreamer was examined, reading was not good, even with reading glasses, and in the other dream, the dreamer was astonished that he could read quite well without reading glasses. In one other dream, he did not see well (TV screen) what was far away while wearing the reading glasses. In the rest of the dreams, the dreamer was looking for the reading glasses or forgot them. Explicitly mentioned reading as activity occurred in 293 dreams (2.29%), which is relatively low, given the amount of time spent with reading during the day. However, very low figures for the percentage of reading dreams were reported previously: 0.2% in sports students and 1.6% in psychology students (Schredl & Erlacher, 2008). Hartmann (2000) offers the explanation that the brain while dreaming is not well suited for focused cognitive activities like reading (and writing, arithmetic) and, thus, these activities occur very rarely in dreams (Schredl & Hofmann, 2003). On top of that, reading glasses never occurred in a realistic context in dreams; that is, the dreamer is reading something with explicit mention that he wore his reading glasses.

Similarly, there was only one dream in the whole series that included a reference to contact lenses: a women who was sympathetic with the dreamer about a problem he had with his glasses told him that she has glasses too, but they also were contact lenses from time to time. That is, the dreamer, who never wore contacts in his waking life, never wore them in his dreams.

The next few dreams are included in order to illustrate different contexts of glasses in dreams.

Dream example (broken glasses):

I am in a kind of gymnasium. A woman is performing a rehearsed number with quite small children. It is really funny. Some adults join in, mirroring her movements standing across. I'm there too, opposite the leader. One part is rough because you get your neighbor's arms in your face. I stop. To my misfortune, I find that my glasses are bent, and they break when I want to re-bend them. This makes me sad, because then I can no longer participate.

Dream example (others break the dreamer's glasses):

I'm sitting in a bus that's pretty full, in the third row. In front of me, two black U.S. soldiers are harassing other passengers. When I say something, one flicks my glasses away so that they crash against the windshield with great momentum and the other tries to hold me tight, a very unpleasant situation.

Dream example (blurred vision):

I go into my room. The radio that could be heard from above is coming from a clock radio on the top shelf in my room, right side. The clock radio is square, my mother used to own one like that. The bed is gone and there are big dust fluffs under the shelf where the old guitar is standing at an angle. I want to clean some of it off, but somehow I get some in my face when I bend down. Since the fluff is crawling, I fear it might be a spider. I see out of focus – as if without glasses, I'm a bit panicked, spit out because it might be crawling in my mouth, manage it, the spider is on the floor. I still see out of focus and cannot hit the spider with my fist to flatten it.

Dream example (glasses of another person):

I'm at an optician and near me is a man, rather unappealing at first, trying on a pair of glasses. Apparently, he wants to buy one of two models. After some time (I am watching what is happening), he turns to me and asks me if the glasses suit him. I say that I don't think they look that good on him, he has distinct eyebrows (curved) while the glasses are quite straight on top. I think about the fact that I can give my opinion in great detail. With time, I become more sympathetic to the man. He is about 50 y., slim, face rather flat/broad.

To summarize, looking closely at dreams with glasses (pun intended) clearly indicates that everyday life activities that are somewhat automatized and pose no problems whatsoever – e.g., lying down the glasses on the usual place before going to sleep – do not show up in dreams. Some elements, like blurred vision (foggy glasses), did occur in the waking life of the dreamer, but even if some of the situations including glasses could have occurred in the dreamer's life, never ever did another person break the dreamer's glasses on purpose. On the other hand, really bizarre things – melting eye glasses – are very rare, and only occurred once. That is, this type of dream might point to a metaphoric quality of dreams; problems (cf. the majority of glasses dreams are negative, if emotions were present) stemming from other areas of the dreamer's waking life are illustrated by using the "weakness" of having to wear glasses to have a proper vision of the outside world. This would be comparable to the idea that non-working telephones in dreams are a met-aphor for some waking-life issues that don't "work out" for the dreamer (Garfield, 2001).

8.5 Beds in dreams

If one thinks about everyday objects that might be the most closely related to sleep and dreaming, beds come immediately to mind. Therefore, the first question is how often beds do occur in dreams, and the second question is about the context in which the bed is occurring in the dream; what func-tion the bed has within the dreams. In the study of Hall and Van de Castle (1966), 4.10% of the dreams included beds, but this study did not pro-vide any context regarding the bed. Interestingly, in a long dreams series ("Barb Sanders"; N= 3,116), beds occurred in 315 dreams (10.19%); this dream series is available on dreambank.net and a description can be found in Domhoff (2018c). In a sample of 1,612 diary dreams reported by 425 students, 7.20% of the dreams included references to beds (Schredl & König, 2016). In about one-fifth of the bed-related contexts (N = 136 in 119 dreams), the bed was associated with the sleeping and waking up of the dreamer; in 8%, erotic activities were pursued in the bed; but in most of the dreams, the bed was just an object (dreamer sees a bed) or something to sit on (see Table 8.12). One would expect that the bed and the bedroom would be most often those the dreamer actually used while dreaming, but only 21 out of the 116 bed dreams (18.10%) depicted the actual sleep environment (Schredl & König, 2016).

To summarize, beds do show up in dreams, but not very often the actual bed and bedroom the dreamer used. The analysis of this dream series is similar to the method applied in the previous study of Schredl and König (2016). Special attention is directed to the dreams featuring the dreamer's bed and bedroom, especially the question of how close to waking reality are bed dreams.

Overall, 1,001 dreams included a reference to beds (7.84%), comparable to the finding of Schredl and König (2016), which was 7.20%. The distribution of bed-related activities is depicted in Table 8.12. Compared to the student sample, the present dreamer more often dreamed about erotic activities (cuddling, intercourse, masturbation) than the students did. One explanation might be that men typically report more erotic dreams (cf. Geißler & Schredl, 2020), as the sample of Schredl and König (2016) consisted mostly of women. Secondly, it might be a recording bias, as detailed erotic dreams might not have been recorded for the purpose of a scientific study with handing over the

TABLE 8.12 Contexts in dreams with beds

Bed-related activities	Present dream series			
	All bed dreams (N = 1,001)		Dreams with dreamer's bed and bedroom (N = 22)	Bed dreams of a student sample (N = 136)[1]
	N	Percent	Percent	Percent
Seeing a bed	266	26.57%	18.18%	30.15%
Sleeping/waking up in a bed	144	14.39%	27.27%	18.38%
Erotic activities in the bed	308	30.77%	22.73%	8.09%
Sitting/lying on the bed (no relationship to sleep)	208	20.78%	18.18%	25.74%
Other activities (e.g., making the bed, get something from beneath the bed)	75	7.49%	13.64%	17.65%

[1]Schredl and König (2016).

dream diary to the experimenter (see section on erotic dreams in this book). In both samples, not even 20% of the bed dreams refer to sleeping and waking up (see Table 8.12); that is, referring to the dreaming context; namely, sleeping in a bed and waking up in order to recall the dream. Just seeing a bed without using it and using the bed as furniture (sitting, lying) is quite common in dreams (see Table 8.12).

If the bed in the dream was specified, it was rarely the bed of the dreamer (see Table 8.13); in most cases, it was not the bed in which the dreamer produced his dreams. For example, there were very large beds (N = 91), double beds (N = 75), old-fashioned beds (N = 17), or bunk beds (N = 17). The following dream is an example of a bed that did not belong to the dreamer in waking life (and a bed type the dreamer had definitely not used that night or in other nights for years).

I lie in a camp bed, which is quite hard. My shoulder hurts after a night sleeping in the side position. It is a large room, probably a self-awareness seminar; there are two or three people in the room, possibly my brother. It is morning; the seminar goes on for several days. I don't like the fact that the bed is so hard. I turn back and forth.

The ratio of the bed standing in the dreamer's bedroom to beds found elsewhere is very large: about two-thirds of the bedrooms are clearly not the dreamer's bedroom, whereas only 6% of the bedrooms in the dream are the actual bedroom the dreamer slept and dreamed in. The most common setting was the apartments of other persons (N = 383), hotel rooms (N = 115), apartments in which the dreamer used to live (N = 55), and hospitals (N = 50). The dreamer has spent nights in hotels and even hospitals, but the proportion of these settings is clearly much higher in the dream compared to the dreamer's waking life, as he spent most of his nights in his own bedroom.

Putting both criteria together, only 22 dreams (0.17%) included the dreamer's bed in his bedroom. These dreams are shown in Table 8.14, the dream scenes that are related to the bed and the bedroom.

TABLE 8.13 Specification of the beds and bedrooms in bed dreams (N = 1,001)

	Bed		Bedroom	
	Dreams	*Percent*	*Dreams*	*Percent*
Dreamer's bed/bedroom	78	7.79%	61	6.09%
Not specified	575	57.44%	263	26.27%
Not the dreamer's bed/ bedroom	348	34.77%	677	67.63%

TABLE 8.14 Dreams with the dreamer's bed in his bedroom (N = 22)

No.	Dream
T00625	The children come into my room and climb under my bed. At first, I think there are three of them. Then it turns out that the third is out in the hallway and there's a rabbit still under the bed. At some point, I get up and put the stuff they dragged in front of the door and tell them to carry it down. I also tell M. to catch the rabbit and carry it back down.
T00752	I am in my Mannheim room, sitting on the bed. There are many other people there besides me. They stand between the desk and the door. Two men, who I don't like, are practicing steps to a male ballet.
T00947	I was out for the night with my girlfriend. We've only known each other for a week. . ... At some point we embrace. It is wonderful, I feel very comfortable. We go to my apartment; I have to leave again in an hour. We go to my room and cuddle on the bed.
T01045	I lie in bed, there is no one (family) there in the apartment. A woman I saw yesterday at the club is also in the apartment. Yesterday I changed money, in one place there are 50 DM in a cloth bag on the wall. Now I hear the door. The woman comes from downstairs.
T01129	An old schoolmate visits me in my apartment, dark, large, there are other persons living there. He had only come for a short visit. I lie on my bed. He seems to be a little drunk.
T01145	I lie on my bed in my Mannheim room and start masturbating. For this, I use a picture of a woman with beautiful breasts. I lie on my stomach and rub myself on the pillow. Then my brother comes into the room, I turn to my left side and grin at him a little exaggerated. It is clear that he guesses what I did.
T01867	Apartment Alphornstraße. I am sitting at my desk in the back room. I hear my relatives approaching. My mother is lying on my bed and resting.
T02309	I am in my room at home. Oddly enough, there is a stream running through it. That's what my brother did, lowered the parquet, etc. . ... The water can't go well in the long run, because everything is made of wood. The bottom part of my bed is also a bit in the water.
T03803	When I wake up, a male friend is lying to my right in my bed. Apparently, I let him in while I was half asleep.
T03807	My former partner and some others are dancing in my apartment. I'm thinking about just leaving and going to my favorite dance club because it's Wednesday night. But I don't know who will go last. In any case, I can't handle my former partner being here and throw myself on the bed. I wish that she would come up to me. She does. She sits down with me and touches me lightly. It is so beautiful.

No.	Dream
T04022	A little mouse is sitting under my bed. It has been living in my room for quite some time. I want to take the opportunity and throw it out the window. Somehow, I can't bring myself to do it. It's so cold outside, she won't be able to find her way. Later, she sits in my bed and is quite distraught. I look at her, she looks at me.
T04380	A distant acquaintance comes to me in the apartment and sits down on the bed. Somehow, she has come of her own accord.
T04657	I am in my room, two members of my dance group have moved in. It is narrow, three beds. One has put stuff on my bed. I tell her to put it away. I am surprised that they are moving in here, although they each had their own room before.
T05928	Lucid dream. . . . Then I dive headfirst into the cool water and swim. I feel the water and turn onto my back. It is a delight, the swimming. Then I push my swim trunks down a bit because I want to take them off to swim more freely and possibly approach a woman. Then I feel myself waking up. I lie in bed next to my partner on my stomach and realize that I actually pushed my underwear down a bit in my sleep. I pull them back up. Later, the two nieces of my partner are in the room. My partner wants to give them cups, which she herself got in larger quantity from her parents. They are monochrome, 60ties cups. Then I really wake up.
T06941	My partner comes into my room and dumps about a small bucket full on the floor to provoke me. She also dumped some water in the hallway. I quickly I get terribly upset and jump up, I was lying on my bed, and pinch my partner two or three times to inflict pain. Then I say as I lay on the bed again, I'm going to punch her in the face next time.
T07603	Pre-lucid dream: . . . Then I see that I'm in my apartment and want to go into the bedroom. But, at the first attempt I get stuck on the door frame. I wonder, but then it works. I lie down in bed and think about whether I can imagine a woman. It doesn't work. Again and again, I think that I am awake and have fantasies. When I then really wake up, I notice that I lie differently in my bed than in the dream (turned to the wall).
T08519	Somehow, I ride on inline skates or slide on snow. In any case, I get home quickly. I am late. I see my brother and another man lying in my bed, it's totally tight, my brother's lower body is half hanging out of the bed.
T10966	I lie in my bed (my apartment) and have slept, maybe masturbated, which is a bit embarrassing for me, because in the bathroom is an employee of a computer company. . ... I get up and think about offering something to drink; he has been there for about two hrs. There is a second employee of the company in my apartment; we are all standing in the bedroom.

(Continued)

TABLE 8.14 (Continued)

No.	Dream
T11131	I go from a room of the apartment, with bed in which I slept, to my room. It is afternoon. My mother has cleaned up my room, also made the bed. This is unusual.
T11368	I lie in my bed, my apartment, but it looks different. In a room upstairs (diagonally offset) the two children (neighbors) run around and trample quite loudly. I'm still half dozing, it's about 7:30, Saturday morning.
T11654	I am alone at home (apartment with my mother and siblings). I lie in my narrow bed (as my real bed), have a thin A4 brochure with pictures of women and want to masturbate. But the blanket is all scrunched up, I get up to pull it right, I see that there are many dust fluffs under the bed.
T12157	I walk around barefoot in the early morning in my apartment. I want quickly go back to bed, but in the living room in front of the kitchen is a lot of water, about 10 cm high, but in a hollow. I am a bit scared, think about what to do. There is also some water in the bedroom by the door. How do I get it cleaned up? I think about whether I have forgotten some water tap, but that is not the case. Apparently, it came from the rain from the outside. I will have to discuss this with my landlord.

A closer look at these bed dreams indicates that, even though the dreamer's real sleep surroundings are present in the dream, they are not a simple representation of the dreamer's everyday life. There were never animals like rabbits (T00625) or mice (T04022) under the dreamer's bed. Similarly, other persons, like the dreamer's mother (T01867), the dreamer's brother with another man (T08519), a male friend (T03803), used the dreamer's bed. In a similar way, some characters showing up in the dreamer's bedroom have never been there – e.g., men practicing ballet (T00752), employees of a computer firm (T10966), other persons in addition to the partner (T03807), other persons (T04657), an unfamiliar woman seen in the club the night before (T01045), the old schoolmate (T01129), and a distant acquaintance (T04380). The times that the mother of the dreamer made his bed (T11131) are also long gone when the dreamer started recording his dreams. The false awakening from a lucid dream (T05928) is also very interesting, as the setting is quite realistic, as that night, the nieces of the dreamer's partner slept elsewhere in the apartment, but the action of pushing down the underwear during sleep never happened. Similarly, the pre-lucid dream (T07603) depicts something that never has happened. Moreover, the brother never saw the dreamer masturbating (T01145). The closest dreams are the instances with the dust fluff under the bed (T11654), but the amount of dust fluff in the dream clearly exceeded the quantities that gather in real life. Bringing home a girlfriend (T00947) also happened in the dreamer's waking life, but the circumstances of these occasions were completely different from those depicted in the dream.

To summarize, beds show up in dreams, as expected. However, the dreamer's bed within the dreamer's bedroom occurred rarely in his dreams. And a closer look at these dreams indicates that even the dreams with the "real sleep environment" are far from simply reflecting something that has really occurred in the dreamer's waking life. Thus, studying bed in dreams, once more, illustrates the creativity of dreaming.

8.6 Clothes and weapons in dreams

In 1966, Hall and Van de Castle (1966) published an analysis of 1,000 dreams collected between 1947 and 1952: 500 dreams reported by 100 female students and 500 dreams reported by 100 male students. They were able to demonstrate several gender differences – e.g., more physical aggression and sexuality in men's dreams compared to the women's dreams – a gender difference that has been stable over the years (Schredl, 2007). Another gender difference was that women tend to dream more often about clothes, whereas men more often dream about weapons (see Table 8.15). Even though the percentage of dreams including references to clothes decreased over the years (Hall et al., 1982; Mathes & Schredl, 2013), the gender difference was still present; that is, dream reports collected in the year 2000 also showed higher percentages of clothes dreams in women compared to men. The gender difference regarding weapons was very pronounced in the two American studies but less pronounced in the German sample (see Table 8.15). As men – like women – typically don't carry weapons with them in waking life (at least in Germany), this difference in dream content might reflect gender-specific preferences in media consumption; that is, men prefer first-person-shooter games (Lange et al., 2021) and spent more time during the day watching action

TABLE 8.15 Gender differences in percentage of clothes and weapons dreams in three different student samples

Topic	Study	Women	Men
Clothing	Western Reserve (1947–1952)	54%	28%
	Richmond (1979–1980)	34%	10%
	Mannheim/Heidelberg/Landau (2000)	19%	9%
Weapons	Western Reserve (1947–1952)	3%	12%
	Richmond (1979–1980)	4%	15%
	Mannheim/Heidelberg/Landau (2000)	3%	6%

movies and playing action games (Moverley et al., 2018). The direct effect of media, especially violent media, on dreaming has been demonstrated (Van den Bulck et al., 2016); similar effects of media in general (Gackenbach & Gahr, 2015; Lambrecht et al., 2013; Moverley et al., 2018) and video game playing (Gackenbach, Rosie, et al., 2011) were found. Thus, the gender differences in weapons dreams might reflect gender-specific media consumption in waking life.

All the three studies (Hall et al., 1982; Hall & Van de Castle, 1966; Mathes & Schredl, 2013) have been carried out in student samples; that is, not much is known about whether these topics change with age. The present dream series over a period of more than 30 yrs presents a unique opportunity to study possible changes over the years.

Overall, references to clothes were coded in 1,545 dreams (12.10%), whereas weapons were much rarer (N = 372 dreams; 2.91%). Even though, there are years with higher and lower percentages, there is a significant linear trend (r = .523, p = .001; Spearman Rank correlation) indicating that the percentage of clothes dreams increases over the years (see Figure 8.7). In the dreamer's fifties, the percentage of dreams with references to clothing is about 18% – almost as high as the figure for female students in 2000 (19%). It would be very interesting to carry out dream content analytic studies in samples with a large age range in order to learn whether this gender difference is decreasing or – another possibility – remains stable, as women might also tend to have more dreams with references to clothes as they are getting older – similar to the increase of clothing dreams in the present dream series.

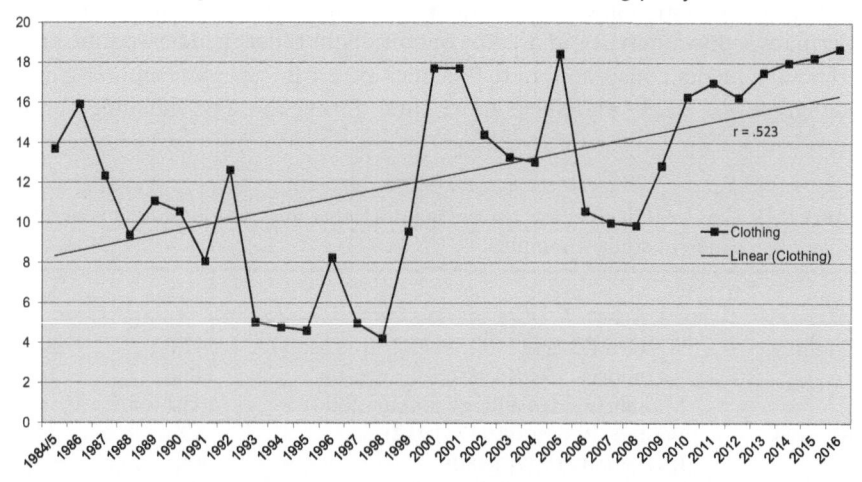

Percentage of dreams with references to clothing per year

FIGURE 8.7 Dreams with references to clothes per year from 1984/5 to 2016

Regarding the percentage of dreams with references to clothes, it is important to keep one methodological issue in mind: clothes in dreams are only coded if something like a hat, shirt, shoes, etc., are explicitly mentioned. This does not imply that, in the 87.9% of the dreams with no references to clothing, the dream characters ran around naked. If this would have been the case, the dreamer would have very likely included some remark about that in his dream report. On the other hand, if clothing is not relevant for the dream action, these "minor" details are often not explicitly mentioned. Thus, the findings should be interpreted with caution; that is, the gender difference does not imply that men have more dreams with naked persons; it much more likely reflect that clothes are more important to women and, thus, were mentioned more often in dreams.

In contrast to the dreams with references to clothing, the weapons dreams decreased over the years (r = -.550, p = .001, Spearman Rank correlation; see Figure 8.8). This might reflect the waking life of the dreamer, who spent considerably less time playing video games and watching action movies when he got older.

The following dream examples illustrate the contexts in which weapons can occur – clearly not everyday life experiences of the dreamer, but not uncommon in action movies or even the news (wars in other countries).

Everywhere around me there are fights to the death. After an event in Karlsruhe, a foreigner takes my clubs and juggling backpack. I turn to him and take my things back. In my imagination he pulls a knife and threatens

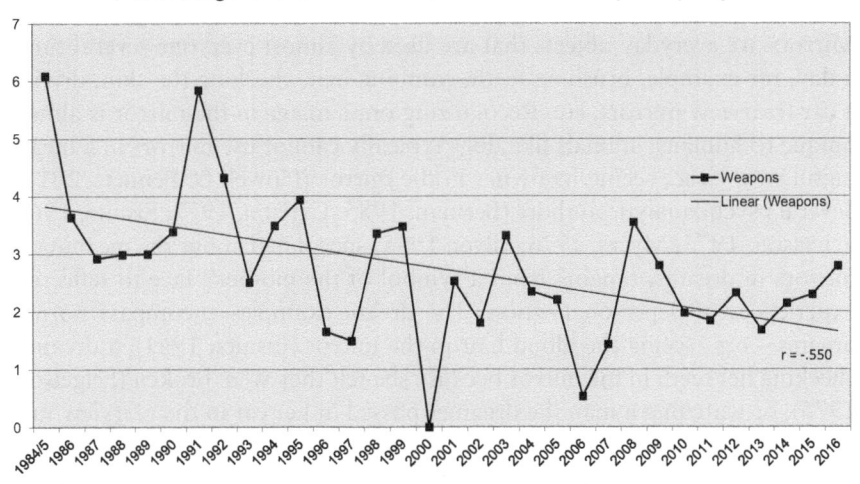

FIGURE 8.8 Dreams with weapons per year from 1984/5 to 2016

me by grabbing my wrist. I hold out a strange policeman to him, whom he stabs. Everything is strange, unreal. Fear.

Many refugees come to an island. Too many. They are to be decimated by only allowing them to marry among themselves and, thus, bringing many children into the world who are unfit for life in the long run, so that the number decreases. I think that this is a huge presumption on the part of the decision-makers. There is a battle going on in front of our house between refugees and the military. The "enemies" throw bombs, but they are always outnumbered. I am quite scared. From behind, they throw smoke bombs into the house. I keep the door closed so that it doesn't get to the front rooms where they are fighting. I use candles to eat the smoke. At some point the fighting stops and I go, unsuspecting at first, into one of the front rooms. There I get scared again and crawl on the floor so that I can't be seen from outside. It is tedious and exhausting.

To summarize, looking at mundane things like clothes and weapons can offer some insight into the nature of dreaming. For the clothes topic, the frequency of dreams with references to clothes might not reflect the actual number of clothes in the dream but the importance the dreamer gives to clothes. On the other hand, weapons in dreams seems more reflective of media consumption or video/computer game-playing and not of real-life experiences. That is, studying these two topics can offer insights into how the continuity between waking and dreaming works.

8.7 Mirrors in dreams

Mirrors are everyday objects that are used by almost everyone several times a day; for example, brushing teeth, combing hair, checking the skin, driving a car (rearview mirror), etc. Recognizing one's image in the mirror is almost unique to humans; animals like dogs typically cannot use mirrors in a meaningful way – e.g., seeing its owner in the mirror (Howell & Bennett, 2011). Several psychoanalytic authors (Berman, 1985; Carlson, 1977; Eisnitz, 1961; Feigelson, 1975; Myers, 1976; Silver, 1985) speculated about the meaning of mirrors in dreams, ranging from a symbol of the mother's face to reflecting experiences of depersonalization. The dream examples encompass normal dreams – e.g., seeing the blond hair in the mirror (Eisnitz, 1961), a dreamer checking her teeth in the mirror because she felt they were broken (Feigelson, 1975), or watching a man the dreamer passed in her car in the rearview mirror (Berman, 1985), but also bizarre reflections in the mirror – e.g., looking down at herself, the dreamer sees her nightgown, in the mirror image, she is naked (Feigelson, 1975); a dreamer looking in the mirror sees that his beard is shaven off, but he can feel the beard with his hand (Carlson, 1977); while the dreamer looks into the mirror, her face is getting smaller and smaller (Myers, 1976). Systematic content analytic studies looking explicitly at mirrors in dreams are still lacking.

The research team of the Lucidity Institute, founded by Stephen LaBerge, carried out a survey asking their members to explore the limits of dream consciousness, and one task was to look into a mirror (LaBerge, 1989). Overall, 43 tries performed by 22 participants were successful; however, only in about one-third was the reflection normal (like in waking life), and in two-thirds, the mirror image was weird – e.g., changing while the lucid dreamer was looking into the mirror (Levitan & LaBerge, 1993). The authors concluded that dream consciousness might have severe difficulties to produce mirror images the dreamer knows from his or her waking life. Again, this study raises the question of how frequent mirror dreams are and whether mirrors in dreams work properly.

In the large-scaled content analytic study of Hall and Van de Castle (1966) based on 500 dreams reported by 100 male students and 500 dreams reported by 100 female students, mirrors showed up in six dreams – slightly more often in women (N = 4, 0.8%) than in men (N = 2, 0.4%). However, it was not specified whether the dreamer looked into the mirror. The topic "seeing oneself in a mirror" was found in 0.93% of 1,612 diary dreams reported by 425 psychology students (Mathes & Schredl, 2014) and in 0.52% of 2,893 most recent dreams (Mathes et al., 2014). Using the dream series of "Barb Sanders" (combining series 1 with 3,116 dreams and series 2 with 1,138 dreams) that are available online (dreambank.net), the author found 57 dreams with mirrors (1.34% of the total dreams). In 36 dream reports, there was mention that the dreamer sees a reflection (63.15% of the mirror dreams), sometimes "normal" like in waking life – e.g., looking in the rearview mirror of her car, seeing her curly hair in the mirror, putting on her stage make-up on – but also bizarre images – e.g., Bugs Bunny, trick mirror images.

In the present dream series, 28 dreams included mirrors (0.22%). Similar to the "Barb Sanders" series, about 60% of the mirror dreams included the description that the dreamer is seeing a reflection (see Table 8.16). Most of the reflections are like those you would expect in waking life (even though the originals of the observed images are bizarre).

In the following dream example, the mirror image is perfectly normal; however, the dream action is completely bizarre; new teeth do not grow in adult jaws.

I feel that something is wrong with my teeth and look in the mirror. There I see that in front of the teeth flatter, new teeth want to burst out. I think about where to go (medical service) because it's Saturday. It looks quite

TABLE 8.16 Mirror dreams (N = 28)

Mirror dreams	Dreams	Example(s)
All mirror dreams	28	
- without reflection	11	Dreamer carries a mirror; dreamer sees a man walking by a mirror; dreamer is seeing a rotating mirror
- with reflection	17	
- "normal"	13	Dreamer checks in the mirror whether he had nose bleeding; dreamer sits in a train and sees his reflection in the mirror; dreamer sees the reflections of other men (bad guys) on the shiny furniture
- bizarre	4	Dreamer sees the reflection of highway with cars in mid-air

terrible and towards the end of the dream, I spit many fallen out teeth into the sink.

The next dream example is a very graphic one. Even though the mirror is working perfectly normally, once again, the question arises why we humans dream such stuff.

I go into the bathroom with toilet, on the 1st floor of the house (belongs to the mother of my partner). The loo itself is a tub; the pooping reminds me of the sitting toilets in France. I hang my butt over the tub and look at my poop via a mirror on the inside of the tub (which I'm surprised there is one). It goes through my mind that this is the first time I've watched myself poop like this. It's a large amount, and at first I think that the food is barely digested and something is wrong with my bowels. But then I realize that it is imagination, and the feces are rather digested food. With the shower hose, I want to flush the poop away, but the basin opens onto the floor (drain) and then flows into a drain in the bathroom floor. However, some feces get on the bathroom floor and I try to drive them with the shower jet in the direction of the drain.

The last mirror dream example shows some similarities to the mirror of Erised in the Harry Potter Book series; however, the dream was recorded on April 2, 1992, about seven years before the first Harry Potter volume was published.

The old, wise man leads me to a house with an old gate. There is a large hall, a lot of stone, some gold, quite noble. A door, gold-framed, stands

*out. It leads to the actual church hall. I look inside. It is quite dark and sol-
emn, a beautiful room. Then my partner and her friend are there. One of
them always turns on the light, but it is supposed to stay dark. This causes
a bit of a tussle among the three of us, until our attention is drawn to a
large mirror. I draw attention to it. We are to be seen in it, however, they
are no simple mirror reflections, but pictures from the past, e.g., a party,
where we have spilled ourselves, above all my partner. We wonder about
this mirror with the unusual property.*

To summarize, mirror dreams are very rare, but the dreaming mind is fully
capable of producing mirror images – the question that was asked by Levitan and LaBerge (1993) for lucid dreams but also seems valid in non-lucid
dreams. Interestingly, it looks like mirror dreams are more frequent in
women compared to men, suggested by the gender difference in the Hall
and Van de Castle (1966) study and the difference between the "Barb Sanders" dream series (1.34%) and the present dreams series (0.22%). However,
larger dream samples would be necessary to corroborate this. The rationale
behind this would be the assumption that women use mirrors more often in
their waking life compared to men. Even though the mirror images themselves were mainly normal, the question is why mirrors and/or mirror images
do occur in dreams.

9

EXTRAORDINARY DREAMS

9.1 Dreaming about dreaming

From a methodological viewpoint, the question arises whether and how much the dreams were affected by keeping a long-term dream journal; that is, does the dreamer dream about recording his dreams? In sleep laboratory studies in which REM awakenings were carried out in order to obtain dream reports, the setting strongly affected dream content: about 20% of the dreams (N = 2,464 dreams from ten different studies) included a direct reference to the laboratory setting, the electrodes, the lab, or the experimenter (Schredl, 2008b). On the one hand, these findings provide direct support for the continuity hypothesis of dreaming (Schredl, 2018b) but also limits the generalizability of dream studies carried out in sleep laboratories, as the participant would not have dreamed about the lab (except if he or she works in a sleep lab) in the normal home setting. Participating in a dream diary study affected dream content much less often; only 0.8% of N = 264 diary dreams included a reference to the experiment (Hall, 1967).

In Table 9.1, different categories in which dreams play a role within a dream are depicted. As the dreamer is a dream researcher, professional topics like working on a dream project, interviewing participants about their dreams, writing dream-related papers, reading scientific papers or books about dreams were not included. The overall context had to be nonwork-related or, if occurring in a work setting, not typical for the work setting – e.g., the dreamer is telling a co-worker about his own dream.

Given the immense amount of time the dreamer has spent recording and, later, typing his dreams, it is astonishing that references to recording dreams

DOI: 10.4324/9781003300373-9

TABLE 9.1 Dreaming about dreaming – different aspects

Topic	Dreams	Percent	Example
Recording dreams	30	0.23%	"Looking for my dream journal to record a dream"
Telling a dream	36	0.28%	"Waking up" from a lucid dream, telling the dream to another person
Recalling a dream	4	0.03%	Try to recall the dreams of last night for an exam
Other person tells a dream	44	0.34%	Known child tells dreamer about having nightmare
Other person dreams about the dreamer	3	0.02%	Female friend tells the dreamer that she had an erotic dream featuring the dreamer
Dream within in a dream	18	0.14%	Dreamer sees a dream of another person
Dream interpretation within in the dream	17	0.13%	Xerox machine in the old school hints at dreamer have not been a creative person as student
Dreamer interpreting dream of other person within the dream	10	0.08%	Dream about tidal wave was interpreted by the dreamer as indicative of a lot of waking-life stress
Dreams as a topic in a conversation	35	0.27%	Talking about dreams in a classroom setting
Recalling something from previous dream(s)	33	0.26%	While being in an elevator doing crazy movements, dreamer remembers having had bizarre elevator dreams previously
Dreamer's dreams are topic	16	0.13%	Dreamer tells someone about his large dream collection

are so rare – about 0.23% of all dreams (see Table 9.1). There are four additional dreams that are related the recording dreams and were coded as belonging in the "Dreamer's dreams are topic" category, as they include conversions or thoughts about recording but not actually the activity itself. In three dreams, the dreamer talks about recording a lot of dreams, even mentions numbers like 8,100 and 11,000 in two dreams – numbers that were appropriate for the time the dreams occurred. In one dream ("I am thinking about introducing a new coding category into the Alchera system, high speed/turf. That's certainly an interesting topic."), the dreamer is referring to the dream journaling software Alchera (see method section), but – interestingly – these thoughts never occurred in waking life, as the dreamer very rarely has dreams about racing a car; even though, some driving problems in dreams occurred, for example, cars with not fully functional brakes (Schredl, 2020a).

Another interesting dream-related activity within dreams is telling a dream or listening to the dreams of another person (see Table 9.1). Although, the dreamer talked about his own dreams or dream of others, the amount of time spent with this activity in waking life is much, much lower compared to the recording and typing of dreams. Nevertheless, the recording of dreams is less frequent compared to dreams in which the dreamer tells his dreams, supporting the hypothesis that some waking-life activities like reading, writing, arithmetic (the three 'R's) are very rare in dreams, mainly because the brain is in a different working mode while dreaming compared to waking life (Hartmann, 1996; Schredl & Hofmann, 2003). It would also support the sociality bias assumption – being a part of the social simulation theory (Revonsuo et al., 2015) – that the dreaming mind more likely features social interactions than intellectual topics like writing something down for oneself.

Sharing dreams is quite common in waking life; more than 25% of the participants of two large surveys reported that they share dreaming at least once a month (Graf et al., 2021; Schredl & Bulkeley, 2019). Dreams were most often shared with partners, friends, or family (Curci & Rime, 2008; Schredl, Buscher, et al., 2015; Schredl, Fröhlich, et al., 2015). However, this seems different for dream sharing in dreams, at least for this dreamer; the largest group are unknown persons that tell the dreamer a dream or listen to a dream of the dreamer (see Table 9.2). In one dream, the dreamer tells his dream to a fantasy figure (*Traumfresserchen*, a children's book by Michael Ende) and, in another dream, he listens to a dream of Heinz Rühmann, a famous German actor.

TABLE 9.2 Dreamer tells a dream within the dream and dreamer listens to dreams of others in the dreams

Person	Dreamer is telling a dream (N = 36)		Dreamer is listening to a dream (N = 44)	
	Dreams	Percent	Dreams	Percent
Family	5	13.89%	2	4.55%
Partner	3	8.33%	2	4.55%
Friend	7	19.44%	8	18.18%
Colleague	3	8.33%	6	13.64%
Therapist/dream group	4	11.11%	7	15.91%
Celebrity/fantasy figure	1	2.78%	1	2.27%
Unknown	13	36.11%	18	40.91%

One of the extraordinary topics is that the dreamer was told a dream dreamed by another person featuring him. One example is mentioned in Table 9.1, the second dream is the following one:

Sleep lab. Top-class people are there, they are interested in my thesis, which I discuss with others at the table. There is something to eat. Someone brought something. My boss tells that he dreamed about me, in a positive context. This is good for my position in the sleep lab. Then, two secretaries come and put bowls of salads, etc., on the table where I am sitting. I walk around a bit and bump into the desk drawer that a colleague has pulled out to put a hard drive unit into the drawer. Others are annoyed that they didn't skip the first meal and are now not very hungry.

Both of these dreams might belong in the "wish fulfillment" category; other people have nice dreams about oneself, even with a positive aftereffect (see previous dream example). The third dream that was grouped into this category was the following one:

I lie in a large bed and place a large coin (lucid talisman) on the temple of P4. She is sleeping and I want to influence her dreams, but this requires another coin, which I cannot place, because P4 is moving. I want to try again; P4 briefly opens her eyes, but does not really wake up. The others (there are still some other people in the huge bed) advise me against it, I should rather snuggle up to P4, which I do (spooning).

The dreamer never did that in real life but heard a talk given by a well-known dream researcher who did some experiments (with the consent of his wife, hopefully) using tactile stimuli to influence her dream content.

Another very interesting category is the dream interpretations that happened within the dream; thus, dreaming about a dream interpretation (see two examples in Table 9.1). In another dream, the dreamer is surrounded by a large number of women and thinks about the possible meaning (within the dream) that portrays a waking-life situation in which a decision is necessary but not easy to make. In yet another dream, two unpleasant men demand money from the dreamer, and the dreamer thinks these men represent unwanted parts of himself (the "Shadow" in Jungian terminology). Another dream involved a dangerous earth tunnel leading to another world; the interpretation within the dream was that some old personality layer was blasted off, so the dreamer gets into closer contact with the people around him. A macabre dream interpretation was that the shrunken heads the dreamer is carrying with him represents the deadened emotions for former romantic partners. Even a Freudian dream interpretation was present in one dream;

stiff cigars were interpreted as sexual symbols. In another dream, a colleague tells a dream about a famous actor, and the dreamer said that this actor represents her creative side.

The concluding example of this topic is a dream in which the dreamer used an analogy regarding emotions to interpret a sexual act within the dream in a non-sexual way.

> *A friend tells me a dream she had. She goes to Tibet with her partner. A rape of a woman occurs in the dream. There are some people sitting around her. They talk about the dream. Someone brings up the Tibet topic. K. says that they have thought about this in waking life. I have the idea that the rape is not to be seen sexually (feeling I am sounding a bit intellectual), but stands for the physical rape through the meditation practice. That's how I feel.*

These dreams reflect – at least partly – the waking-life attitude of the dreamer toward working with dreams, comparing the emotions and basic action patterns of the dream experience with experiences occurring in the current waking life (Edwards et al., 2015; Malinowski, 2021a; Schredl, 2015a).

Another example of dreams with talking about dreams as a topic is a dream in which the dreamer asks two women whether they had dreams in which they can fly while holding on to their luggage.

In 33 dreams, the dreamer experiences something or see something and thinks that he already dreamed about it (déjà rêve = already dreamed). For more information about déjà rêve experiences occurring in waking life, see Funkhouser and Schredl (2010) and Schredl, Funkhouser, et al. (2017). These 33 dreams, on the other hand, included dreamed déjà rêve experiences. The long dream series facilitates the differentiation between the impression of having dreamed about it without actually having recorded a dream with such a topic or whether recalling a specific dream topic has already occurred in a dream previously recorded. However, it is never possible to be perfectly sure whether something might have been dreamed but not previously remembered and recorded. In 20 of the 33 dreams including the topic of recalling that something has already been dreamed, these topics were familiar to the dreamer in the dream, sometimes even triggered lucidity – e.g., three times, the dreamer recognized that jumping very high (not physically possible) did occur in previous dreams and became lucid. In two flying dreams, the dreamer was aware that he had previously had flying dreams with the fear about what will happen if the flying ability is no longer present (see flying topic in this chapter). In a few dreams, the dreamer remembered how many lucid dreams he had had this particular year. In addition, there were several dreams in which the dreamer knew that he had had specific dreams before – e.g., getting a large amount of money from a slot machine or trying to get from Heidelberg (city) to Wiesloch (city) (distance about 20 kilometers) with no public transportation available. The déjà rêve experiences without any clear reference to earlier dreams were related to having already visited a music store, knowing a certain route from a previous dream, or a specific situation with the brother. Knowing previously recorded dreams very well (recording plus typing and coding), the situations the dreamer thought he dreamed were not found in previous dreams. In one case, it is evident (very low likelihood), as the dreamer sees a woman (stranger to the dreamer) and thinks that he had a dream about the two of them having a date.

The last two dream examples include a confusion about being in a dream and being awake.

I'm walking in a residential area, with a lot of plants, somewhat hilly. Somehow, I realize that I am dreaming. I try to jump up to a balcony, but don't make it. I already suspect that I am not dreaming after all and let myself drift without wanting to influence the dream. Then I float (have not really arrived on the ground after jumping up) to a garden (large). On a stair sits a woman of whom I think at first that she is not pretty enough. However, this is not the case and she is very interested, warm and soft. We lie on the grass and take off her pants. She resembles P5. I have a great desire and want sex. There I wake up, not fully, because P5 (lying in the bed I am lying in) complains what I do on her. I lie on her and act out the dream. Only then do I wake up properly.

If this type of behavior had occurred in waking life, it would have been a case of sexsomnia – a NREM parasomnia in which the not fully awakened dreamer performs sexual acts on the bedpartner (Idir et al., 2022). Dreaming about it (dreamer wasn't actually doing something in real life) is, of course, a different phenomenon but, nevertheless, very interesting.

In the next dream, a woman is telling a vivid dream that the dreamer sees like a movie – a "dream" of every neuroscientist in the dream field (e.g., Horikawa et al., 2013). At the end, the dreamer is so immersed that he is part of the woman's dream.

I sit next to a young woman who tells me a dream. Immediately I see the images of the dream, she is a kind of Chinese lion with a mane of fire, fleeing from a kind of Chinese dragon, consisting of four people under a large costume. It is a savannah type area. She hides from time to time to make the chase more difficult. Then she manages to shake off the pursuer(s). She goes back to the starting place, knocks a guard off a "", which again consists of several people under a colorful costume, and wants to go back to her hometown. There are other people in this place who are connected to the Chinese dragons and want to stop the woman. A man (mustache, small, Asian/Mongolian looking) ignites a rocket that flies to a city ruler to warn him. I see how the rocket (firework rocket) is ignited, at first nothing happens, I hope, but then it flies off. The woman and I are on a high vehicle, tram-like, and see someone being interrogated below. It is not entirely clear, but the ruler seems to have fallen from grace, so the missile sent as a message has no effect. A man is being executed in which the vehicle we are on is pushed forward a bit on the tracks and so goes over his head. I feel a slight crack (we don't see anything as we are looking down the front and the execution is on the side) and say to the woman that it is a well-made film, that despite the death only being acted, something has been put on the rails to give a real impression. The woman and I are very boisterous and familiar. We jump off the vehicle (about 10 feet high) into the water (dock). I swim to the ladder; she comes after me. It is very pleasant with her.

It is also very important to note that none of these dreams reflect experiences the dreamer had in his waking life – even the mundane ones like recording a dream, which happened in totally untypical situations – e.g., the mother of the dreamer disrupting the recording. Or, the telling of dreams to strangers or doing the kind of interpretation done in the dream in real life. Even the boss never told the dreamer that he had had a dream about him (a colleague of the dreamer once did this in real life; she hesitated because it was an erotic dream).

9.2 Flying dreams

Flying dreams are a prime example of a dream topic that is not continuous to waking life, as flying dreams are defined as dreams in which the dreamer can fly without any or with inadequate aids. On the other hand, there are "real" flying dreams – e.g., dreams in which the dreamer is sitting in a plane or another means of transportation that can fly. These are typically not included in the studies focusing on flying dreams. Depending on the study, about 30% to 73.9% of the participants reported that they had experienced flying dreams at least once in their life (Schredl, 2019b). On the other hand, the actual frequency of flying dreams in diary dream sample is quite low: 1.2% of the total dreams (N = 1,910 dreams) (Barrett, 1991). Interestingly, flying is the most common chosen activity in lucid dreams; 62.6% of the respondents reported that they planned flying if they became lucid in their dreams (Stumbrys et al., 2014).

The main objective of looking at flying dreams in this series is to emphasize the large diversity of flying dreams, even in one dreamer; that is, not all flying dreams are alike. In addition, the analysis also looked into changes in non-lucid flying dreams due to the waking-life experience of flying (airplane travels).

Overall, 237 dreams (1.87%) of the dreams included flying without adequate means. Of this total sample, 71 dreams were lucid; 22, pre-lucid; and 144, non-lucid, resulting in a percentage of 1.14% of non-lucid flying dreams. On the other hand, the dreamer had 52 dreams in which he was on a plane flying, eight dreams with a helicopter, four dreams with a spaceship, and two dreams with a hang glider; that is, 0.52% of the dreams in the series included references to flying that also would be possible in waking life.

As the dreamer had his first real flight (overall four flights) from Germany to the US in 1996, a statistical analysis was carried out to test whether the frequency of "real" flying dreams – that is, flying in a plane – increases, comparing the dreams of two years prior to the first flight and the dreams of the two years after the first flight. As predicted by the continuity hypothesis, the dreams with flying in a plane increased significantly (see Table 9.3), whereas the frequency of non-lucid flying dreams – those that are not related to flying experiences in waking life – was not affected.

The percentage of non-lucid flying dreams varied between 0% to 2% per year (see Figure 9.1), with no upwards or downwards trend regarding time ($r = -.033$, $p = .858$, Spearman rank correlation). There is a massive increase in flying dreams in total due to the increase in lucid flying dreams, starting in 1996, with a peak in 1998. This is explained by the simple fact that the dreamer attended a lucid dream seminar in 1996 and practiced reality checks in order to increase his lucid dream frequency (see lucid dream section in this chapter); before that, almost no lucid flying dreams occurred, but some lucid flying dreams occurred, even though lucid dreaming frequency dropped dramatically after the dreamer stopped performing reality checks during the daytime (see lucid dream section in this chapter).

The next analysis looked at the social aspect of flying dreams (see Table 9.4). In almost half of the flying dreams, interaction between the

TABLE 9.3 Non-lucid flying dreams and dreams with "real" flying in an airplane for the period before and after the first flight (Europe – USA) of the dreamer in waking life (July 9, 1996)

	Period from July 9, 1994 to July 9, 1996 (N = 936 dreams)		Period from July 9, 1996 to July 9, 1998 (N = 446 dreams)		Statistical analysis (Klingenberg, 2008)
	Dreams	Percent	Dreams	Percent	
Non-lucid flying dreams	13	1.39%	6	1.35%	t = −0.1 p = .9482
Dreams with flying in an airplane	2	0.16%	5	1.12%	t = 2.0 p = .0472

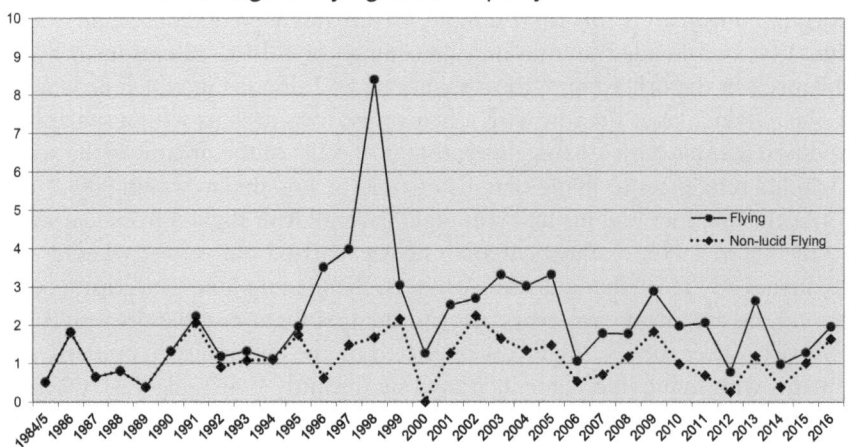

Percentage of flying dreams per year

FIGURE 9.1 Flying dreams per year

TABLE 9.4 Flying dreams (N = 237) – different characteristics

Topic	Dreams	Percent	Example
Other persons seeing the dreamer fly	105	44.30%	Dreamer demonstrates his ability to fly to a friend
Other persons present but not specified whether they see the dreamer flying	76	32.07%	Dreamer starts flying in a concert hall with other pre
Dreamer alone in the dream	40	20.68%	Dreamer is flying over a deserted landscape
Dreamer actively avoids being seen flying by others	7	2.95%	Dreamer does not want other people (city) that he is flying
Other persons in the dream fly	44	0.14%	Group session, about 50 persons (including the dreamer) are floating in a circle

dreamer and others occurs – at least the dreamer is noticing that others can see him. In about one-fifth of the flying dreams, there is no social interaction; the dreamer is alone. In very rare cases, the dreamer avoids being seen and does not want attract attention. In the other dreams, it was not clear whether other dream characters see him flying or not (see Table 9.4).

In 116 flying dreams, the dreamer included an explicit reference to enjoying flying; this does not imply that the other dreams were neutral or negative;

TABLE 9.5 Flying dreams (N = 237) – anxiety related to flying respective not being able to fly anymore

Topic	Dreams	Percent
Lucid flying dream (N = 71)	17	23.94%
Pre-lucid flying dream (N = 22)	3	13.64%
Non-lucid flying dream (N = 144)	32	22.22%
Total (N = 237)	52	21.94%

they do not include any reference to emotions. However, 52 flying dreams included the anxiety of not being able to fly anymore (see Table 9.5). A typical theme is that the dreamer does not dare to fly too high in case the unusual ability to fly might stop at any moment. Even in lucid flying dreams, extreme anxiety can occur:

Then I'm outside, on the top floor of a shell (about 8th – 10th floor, concrete, with pillars, large outline) and call my friend for help, I want to build something there. In perspective, I am first feeling like this friend, later I am completely myself. Since it's urgent, I call out that he should just jump. He/I (Bud Spencer type like guy) jumps up, flies into the air, overshoots and flies very high. Now it's me, I get very scared that I might crash, remind myself that nothing can happen even if I hit the ground, which I almost did at one time. Then I land bumpy (prone position) on the concrete building.

Being lucid helped to conquer the fear, but at first, the panic level was high. It is interesting that fear occurring in about 22% of all flying dreams occurs equally often in lucid and non-lucid flying dreams.

In most of the flying dreams, the specific flying technique is not explicitly mentioned. If explicitly mentioned, the most common technique is concentration (N = 42 dreams); that is, flying involves some kind of cognitive effort. In 23 flying dreams, the dreamer moves his hands and/or arms like swimming or waggling. Similarly, the exact body posture while flying was quite rarely explicitly mentioned in the dream report: prone position (N = 26), lying on the back (N = 8), flying in a sitting position (N = 13), flying in a standing position (N = 10), and two dreams with being in a horizontal position but not specified whether it is prone or back position. Lastly, the dreamer flew most often without any aids, but in 38 dreams, he had some prop that helped him fly – even though this would not work in waking life – e.g., car, bus, holding a small ball in hand, carpet, a small jet in one hand, sitting on a metal plate, fluttering with the shirt, piece of wood, unicycle, and, once, even flying with a whole house.

A few dream examples will help to illustrate the diversity of the flying dreams. The first example includes other persons flying, the dreamer enjoys flying, a bit like showing off his skill.

Dream example:

> *I am in a school. It's break and I walk into the classroom where the next class will be. There is a lot going on, many students on their way. The classroom is also crowded, it is a square of desks around which people (me too) are sitting tightly. A discussion develops, possibly about teaching style. I see two young women floating through the air; this immediately animates me to join in, although I am participating in the discussion. The room is now open to the ceiling, I lift off from my chair with little effort and fly after the two young women. They can't yet fly as well as I can (because they are in a lower grade). Flying is great fun; I hover like this at a height of about 10 meters. It is dark, evening. After some time I land again carefully on my chair. The others have noticed my flying. Even though it is something special, it is nothing out of the ordinary.*

In the next dream, the ability to fly serves as an unreliable reality check for lucidity.

Dream example:

> *Outside is a huge entrance hall, a woman (young) tells another person that she has swept large parts of it, she is in training. I feel physically fit and walk, jog around a bit. It's fun to move around. I also try to move forward without touching the ground, I succeed, waving my arms, like swimming. A hunch rises that it might be a dream. At one point, I'm just above the floor in breaststroke, then again almost under the ceiling. But overall, I still don't think it's a dream because I can't really fly well.*

In the following dream, the dreamer "learns" a new flying technique, showing off his skills.

Dream example:

> *I dash up the stairs, it's an old building, third floor or so, and quickly realize that I can fly. I keep my left arm bent and pull on it with my right hand, a bit like a throttle stick. It's fun. It goes up at great speed. In the apartment, I demonstrate the flying technique to my mother and emphasize that I am flying with a new technique (arms). There is also a young, pretty woman there, taking care of a baby (not hers) that I want to impress. We*

are in the process of getting to know each other, something could develop. Finally, I end up on the couch and am a bit exhausted, have to orient myself, what's going on.

The last dream recounts an extraordinary starting point for the ability to fly. Dream example:

Now I am alone with my sister, we walk a small path up a slope. It is an impressive view of the Danube and some tributaries; one is lower, so that the water of the Danube initially flows in there, but soon (right side) it is reversed, the water flows back into the Danube, partly with considerable speed. I make a remark that we are quite high (we look far down). Then we are on one of the tributaries. Now the other person is a colleague of mine. A man makes a joke and recites some kind of spell, touching my neck. The spell is supposed to make me fly. At first, I do not believe in it, but when I do a few small jumps, I realize that I can fly, not high, with swimming movements, breaststroke and backstroke. I demonstrate it to my colleague; also say something to the effect that such things are possible in dreams. We want to go back to the others.

9.3 Lucid dreaming

Lucid dreams are defined as dreams in which the dreamer is aware that she or he is dreaming while still dreaming (LaBerge, 1985). Keep in mind that non-lucid dreams – that is, the majority of the dreams – are characterized by the distinct impression that the dream action is "real"; the dreamer experiences the dream – even if bizarre things happen – as real as waking life (Schredl, 2018b).

Prevalence data stemming from 34 studies yielded a mean estimate of 55% of the participants stating that they had had at least one lucid dream in their lifetime (Saunders et al., 2016). In a representative study carried out in Germany, the lucid dream incidence was about 50% (Schredl & Erlacher, 2011), but the percentage of persons with high lucid dream frequencies of once a week or more was low: about 5%. Large-scaled studies (Hess et al., 2017; Schredl & Erlacher, 2004; Schredl et al., 2016; Schredl, Zumstein, et al., 2022) indicated that trait factors like openness to experience, boundary thinness, and high sensory-processing sensitivity are related to lucid dream frequency. As lucid dreams are often fun (e.g., Stocks et al., 2020), research focused on so-called induction techniques aiming at increasing lucid dream frequency (Stumbrys et al., 2012; Tan & Fan, 2022). This area of research indicated that techniques like practicing reality checks during the day (Purcell et al., 1986) or the wake-up-back-to-bed technique (Erlacher et al., 2022; Schredl, Dyck, et al., 2020) can be very effective. However, these studies did not look at possible long-term effects of practicing induction techniques because they stop after a few weeks of training (typically compared with a control group without training). So far, only one study (LaBerge, 1980a) looked at a time interval of 36 months: the author, who was also the dreamer, stated that, prior to using the first induction technique, he recalled lucid dreams less than once per month. The first method he applied was autosuggestion: the person suggests to himself or herself to have a lucid dream during the night before falling asleep (Garfield, 1974). LaBerge (1980a) was able to increase his lucid dream frequency to five per month. Within these first 16 months were two months with more than ten lucid dreams – the first one when he wrote his doctoral proposal (a study on lucid dream research), and the second peak occurred when he doubled his efforts to have a lucid dream because he slept in a sleep lab with full polysomnographic recording. Then he started to create his own induction technique called MILD (Mnemonic Induction of Lucid Dreams), which requires one to rehearse a dream before falling asleep and visualize becoming lucid while focusing on the intention to remember that one is dreaming. This worked very well for him, as he was able to experience about 21 lucid dreams per month. However, discontinuing the training for four months led to a considerable drop in lucid dream frequency (12 to 15 lucid dreams per month, which is still a large number), but taking up the training restored the high levels of the first training phase. So far, this case study is the only one showing that lucid dream frequency might decline after stopping training; thus, lucid dreaming is a learnable skill that requires constant training. Here again, the analysis of a long dream series can be of value.

Overall, the dream series included 172 lucid and pre-lucid dreams (1.35% of the total dreams). Forty-seven were classified as pre-lucid: the dreamer asks the question whether he might be in a dream but ultimately concludes he is still awake (see the following examples). Thirty-four dreams were lucid dreams but without the dreamer having control and the ability to perform actions he would like to do. The rest (N = 91) were lucid dreams with having the ability to deliberately carry out actions, like jumping in the air and flying away. The percentage of lucid dreams in relation to all dreams was 0.98%.

The time course of the lucid dream frequency is depicted in Figure 9.2. Until 1995, the frequency of lucid dreams was very low; the abrupt increase in 1996 was a result of practicing reality checks after attending a seminar on lucid dreams given by Paul Tholey and Brigitte Holzinger in February 1996. It took almost three months to experience the first induced lucid dream. In the following two years, the percentage further increased, even though the dreamer was not practicing reality checks as regularly as in the beginning. After discontinuing the training, the frequency of lucid dreams dropped, and after a few ups and downs, the frequency of lucid dreams in 2015 and 2016 dropped to the pre-training level. Thus, this is the first long-term study indicating that lucid dreaming is, indeed, a learnable skill

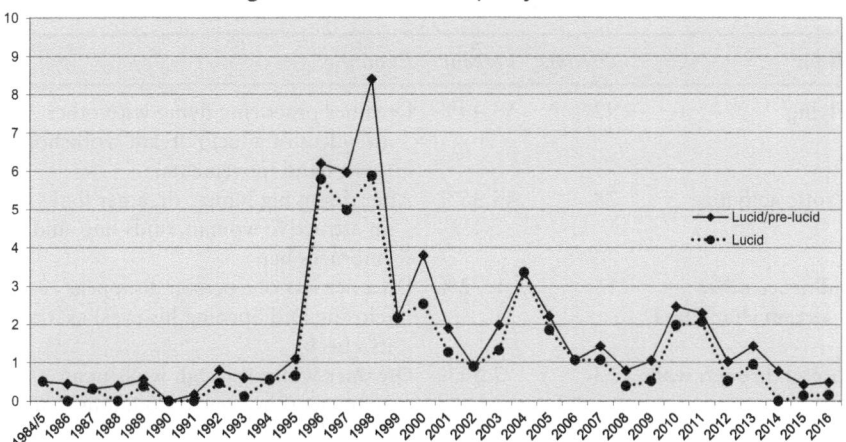

FIGURE 9.2   Pre-lucid and lucid dreams per year

(LaBerge, 1980a; Purcell et al., 1986), but it can be lost if regular training is stopped – even though it takes quite a time (about 20 years) to fall back to the pre-training levels.

Similarly to the findings in a larger sample (Stumbrys et al., 2014), the most frequent topic in the pre-lucid and lucid dreams have been flying and erotic activities (see Table 9.6). It is even more obvious if the pre-lucid and lucid dreams were classified into four groups (see Table 9.7); only about a quarter of these dreams do not include flying and/or erotic activities. On a personal note, the dreamer enjoyed very much the ability to go through walls in a lucid dream; for him, that is more out of the ordinary than flying (having had a considerable number of non-lucid flying dreams). About 14% of the pre-lucid and lucid dreams (N = 17 pre-lucid dreams, N = 7 lucid dreams) did not include an action that the lucid dreamer wanted to carry out; this supports the idea that lucid dreams did not always include the ability to change the action within the dream (Mallett et al., 2021; Schredl, Rieger, et al., 2018). Interestingly, the dreamer only had one lucid dream from which he deliberately wanted to awaken but was not able to do so. This is a common characteristic of lucid nightmares: being in a nightmarish situation, wanting to get out by waking up, and not being able to do so (Schredl & Bulkeley, 2020; Stumbrys, 2018). The low number of those dreams might be explained by the fact that the dreamer never had nightmares, even though some dreams are very distressing, including the lucid one he wanted to wake up from. Within the concept of nightmare treatment, the idea to wake up from a distressing dream seems counterproductive, as it is an avoidance strategy (Schredl & Bulkeley, 2020). The most effective therapeutic

TABLE 9.6 Actions deliberately carried out in lucid dreams (N = 240 activities in 172 pre-lucid and lucid dreams)

Topic	Dreams	Percent	Example
Flying	92	53.49%	Dreamer practicing flying with other attendees of a lucid dream workshop (with hand movements)
Erotic activities	78	45.35%	After doing big jumps, dreamer looks for an attractive woman, finds one, and embraces her
Influence other dream characters	15	8.72%	Dreamer lets one person disappear (closing and opening his eyes) as a reality check
Going through walls	13	7.56%	Dreamer walks through walls in an apartment; it is more strenuous than normal walking
Influencing the ability to move/act	9	5.23%	Picking up an adult man to demonstrate my strength
Seeking social contacts	5	2.91%	Dreamer contemplated seeking out other people because he felt lonely in the lucid dream
Experimenting	2	1.16%	Dreamer tests whether he will burn his finger touching a lit cigarette (it was hot)
Doing dream interpretation	1	0.58%	Dreamer is becoming lucid and starts to interpret the dreamer (the xerox machine reflecting his lack of creativity in school (arts subject)
Wake-up from the dream	1	0.58%	Scary flying dreams, the dreamer did not manage to wake up (but spontaneous awakening occurred)
Lucid dreams without actively doing something	24	13.95%	Dreamer becomes lucid, thinks about what he might do, but wakes up

TABLE 9.7 Actions deliberately carried out in lucid dreams in 172 pre-lucid and lucid dreams

Topic	Dreams	Percent
Flying and erotic activities	38	22.09%
Only flying	54	31.40%
Only erotic activities	40	23.26%
All other pre-lucid and lucid dreams	40	23.26%

intervention – Imagery Rehearsal Therapy (IRT) – is tackling this problem by actively confronting the nightmare situation *in sensu* and imagining a coping strategy with a positive ending (Krakow & Zadra, 2010). Thus, practicing IRT during the day would be the first advice to persons with lucid nightmares.

In this dream series, money as a dream topic was studied; almost 9% of all dreams included a reference to money (see Chapter 8.2). On the one hand, this would be in line with the continuity hypothesis of dreaming (Schredl, 2018b), but, on the other hand, why does the dreamer need to pay for something in a lucid dream? And, indeed, the frequency of money references was markedly lower in pre-lucid and lucid dreams (5.81%) compared to all other non-lucid dreams (8.98%); the resulting effect size was $h = 0.121$. The difference is even more remarkable as the lucid dreams were longer (230.09 ± 118.87 words per dream, on average) compared to the non-lucid dreams (136.33 ± 84.12 words per dream) due to the fact that, in longer dreams, all topics (not only money) have a higher probability of occurring.

The next two examples are included to illustrate the in-between category of pre-lucid drams; there is an idea that this is weird, dream-like, but somehow (not applying waking-life logic), the dreamer concludes that he is awake.

Dream example (pre-lucid):

> *I'm at some sort of conference and I'm walking around the grounds, a university. I meet some men with whom I scuffle a bit. We are now in a room with many people. Then I demonstrate that I can fly. I flap my hands a bit, unusual for me, and float back and forth. People are totally impressed. It goes back and forth for a while, and then I land again. I explain to a young man how I learned to fly in reality. Two things are necessary for this, daydreaming and the night dreams, I have already flown 30–40 times in dreams. If I succeed in imagining this feeling in waking life, then I can fly.*

Dream example (pre-lucid):

> *I am in a very large department store. . . . I pass a large fur department, mainly women choose coats here and try them on behind fur curtains. In addition, the floor is covered with furs, a pleasant feeling while walking. At the end of the department, the furs are a bit out of place, as they have no grip on the floor. From a fast run, I get the idea to jump off and float a bit. It works quite well; I can float up to the ceiling (about 5–6 meters high, it is an old-fashioned house). However, when I do this I think I am awake and wonder all the time that flying while awake works. I am also very careful as I fly towards a crowd of people to draw attention to myself. It's not so strange for people*

though, they hardly pay attention to me. Another man, more of a bad guy, is to be caught, but I suspect he wants to fly away. The flying was great fun.

Even accomplished lucid dreamers stated that, in about 50% of their lucid dreams, they were not able to accomplish their intended plans (Stumbrys et al., 2014). In this dream series, 12 dreams included a rejection of the dreamer by a female dream character because the dreamer was approaching her to have sex. The second dream provides a hint at how this unexpected turn of events in the lucid dream might be explained; it depicts, in a very illustrative way, the dreamer's fear being rejected – even in a lucid dream.

Dream example (rejection):

I am at some kind of party in a large, modernly furnished room. There, to my astonishment, I see a female friend and a former schoolmate (female). I immediately go up to them and want to talk to them, especially to the female friend. However, at first the two of them ignore me. Somehow, I realize that it is a dream and I approach the former schoolmate to cuddle with her. She fends me off a bit. I reply that it is a dream after all, take her in my arms and we fly. She is still a bit dismissive, but lets me take off her bodysuit. I am very aroused and feel my erected penis. It is a very intense erotic closeness with her.

Dream example (rejection):

I walk in a dark park. I'm already a little scared as I walk through dark places. It is a long way and I realize that I do this every day or evening. Since it is so unusual (compared to waking life), I realize that I am dreaming. I fly and immediately think of sex. Here is no other person far and wide, but after a short time I come into a hall where there are many people. I see an attractive woman sitting nearby and end up in front of her. However, she is vehemently against sex with me (I already feared it.) So, I look around. It is not easy for me to endure the looks of the others, since they know what I want. A former schoolmate (male) shows up, I am asking myself if he is homosexual (and want to approach me). Somehow I am frustrated that the woman I wanted rejected me.

To summarize the lucid dream topic: the experiences of this dreamer clearly indicate that lucid dreaming is a learnable skill but also demonstrate that this ability gets lost over the years if the lucid dreaming skill is not practiced regularly. However, one should keep in mind that lucid dreaming skills vary considerably from person to person (Schredl, Rieger, et al., 2018), and given the pre-training frequency of lucid dreaming, the dreamer is on the lower end of the lucid-dreaming-skill continuum. Thus, it would be very interesting to re-evaluate participants who increased their lucid dreaming frequency during an induction study, whether they were able to maintain their lucid dreaming skills even without training or whether similar drop-offs like in the present dreamer occurred.

10

TYPICAL DREAMS

10.1 Examination dreams

Patricia Garfield (2001) included examination dreams in her book *The Universal Dream Key: The Twelve Most Common Dream Themes Around the World*. Indeed, in student samples, 40 to 80% of the participants stated that they had examination dreams (Arnulf et al., 2014; Griffith et al., 1958; Nasser & Bulkeley, 2009; Nielsen et al., 2003; Schredl et al., 2004; Yu, 2008). The actual percentage of examination dreams related to all recalled dreams was 2.2% in diary dreams reported by students (Mathes & Schredl, 2014) and 0.7% in most recent dreams reported by adults (Mathes et al., 2014). That is, almost everyone had had examination dreams, but they are not very frequent. Asking school-aged children for the most recent bad dream only 3% of these dreams were examination dreams, but in a representative sample, 12.7% of the participants who experienced nightmares and/or bad dreams, at least from time to time, reported having examination dreams (Schredl, 2010a). Prior to an important exam, 171 out of 308 students who recalled a dream on the morning of the examination day reported that the examination played a role in the dream (Arnulf et al., 2014). Similarly, 12.7% of athletes experienced distressful dreams prior to a competition or an important game (Erlacher et al., 2011). Interestingly, persons who failed and persons who passed with excellence did not report as many examination dreams as those who were just able to pass the examinations (Ekeh, 1972). The finding that reporting an examination dream prior to the exam is related to a slightly better outcome (Arnulf et al., 2014) points in a similar direction. Sigmund Freud (1900/1991), who had examination dreams himself, remarked that he never dreamed about the one exam he failed but only of successfully passed exams and interpreted his examination

DOI: 10.4324/9781003300373-10

dreams as a form of consolation ("despite the anxiety you are able to pass the examination"). Arnulf et al. (2014) interpreted their finding in view of the Threat Simulation Theory (Revonsuo, 2000b): the student practiced the exam and, thus, performed better. From the viewpoint of the continuity hypothesis (Schredl, 2003), one would argue that persons who are anxious about their exam might dream more often about it, but those would also be individuals putting a lot of work into the preparation, and thus, they perform better.

The typical examination dream is conceptualized as being nightmarish – e.g., being too late, not prepared at all, not understanding the questions, and eventually failing the exam (Garfield, 2001). Systematic research into the content of examination dreams, however, is scarce. Arnulf et al. (2014) asked several questions about the characteristics of examination dreams and found that only 41.5% of those dreams were disagreeable, an equal amount were neutral, and 17% were even agreeable. About 14% stated that the dream examinations were easy (Arnulf et al., 2014). This clearly indicates that not every examination dream is a nightmare. The present analysis – an expansion of the analyses presented in Schredl (2017b) – was carried out to take a closer look at the frequency of examination dreams in a longitudinal design and at the content and characteristics of examination dreams.

Overall, the dreamer was undergoing some form of examination in 122 dreams (0.96%). An additional 35 dreams included the topic of examination, like other dream characters undergoing exams (N = 20 dreams), talking about exams (N = 8 dreams), and the dreamer himself being an examiner (N = 7 dreams). In the five time periods (see Table 10.1), the frequency of

TABLE 10.1 Examination dreams in different time periods

Period	Total number of dreams	Number of examination dreams	Percent of examination dreams	Percent of dreams with reference to waking-life examinations
Studying electrical engineering (till 4-26-1986)	279	11	3.94%	0.36%
Studying v (10-13-1986 to 9-24-1991)	2320	31	1.34%	0.34%
PhD studies (9-25-1991 to 5-18-1998)	3605	29	0.80%	0.03%
Habilitation (including CBT exam, sleep medicine exam) (5-19-1998 to 7-16-2003)	938	4	0.43%	0.00%
Professional life (without any exams) (since 7-17-2003)	5540	43	0.78%	0.04%

CBT = Cognitive-Behavioral Therapy.

TABLE 10.2 Topics of examination dreams (N = 122)

Topic	Number
Psychology	29
Electrical engineering	16
Bizarre topics	5
Physics	3
German	3
Arts	3
Sleep medicine	3
Geography	3
Mathematics	2
Juggling (practical)	2
Physiology	2
Not specified	45

N = 1: business studies, martial arts, Latin, chemical engineering, ice skating (practical), vision test.

examination dreams varies; that is, the percentage is highest during the engineering studies (very demanding curriculum with a high number of written and oral exams), second highest is psychology, with the habilitation period as lowest. Statistical analyses are presented in Schredl (2017b), indicating the differences between the studying periods and the later periods were significant, with higher percentages in the periods the dreamer was actually undergoing a lot of exams. But, even after all exams had been passed (in 2003) examination dreams showed up, but the number of examination dreams that were related to actual exams the dreamer passed was extremely small (N = 2).

If the topic of the examination was mentioned in the dream, most topics are subjects the dreamer had had examinations in – e.g., psychology, electrical engineering, high school graduation (mathematics, physics, geography, German), sleep medicine (see Table 10.2). Interestingly, the subject the dreamer faced in high school graduation in waking life and was totally unprepared for (due to a misinformation given by his teacher) never showed up in a dream (history, with the theme of the Nazi takeover in Germany). Similarly, the only exam the dreamer failed (with 56% of his fellow students) also never showed up in dreams (advanced mathematics) – in line with the observation of Sigmund Freud (1900/1991). In addition, there are several examination subjects the dreamer never studied or took an exam in, like Latin, arts, martial arts, juggling, chemical engineering, and ice skating. Even several completely bizarre examination topics showed up – e.g., a dog trying to prevent an oil spill disaster (see the following dream example), a question

TABLE 10.3 Emotional tone and preparedness of examination dreams (N = 122)

Topic	Number	Percent
Negative emotions	28	22.95%
Neutral	79	64.75%
Positive emotions	15	12.30%
Lack of knowledge	24	19.67%
Not specified	43	35.25%
Well prepared	55	45.08%

about different types of meat and sausages or the function of eggs in an electrical circuit, questions about color spots of cows, questions about places from an island in the ocean off America, and a qualitative task in which a text is given in which a man turns on a woman and sleeps with the woman and the dreamer does not understand the question at all.

Similar to the study of Arnulf et al. (2014), the negative emotions outweigh the positive emotions, with most examination dreams being neutral (see Table 10.3). One can add that none of the examination dreams were of a nightmarish type. Dream examples can be found following Table 10.3. In most examination dreams, the dreamer is well prepared (also reflecting the dreamer's waking-life style to deal with upcoming examinations). Interestingly, there were several dreams in which the dreamer received a grade that did not reflect his performance, so he was annoyed in the dream (a source of negative emotions in the examination dreams). This happened to him three times in waking life; luckily for him, the complaint was heard and the grade was corrected.

The first dream example is a dream with a real-life examiner starting with questions about optical communications engineering (the topic the dreamer specialized in while studying electrical engineering) but then drifted into a completely bizarre direction that put the dreamer under pressure.

Dream (bizarre examination topic):

I take an exam with Professor X (Electrical engineering) in the institute library. First, he asks me some questions, all of which I can answer well. It's about optical components, e.g. spacers, fiber connections such as splices, flaring optics, boron-doped fibers coated with erosion-resistant plastic. Then he hands me a piece of paper with a task on it. It's about a ship leaking oil. A dog is trying to save the situation. The question for the task is: "Which way is the dog swimming?" Since the instructions are quite long, it takes me some time to read through the task. In the process, I knock a bottle off the table, which was somehow important for the task. Now, later on, one can't tell from the bottle what comes out. Prof. X gets a little impatient because I read slowly and asks me for the solution. I answer, the dog swims in the direction, which normal humans would swim, but I must read first the task completely.

The second dream example again included a real-life examiner and a subject the dreamer did not like very much during his psychology studies. That is the reason why he was glad to pass with an A, but unfortunately, the dream was not precognitive, the grade he received in real life was not as good.

I am sitting with Prof. Y in the examination on psychology of speech. He is without an assessor; this one sits a bit apart. He asks again questions about Chomsky and wants to know another name. I admit that I don't know all the names from the psychology of language, but I could put the facts into a bigger picture. Then he wants to know names from Gestalt psychology, Max Horkheimer, then I steer on, but I notice that my associations are running away. I say that, the examination situation is not so suitable, my associations run away. Then I remember, Kafka, Franz, aha, Koffka with 2 f. That was the end, he sends me out to make the grade. He smiles a little. I am very unsure. After a short time he calls me, there are other people standing in the hall. I get an A. I say, "Too bad I was dreaming" and go away.

Dream example (positive emotion):

Seminar room. A lecturer is examining people. Two friends of mine are handing out notes. One woman knows a lot. The two of them immediately think that these are 7 points. I make fun of them by indicating that I am holding up a sign like a contest judge. I sit there quite casually, don't know that much, but I could figure it out by thinking about it. I have already made a good grade in an oral exam. In between, someone tells me about a rattlesnake that he once wanted to catch, a dangerous undertaking.

Dream example (negative emotion):

I am in a hospital, it is evening. A doctor has taken blood from a thick, protruding vein of mine. The doctor wants to give me another benzodiazepine (brotilazam or something like that). I immediately say that I don't want that, also because I have to write an exam the next day. I tell him that he does not want to undermine my performance (cognitive). He wanted to foist it on me without my knowledge, but explained it to his colleague, not knowing that I know my way around a bit. Once at home, I rummage in a desk drawer where there are papers for the exam. I have studied, but it has been a while (weeks). I'm a little anxious about whether I'll do well on the next day, and I'm thinking about reading through all the stuff again. However, I decide against it, it will work out.

Dream example (topic never studied):

I go to a large lecture hall where Ole Nydal (Buddhist teacher) is to give a lecture. I am a little late and think about whether I should go to the bathroom quickly beforehand. Then I go in and sit down in the back. There is still relaxation music playing. Then I go out again and go to the bathroom. When I come back, someone is talking. He is hectic, nervous and constantly looking for the German words. I say to another woman that I could explain to him what meditation is. Later I tell someone that I have to take an exam in Latin, even though I've never had Latin before. That will be quite hard, I think about doing a crash course over three weeks.

The following examination dream occurred long after the last examination (that examination was in 2003) and featured a subject, the dreamer faced in his high school graduation exam. Back then, he was prepared fairly well, but had the experience of being asked something he knows nothing at all about it (the original topic in real life was history), so the worries in the dreamer might reflect this past experience in a creative way.

Dream example (reference to a real-life examination, dream date: April 8th, 2012):

I'm in a large room, almost like a ballroom, with the people from my graduation class (school). I'm talking to an old schoolmate, who is taller than me, though, which I notice, because only two other schoolmates are taller than me (in real life). We talk about the graduation. Later, I realize that tomorrow or so I have geography exam (oral) and I haven't studied anything for it because I was so busy with my social issues. On the one hand, I am sure that I know something, but on the other hand, it could be that something comes up where I know absolutely nothing. I'll tell someone else nearby about this. I'm somewhat worried about how I'm going to get through this.

As the dreamer is an associated professor mainly focusing on research, he was not very much involved in setting up and doing exams with students. Therefore, it is plausible that the number of dreams about the dreamer being an examiner himself are very rare (N = 7). The following dream is an example.

Dream example (dreamer as examiner):

> *I walk past a small lecture hall building where an exam is being written that I designed. Since I have time, I go in to help with the evaluation. The main examiner is another professor; there are assistants who are already evaluating. I take some exams from the pile, not quite sure if I know all the solutions by heart. We can't shout the solutions to each other, because there are still quite a few students writing, about 30–40. I read the first questions (multiple choice) and find that they are not easy. Probably there is a solution sheet, which the other correctors also use.*

To summarize, examination dreams are relatively frequent, especially in times with a lot of exams in real life, thus reflecting waking life according the continuity hypothesis (Schredl, 2018b). But they also occur in times without any examinations ahead, thus suggesting that those dreams might have a metaphorical meaning (evaluation of one's performance by others, e.g., within one's profession). Simple reflections of examinations the dreamer had in his waking life are extremely rare. An open question is the creativity of the examination dreams – e.g., why do they include subjects that don't make sense at all?

10.2 Toilet dreams

Nielsen et al. (2003) included the topic "Have you ever dreamed of being unable to find, or embarrassed about using a toilet?" in their Typical Dream Questionnaire (TDQ). Indeed, 19.2% of the participants (student sample) responded with a yes to this question. The percentage of participants with this dream theme was even higher in Germany (30.0%; Schredl et al., 2004) and Hong Kong (59.5%; Yu, 2008), but lower in Jordan (7.4%; Nasser & Bulkeley, 2009). These were all student samples; as nocturia increases with age (Yoshimura et al., 2004), it would be interesting to study whether this theme increases with age. In the 19th century, the idea was that dreams about toilets are stimulated by the urge to urinate (*"Leibreiztraum"*), and, in order to avoid a catastrophe (wetting the bed), the dreamer wakes up so s/he can use the toilet. But even at that time, Weygandt (1893) reported a dream example in which he successfully urinated but the bed stayed dry. The findings that dreams of patients with enuresis (nocturnal bedwetting) do not dream of urinating (Gastaut & Broughton, 1964; Pierce, 1963; Pierce et al., 1961), again asking the question of whether toilet dreams are simply caused by bodily needs. Systematic dream content analytic studies of toilet dreams are scarce. In a series of 600 dreams reported by a female dreamer from 25 yrs to 76 yrs old, 9% of the dreams included in a reference to toilets (Smith & Hall, 1964). A similar figure of 8% was reported for a dream series of a man who recorded his dreams (N = 271) over a period of two years (Hall, 1981). Unfortunately, the age of the dreamer was not reported, although he had recorded his dreams for many years prior to the study (middle-aged to elderly man), but Hall (1981) added that the dreamer always awakened with a strong urge to urinate during the night, irrespective of the dream content. In a subsample of the present dream series (N = 6,991 dreams), references to toilets were found in 2.52% of the dreams (Schredl, 2011c). The presented analysis expands on this previous publication.

The rationale for taking a closer look at toilet dreams is, first, looking at the frequency of the "dramatic" version – e.g., urge to urinate/defecate at the end of the dream and waking up from the dream without satisfying the need. As every human uses toilets every day (mostly those toilets with whom s/he is familiar), the second question is whether these dreamed toilet visits resemble real-life toilet visits.

Overall, 342 dreams included a reference to toilets, with 297 dreams (2.33%) in which the dreamer wants to use or is using a toilet. The remaining 45 dreams are dreams in which other dream characters are using or want to use a toilet.

The frequency of toilet dreams shows a small (r = .123) but non-significant increase over time (see Figure 10.1); thus, a simple increase of nocturnal toilet use (which also happened with the dreamer) is not reflected in an increase in toilet dream occurrences.

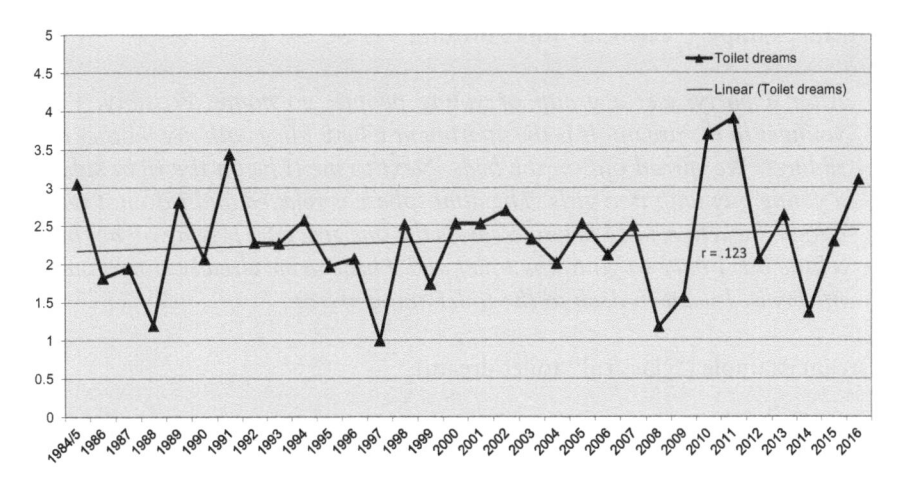

FIGURE 10.1 Percentage of dreams related to toilet use by the dreamer per year

TABLE 10.4 Toilet dreams (N = 297)

Topic	Dreams	Percent
Dreamer wants to use a toilet	55	18.52%
Dreamer urinates	95	31.99%
Dreamer defecates	49	16.50%
Urge to urinate and not relieved in the dream	32	10.77%
Urge to defecate and not relieved in the dream	4	1.35%
Using the toilet without further details given in the dream	62	20.88%

In almost 50% of the dreams, the dreamer urinated or defecated successfully (without wetting or soiling the bed) (see Table 10.4). The "classical" toilet dream (having an urge but not able to find relief) are slightly more than 10% of the dreams. In another classification process, the dreams were grouped into dreams in which the toilet-related activity occurs at the end of the dream (N = 70) and dreams in which, after the toilet activity, other things happen (N = 227). In the 36 dreams with the unrelieved urges, 22 times, this incident occurred at the end of the dreams, thus being a "classical" toilet dream, feeling a clear urge to urinate or defecate but waking up prior to the chance to get relief. That results in a figure of 7.41% of "classical" toilet dreams in relation to all toilet dreams involving the dreamer. The following two dream examples illustrate this topic.

Dream example ("classical" toilet dream):

After a party, we, a group of young people, go home. Possibly, I am younger in the dream. It is the apartment where I live with my mother and siblings. We spread out on the beds. Next to me (I lie on the right side) is a young guy with two girls. The atmosphere is relaxed and I do not really dare to be active, but I begin to caress the one girl, who is lying on her back a little bit. I have to go to the toilet and a little urine already comes out of the penis. I want to dash to the toilet and wake up.

Dream example ("classical" toilet dream):

I am now in a doctor's office. In the corridor, some people are talking to each other; a doctor is also there. I want to pass by to use the toilet at the end of the corridor. In the one patient's room on the left, there is also a toilet, but the room is occupied. I close the door; the toilet is 1950ties style.

TABLE 10.5 Setting of toilet dreams (N = 297)

Setting	Dreams	Percent
Restaurant, pub, hotel	101	34.01%
Apartment of others	70	23.57%
Own apartment	35	11.78%
Office building	24	8.08%
University/school	21	7.07%
Public toilet	17	5.72%
Nature	11	3.70%
Gymnasium/indoor pool	8	2.69%
Train/bus	5	1.68%
Not specified	5	1.68%

I sit down; there is still some junk in the toilet. I feel my urge to urinate, but before I pee, I wake up.

There is a large diversity of settings in which the toilet is located (see Table 10.5). Interestingly, only about 12% of the toilet dreams take place at the dreamer's apartment. Even though the dreamer used his own toilet at home the most often in his waking life, in dreams, other settings, like hotels, restaurants, pubs, apartments of others, occur much more often than dreams featuring his own toilet.

The toilet dreams were also classified into realistic (N = 2), possible in waking life but never occurred in waking life (N = 282), and bizarre dreams (N = 13). The two realistic toilet dreams took place in the dreamer's apartment; in one dream, the dreamer used the toilet prior to going to bed; in the other dream, the dreamer used the toilet in the morning prior to leaving the apartment, but the urge was not that strong and the time critical – he was late. The following dream is an example of a bizarre dream – a full functional toilet on the sidewalk in front of his apartment building.

Dream example (bizarre toilet dream):

I am sitting on the toilet. The loo is on the sidewalk in front of the apartment building I live in. I'm a little embarrassed that people see my penis. There are a lot of people who want to get into the house. I poop, flush and then go up to my apartment.

Overall, in more than half of the toilet dreams (54.54%), some impediment occurs (see Table 10.6). However, these problems often did not hinder the dreamer in relieving himself. In 67.97% of these type of dreams (successful relief), one handicap or another was present; the same figure was obtained

TABLE 10.6 Handicaps within toilet dreams (N = 162)

Setting	Dreams	Percent
Other persons present	82	50.62%
Toilet is dirty	23	14.20%
Urine or feces go wrong	20	12.35%
Toilet is visible	18	11.11%
Dreamer doesn't find a toilet	6	3.70%
Another person is occupying the toilet	5	3.09%
Toilet is out of order	4	2.47%
Technical problems	3	1.85%
No money	1	0.62%

for the toilet dreams including the unfulfilled urges 63.89%; that is, the presence of problems doesn't have a general effect on whether the dreamer can or cannot fulfill his need. The following dream examples illustrate this point.

Dream example (problems related to toilet use):

> I'm in a pub and looking for people I know. In the toilet, I pee in a gutter, two or three somewhat vulgar women try to harass me, but that does not bother me. I am self-confident; they notice that and stop. They are in the men's room, because a section of it is the dance floor. I can also pee quite easily. I go back to the two pub rooms, see only a former schoolmate with her boyfriend, no one else I know. I am a little disappointed.

Dream example (gross dream action):

> I'm in the sleep lab. There is a lot other persons in the large room. A patient, a young man, comes to me; we had made an appointment to talk. However, I still have to change clothes; for this I sit in my corner, I have to poop at the same time, I try to hide that and then want to clean it. This works despite the crowded place. Then I look for the test I want to do first with the patient.

As mentioned earlier, in 45 toilet dreams, not the dreamer but another character or other characters were involved in toilet-related activities. In 24 dreams, the dreamer sees another person urinating/defecating. The following dream is an example.

Dream example:

> Train station area, rather disused station with some tracks. A former boss (female) is nearby in her underwear and T-shirt and pees in a small arc on

the ballast by the tracks. I find the whole thing a bit embarrassing, the others (some people nearby) not so. I also wonder a bit about her anatomy. One friend says later that he has felt stimulating feelings (erotic) in relation to the former boss.

In 18 dreams, the dreamer has to wait because another person has to go to the bathroom – e.g., a salesman in a department store, a travel companion. The following dream is a more dramatic version of a toilet with another character wants to use the toilet.

Dream example:

Now I am in the car of a woman and am taken by her in the direction of the city center. Since I have time, I can drive a bit through the area and go back with the tram. The woman has to go to the toilet and drives quite fast around a shopping center with a gas station. Once, she almost breaks through a barrier. I suggest stopping at a restaurant, but she doesn't want to. In the meantime, she holds me by my wrists, which is rather unpleasant since I don't want anything from her. Then she does break through a fence and rolls over some tables on the terrace of a restaurant. When the car stops, she quickly gets out going to the bathroom.

The remaining three dreams included topics like pouring the urine of the brother in a toilet, a dog is peeing on the dreamer, and hearing noises of defecation.

Overall, the analysis of the toilet dreams indicate that this dream topic is much broader than the "classical" theme of not being able to find, or being embarrassed about using a toilet; only 7.41% of the toilet dreams reported in this series could be classified in this category. This raises the question of whether all toilet dreams are reflections of needs of the sleeping body, and the fact that the majority of the toilet dreams included successful urinating or defecating also questions this general explanation for the occurrence of toilet dreams. Moreover, these dreams almost never replay actual waking-life experiences of the dreamer; on the contrary, the previous examples illustrate clearly that some of the toilet dreams are clearly out of the ordinary. Interestingly, persons with inflammatory bowel disease or irritable bowel syndrome reported more often dreams about soiling themselves (16% and 14% [patients] vs. 2% [controls]) (Lal & Whorwell, 2002). Thus, it would be very interesting to study the frequency of toilet dreams in persons with nocturia (frequent visits to the toilet at night) or intestinal incontinence. Again, studying toilet dreams shows how creative dreams can present a simple, everyday activity and leaves the big question open why we have such creative dreams about something that mundane.

10.3 Tooth dreams

Sigmund Freud (1900/1991) has included remarks on dreams about teeth falling out in a chapter about typical dreams; pointing out a similarity to a slang word for masturbation (*"runterreißen"* ["tear down"]), he saw these dreams as representations of masturbation issues – e.g., fear of punishment. Subsequent authors also pointed out other possible meanings of these dreams – e.g., fear of growing old (a man dreamed that all his teeth crumbled and fell out) (Schneck, 1956) or a more direct symbolization of dental fear (not want to go to the dentist, fear of having toothaches, etc.) (Capps & Carlin, 2011). In one dream, the dentist pulls out four to five teeth against the will of the dreamer; this was interpreted as a representation of the analyst (being the dentist in the dream) who works against the resistances of the patient (Hitschmann, 1931).

Interestingly, quantitative dream research using a questionnaire eliciting typical dream themes found that about 20% to 50% of the participants answered the question "Have you ever dreamed of your teeth falling out" in an affirmative way (Griffith et al., 1958; Nasser & Bulkeley, 2009; Nielsen et al., 2003; Schredl et al., 2004; Ward et al., 1961; Yu, 2008). That is, a substantial number of individuals had, at least once, this type of dream. The actual frequency seems to be rather low, as only 0.56% of diary dreams (Mathes & Schredl, 2014) and 0.59% of most recent dreams (Mathes et al., 2014) included the theme of teeth falling out.

In the present dream series, 97 dreams included a reference to teeth or objects that are related to teeth (e.g., toothbrush). These dreams were differentiated into different groups (see Table 10.7). As can be seen, the contexts of teeth in dreams is manifold, from using the word "tooth" as a metaphor used often in everyday language to the more distressing dreams of a toothache and teeth falling out. It is interesting to notice that a routine carried out daily – namely, brushing one's teeth – showed up very rarely in dreams; only five dreams refer to this behavior. Even the thoughts about going to a dentist occurred more often.

Of the ten dreams in the category "Toothache, teeth falling out," five dreams could be classified as typical dreams of teeth falling out, resulting in a percentage of 0.04%. Whereas all five dream experiences were distressing, in four of those dreams, the dreamer seeks help from professionals – an action you would also carry out if teeth would fall out in waking life. These dreams are shown in the following paragraphs.

Dream example (losing teeth):

> *After this (window) is fixed by hand, I lose teeth, first the upper left canine tooth; it is loose and falls out when pressed lightly, immediately followed by the next one. I panic that I will become completely toothless and need dentures, a third tooth of the top row follows.*

TABLE 10.7 Teeth dreams (N = 97)

Topic	Dreams	Example(s)
Metaphor related to teeth	8	*"Wir wollen ihm auf den Zahn fühlen"* is "We want to get to the bottom of it"; *"Affenzahn"* is "breakneck speed"
Dentist	7	Dentist is a party guest
Dentist visit is topic	17	Dreamer wants to go to the dentist for checking (no pain)
Animal teeth	15	Fishing, the dreamer catches a fish that is 1 meter long and has many sharp teeth; venomous tooth of a snake
Objects related to teeth (toothbrush, toothpick)	13	A woman performs tricks with toothpicks; man talks about his dental prosthesis
Brushing teeth		
• Dreamer	5	Hotel, dreamer and his boss brush their teeth
• Another person	2	One of the dreamer's roommates is brushing his teeth
Toothache, teeth falling out		
• Dreamer	10	Dreamer has severe gum pain and is looking for a dentist clinic; wearing a bite splint made from lapis lazuli affects the teeth in a negative way; one of the lower molars (left) has quite a bit of decay
• Another person	1	A bad guy has severe toothaches
Using teeth to do something		
• Dreamer	5	Dreamer holds a thick glass lens between his teeth (experiment); dreamer catches a small arrow with his teeth
• Another person	2	As part of a song, the singers vigorously rattle their teeth
Looking at teeth		
• Dreamer	1	Dreamer looks at his teeth using a mirror
• Another person	11	Dreamer sees a weird man with odd-looking teeth; man has black teeth; dreamer adores strong and beautiful teeth of a female friend

Dream example (losing teeth plus dentist):

Tooth. I touch a lower, front tooth in the morning, it hurts and parts break off by the touch, it is quite rotten, after a while I have it in my hand, terrible, but the other teeth are solid. I go to the dentist anyway. I show him the tooth.

Dream example (losing teeth plus dentist):

> *I lie in my mother's double bed and watch TV. My father is lying on the left. Suddenly, a tooth breaks out at the bottom front left of my mouth. My mother comes and lies down; I go into the bathroom and rinse my mouth. I am a little afraid of choking. Some tooth debris and blood come out. Also, two other teeth are broken out. They were quite porous. I am quite shocked and want to go to the dentist right away tomorrow. I wonder if I can get an appointment at my practice right away. Maybe I'll get a referral.*

Dream example (losing teeth plus dentist):

> *I am in an apartment (parental or mother). I notice that a tooth is falling out. It is a thick molar tooth. An adhesion has formed between the tooth and the gum, which has pushed the tooth away. I am very afraid that this will happen to the other teeth as well, and I want to go to the dentist right away, possibly with my mother. However, my mother is feeling bad (depressed), so it is better to ask someone from my siblings to drive me. Besides, it is Thursday evening and tomorrow on Good Friday holiday, my dentist is closed. I'm thinking of going to the dental clinic as they treat emergencies, even though it's not that good. I want to take the tooth where the adhesion is so they can see what's going on. I am very careful not to wiggle the other teeth.*

Dream example (losing teeth plus dentist):

> *I feel that something is wrong with my teeth and look in the mirror. There I see how in front of the normal teeth flatter, new teeth want to burst out. I think about where to go (medical service) because it's Saturday. It looks quite terrible and towards the end of the dream, I spit many fallen out teeth into the sink.*

Teeth can occur in varying contexts in dreams; in this series, the mundane tooth dreams – just brushing one's own teeth – is very rare. Also, the classical nightmare tooth dreams are rare, and in most of them, the dreamer thought about seeking help. It would be very interesting to study tooth dreams in larger samples, as they provide a good illustration how the dream ego handles emergencies, ranging from waking up from the dream with panic to calmly (more or less) seeking a solution for the dream problem. A simple tip for tooth dreams was provided by (Faraday, 1976): make an appointment with your dentist.

11
CONTRIBUTIONS TO DREAM THEORIES

The dream series was analyzed regarding different characteristics and topics (see Chapters 5 to 10): dream characters, especially persons known to the dreamer, sensory perceptions, activities like sexuality or hobbies, mundane aspects like time references, money, beds, as well as extraordinary and typical dreams. In Table 11.1, the frequencies of some dream ingredients are depicted, illustrating that all aspects of waking life can show up in dreams. In other papers based on this dream series, topics like animals in dreams (Schredl, 2013a), smoking in dreams (Schredl, 2014), breaking the law in dreams (Schredl, 2021b), being naked in dreams (Schredl, 2021c), means of transportation (Schredl, 2020a), clocks in dreams (Schredl, 2021d), and elevators (Schredl, 2020c) have been analyzed. It should be kept in mind that the analyses presented in previous publications and in this book are far from complete; for example, other interesting topics would be work-related dreams or dream emotions, just to name two. Overall, the analysis of this dream series clearly indicates how abundant dreams are; they include everything that can be experienced in waking life and more.

The next paragraphs will discuss whether the findings based on this dream series are helpful in understanding how dreaming works, respectively, provide some ideas about the current dream theories like the continuity hypothesis of dreaming or the theories about dream functions.

11.1 Contribution to the continuity hypothesis: the CDC theory

The original formulation of the continuity hypothesis stated "The dream world is neither discontinuous nor inverse in its relationship to the conscious world. We remain the same person, the same personality with the same

DOI: 10.4324/9781003300373-11

TABLE 11.1 Frequency of different dream elements/activities/characteristics (N = 12,769 dreams)

		Percent
Social	Core family members	18.48%
	Partner	11.42%
	Friends	5.29%
	Colleagues/fellow students	9.45%
	Acquaintances	6.09%
	Old school friends	5.87%
	Celebrities	1.29%
Animals		7.45%
Everyday objects	Clothing	12.10%
	Colors	9.39%
	Money	8.93%
	Beds	7.84%
	Weapons	2.91%
	Telephones	2.15%
	Glasses	1.11%
	Mirrors	0.22%
Activities	Erotic activities	14.63%
	Hobby (circus art-related activities)	3.27%
	Flying	1.87%

characteristics, and the same basic beliefs and convictions whether awake or asleep" (p. 104; Hall & Nordby, 1972). Based on the analyses in this book and the dream literature (Schredl, 2018b), the hypothesis, in its current form, seems not complete; there is discontinuity (elements that do not fit into the waking-world of the dreamer) and creativity (elements the dreamer never experienced in his waking life) in dreams (see Table 11.2). Thus, the continuity hypothesis with different emphases, whether cognitive or experiential (Domhoff, 2017a, 2017b, 2018a; Erdelyi, 2017; Jenkins, 2018; Schredl, 2003, 2017c), is not able to fully explain dream content in its diversity. For example, the simple question why we dream about being able to fly without adequate means cannot be answered within this theoretical framework.

Evaluating the data of this long dream series presented in this book clearly indicates that there is a lot of continuity between waking and dreaming; for example, family members and partners are by far the most frequent dream characters, clearly reflecting that they were or are still important to the dreamer in his waking life. However, even if there is continuity at first glance, a closer look also reveals a considerable amount of discontinuity (aspects that are not continuous with the waking life of the dreamer). A few examples will be presented to illustrate this.

TABLE 11.2 Relationships between waking and dreams

Type	Supportive data from the dream series
Continuity	Close persons are frequent in dreams, money (current currency), decrease of partner dreams after separation
Discontinuity	Context of money in dreams, context of sensory perceptions in dreams – e.g., pain
Creativity	Flying dreams, elevator dreams

For the topic of money, there is a clear continuity regarding the currency of the dream money. In the year Germany switched from the Deutsche Mark to the Euro, the currency in the dream also changed, with only a few reminiscences of "Deutsche Mark" after 2002. Additionally, the dreamer never dreamed about Euros before they were introduced. On the other hand, even though most dream situations that involved money were not bizarre (see Table 8.5), none of these situations occurred in the life of the dreamer, from buying a bottle of liquor for 23.20 DM to looking at on old pair of trousers for 500 DM to receiving a check over 8 million DM. It should be noted that, for these types of analysis, it is advantageous that the dreamer and the researcher are one and the same person, as this evaluation (if a topic ever came up in waking life) can only be answered by the dreamer himself. The finding that the money-associated dream situations are not reflections of real memories raises the question of why dream experiences are discontinuous with waking life. One explanation could be the so-called "emotional continuity." The idea would be that positive emotions – e.g., work-related success – is affecting other dreams; for example, reflected in a dream of receiving a lot of money. That is, money-related dreams are discontinuous on a thematic level but continuous on an emotional level. Unfortunately, this topic was not studied within this dream series, as the information about the emotional status of the dreamer in waking life was not elicited. Based on the idea that dreams are metaphorical (Malinowski & Horton, 2015; States, 1992), one can hypothesize that the dream with the pair of old trousers for 500 DM could be a depiction of a frustrating experience, as the dreamer liked the trousers and would have bought them if they were cheaper (a lot cheaper). That is, the dream scenario is depicting the more general topic of frustration. Thus, metaphor might not be the best word; a better name would be: the basic pattern of the dream (Schredl, 2015a) – in this case, frustration; the dream might be related to a waking-life experience in which frustration was present but in a totally different context. But it should be stated that this is pure speculation, or using a more scientific term, a working hypothesis that has not been tested systematically in empirical studies. The positive side is that these kinds of hypotheses could be tested.

Another example that fits in this line of thinking are the telephone dreams, especially those dreams in which telephone are not working properly. As the dreamer uses a phone in his waking life regularly, it does reflect continuity that telephones show up in the dreams. The increase of mobile phones over time is also continuous with waking life, as their popularity also increased over time. On the other hand, the high percentage of problems related to using the telephone in dreams (about 20% of all telephone dreams) is not continuous with waking life, even though, on rare occasions, telephone problems have also occurred in the dreamer's waking life. Again, Garfield (2001), for example, pointed out that the dream is not about telephones per se but an illustrative way to depict a more general topic (basic pattern) of having a problem with communication with other persons.

Colors were spontaneously reported in only about 10% of dreams in this dream series – a finding that is in line with previous findings – e.g. 25% dream reports with color mentioned in a student sample (Schredl, 2008d). If dreaming is completely continuous with waking, one would expect that all dreams include color(s). This led some researcher to the idea that dreams are, in this respect, discontinuous with waking life, with no color or only black, white, and gray; for an overview, see Schwitzgebel (2002). However, probing questions – that is, asking the dreamers directly upon awakening about the colors of the dream objects – revealed that more than 80% (Rechtschaffen & Buchignani, 1992) or 90% (Schredl et al., 2008) of the dreams included some reference to color. If dreams were recalled in the home setting, the participants stated that, in about 40% of the recalled dreams, they were not able to recall whether there was any color in the dream (König et al., 2017). Thus, dreams are very likely as colorful as waking life, but it seems difficult to remember colors if they are not central to the dream plot, and, if colors are normal (e.g., a yellow banana), colors are not mentioned in the dream report. The analysis of color dreams in the present dream series indicated that the spontaneous use of color words in dreams is comparable to the use of color words; for example, my black shoes, blue sky, woman with blond hair, red wine, red brick wall, or blue car. That is, the color is mentioned because it specifies the object/element; as for these objects/elements, the color can vary (hair, cars, clothing, etc.). Skin-colored faces or yellow bananas have not been mentioned in the selected dream reports of these series. On the other hand, some dreams also include some bizarre coloring – e.g., a neon pink bird that looks like a small kite. The dreamer even thinks about the causes of this unusual coloring (mimicking the color of a specifically colored surface). Overall, studying colors in dreams also provides support for the continuity hypothesis of dreams but also highlights that the continuity hypothesis, as a sole theory for explaining dream contents, is incomplete.

Another topic that illustrates the mixture of continuity, discontinuity, and creativity happening in dreams is pain perception in dreams. The dreamer suffered from chronic tension headaches for about ten years, a condition that was very distressing for the dreamer; for example, in writing long exams. However, only 6 of the 130 pain dreams refer to this health condition. Although more the 50% of the pain dreams included pain sensations that are known to the dreamer in his waking life – e.g., knee pain, stomachache, etc. – there are a lot of pain sensations the dreamer never experienced in his waking life – e.g., being shot in the belly, getting one's arm chopped off, bitten by small monsters. This is in clear contrast to the continuity hypothesis; one might speculate whether the dreamer saw a movie with comparable scenes and saw the faces of the actor full of pain and experienced pain empathically. But this is quite different from the dream, experiencing the pain of getting an arm chopped of compared to "just" seeing it. It's even difficult to describe such an experience that has never been experienced in waking life.

Another explanation of "discontinuities" in dreams might be the effect of media on dreams (Moverley et al., 2018; Stephan et al., 2012). In this context, it is important not to restrict waking-life experiences to events that take place in real life but also include experiences like watching a movie or inner images that pop up while reading a captivating book. In the present dream series, this is best reflected by the relatively high number of dreams with weapons (see Chapter 8.6). About 3% of the dreams included weapons, even though weapons like guns do not play any role in the waking life of the dreamer but, of course, are present in many action movies. Interestingly, the percentage of weapon dreams decreased over the years (see Figure 8.8), parallel to the dreamer's decreasing consumption of action movies or TV series with a lot of fighting and killing. This finding emphasizes the importance of eliciting "waking-life experience" in research designs aiming at studying the continuity between waking in dreaming very carefully; that is, including experiences related to media and also thoughts and mind-wandering. For example, the finding of Tuominen et al. (2021) that, in times of social isolation, close persons can even turn up more often in dreams than in the normal, everyday settings that include these persons can be explained by the fact that the participants thought a lot about these close persons while they were socially isolated.

A topic that is even more discontinuous with waking-life and fits into the creativity part is the theme of flying. Interestingly, the frequency of flying dreams was not related to experiencing real flights in waking life (travelling by plane); there was no increase in flying dreams after the first flights in waking life. Given that 1.44% of all dreams included non-lucid flying (one can argue that lucid flying dreams are different, as the dreamer often deliberately wants to fly in those dreams), the question arises why such dreams occur. It is clearly not continuous with waking life and never will be; that is, training such a skill in dreams is completely wasted time. One study (Schredl, 2008c) investigated the idea that flying dreams might be continuous with waking life on an emotional level and, indeed, having flying dreams was correlated with lower neuroticism scores, whereas falling dreams were correlated with higher neuroticism scores. This would fit in with the emotional continuity, as flying in dreams is very often associated with very positive emotions. The idea of flying dreams as a metaphor or illustrating a basic pattern is also very plausible; for example, in German, one can use the word "*Hochgefühle*" for elevated mood. Thus, flying dreams reflect positive waking-life emotions that occurred in a realistic context – e.g., falling in love, passing an exam with success, receiving a nice gift, etc. In addition, the other aspect that might be related to having periods with elevated emotions in waking – worrying about how long this will last before a downfall occurs – is represented in about 22% of the flying dreams: what would happen if the ability to fly is suddenly gone; that is, the flying dream would then become a falling dream. Interestingly, the dream series also included elevator dreams, of which about 40% were bizarre elevator dreams (flying elevator, dangling, elevators without walls, etc.) and those were often associated with anxiety (Schredl, 2020c). The basic pattern would be: "There is something not working in the usual way, that's scary." Again, the question arises how to fit this type of dream into the framework of the continuity hypothesis.

Looking again at Table 11.2, it seems clear that the analyses presented in this book – even though they are based on only one dream series – clearly indicate that the continuity hypothesis should be expanded to a broader framework. The author would like to suggest a new concept: the CDC theory of dreaming; C = Continuity, D = Discontinuity, and C = Creativity. Such a framework would allow studying questions like: "What kind of waking-life experiences might be reflected in bizarre dreams?" This would include concepts like metaphorical expressions (Malinowski & Horton, 2015; States, 1992) and illustrating basic patterns (Schredl, 2015a) – e.g., living in a room without solid walls in the dream might be pointing to the waking-life topic of setting boundaries in relationships with others. The CDC theory would also promote the study of the frequency of creative dreams; Schredl and Erlacher (2007) estimated, based on their survey data, that about 7.8% of all dreams include creative ideas that are beneficial for waking life. They also showed that creative dreams not only occur in professionals like musicians, artists and so on, but in "normal" people as well. It would be very interesting to learn what kind of waking-life experiences and/or personality variables, like thin boundaries, might trigger creative dreams.

Even though it is necessary to expand the continuity hypothesis to a broader concept (see the foregoing), it seems that the larger part of dream elements can be explained within the concept of continuity; that is, these dream elements had occurred in the waking life of the dreamer. Schredl (2003) was the first to point out that the continuity hypothesis, in its original form, could be interpreted in a way that all waking-life experiences, concerns, and so on show up with equal likelihood in subsequent dreams, but taking a closer look at the empirical findings, this seems not to be the case. In Table 1.2 (Chapter 1) four factors that might affect the continuity between waking and dreaming have been introduced: (1) time interval between waking-life event and dream, (2) emotional intensity of the waking-life experience, (3) type of waking-life experience, and (4) personality factors. There is empirical evidence supporting that, for example, more distant waking-life experiences were less likely to be incorporated into dreams or emotionally intense waking-life experiences have a higher probability of being reflected in dreams than mundane ones (Schredl, 2003, 2018b). The question at hand is whether the findings based on this dream series corroborates these factors (except for factor 4, as this is not possible to study in a single case study) or might even add new factors that have not been investigated yet (see Table 11.3).

There are several topics that were analyzed in this series that clearly support that the time interval between waking-life experience (event, thought, etc.) and the dream is related to the probability this waking-life experience is incorporated into dreams (Botman & Crovitz, 1989; Vallat et al., 2017). For example, there is a decrease in the percentage of dreams with core family members (see Figure 5.1), which makes sense, as the dreamer spent much more time with his family during childhood, adolescence, and early adulthood than in later years. Another finding that supports the effect of this factor is the decrease of partner dreams after separation (see Figure 5.4).

TABLE 11.3 Factors affecting continuity

Factor	Data from the dream series supporting this claim (examples)
Time interval between waking-life event and dream	Decrease of partner dreams after separation, decrease of fellow student dreams after finishing studying, circus-art dreams, but no decrease in the frequency of dreams about schoolmates
Emotional involvement	Close persons (family, partners, friends) occur much more often that colleagues and acquaintances, frequent dreams including the dreamer's "true love," even after separation
Type of waking-life experience – e.g., sociality bias, ordinariness	Frequent social interactions within dreams, ordinary things (glasses, mirrors) rare
"Good old times" overrepresented?	Positive dreams of the "true love," despite the problems that triggered the separations

Similarly, the frequency of dreams featuring fellow students decreased after the dreamer finished his studies and, thus, did not see the fellow student that often any more (see Figure 5.6). The same pattern was also found for the "circus arts" hobby: high frequency of dreams related to that hobby during intense periods of training but a steady decline after the waking-life involvement with this hobby decreased (see Figure 7.3). These examples illustrate that dreams preferentially include recent waking-life experiences but also – to a lesser extent – include material from long-term memory.

However, there is one exception to the rule, which is the lack of decline over time of the dreams including schoolmates. There is a decline in frequency in the first two years (see Figure 5.5) and an increase in the year with the big reunion party (after 20 years), but overall, there is no detectable decline in frequency. This is astonishing, as something like emotional involvement did not a play a role in this context; the dreamer had only very sporadic contact with a few schoolmates over the 30 years, but no regular contacts after finishing school (with the exception of two schoolmates who also started studying electrical engineering at the same university as the dreamer, but even these contacts decrease even before the start of the dream diary in 1984). First, it would be interesting to know whether this pattern can also be found in other dream series. So far, this type of analysis has not been applied to other dream series. Another approach would be to look at dreams of students who just finished school and test whether the frequency of schoolmates declines over time; that is, decreases with an increasing time interval between finishing school and dream reporting. Speculating about possible factors that might explain this non-existent decrease of schoolmate dreams over time, two topics came to mind. Regarding forming a peer-group, the schoolmates – at least in case of the present dreamer – played an important role; thus, this might reflect some form of imprinting and, thus, these first "imprinted" contacts are very stable over time. Another line of thinking is based on the metaphor concept. Like a movie director casts actors and actresses who fit the roles given by the script, the dream might pick persons known to the dreamer who reflect distinct personality types, so the person fits into the dream plot. In one of the dream examples given in Chapter 5.4, one schoolmate represents a helpful person, but others represent persons who – even knowing the dreamer quite well – do not really care about him, showing this by leaving without saying goodbye. In order to test this working hypothesis, a very detailed recording of waking-life experiences has to be carried out, in addition to the dream journaling – e.g., the question whether, in the current waking life, persons play a role who treated the dreamer in the same way particular former schoolmates did.

The emotional involvement factor (see Table 11.3) was not tested directly – that is, by directly correlating emotional closeness ratings with the frequency of dreams with the respective person – as it has been done in Han and

Schweickert (2016). However, persons close to the dreamer (family, partners, and friends) occurred much more often than persons who are not that close like colleagues and acquaintances (see Table 5.2). Similarly, the high frequency of dreams featuring the dreamer's "true love" – even after being separated and having no contact at all (see Figure 5.3) – support the notion that emotional involvement increases the chances of dreaming about this person. The importance of emotional involvement has been demonstrated in different studies (e.g., Malinowski & Horton, 2014a; Schredl, 2006); for example, high work-related stress levels were associated with a higher frequency of work-related dreams (Schredl, Anderson, et al., 2020).

As the Social Simulation Theory (Revonsuo et al., 2015; Tuominen, Revonsuo, et al., 2019) postulates that prosocial interactions in dreams are preferentially aimed at people with whom the dreamer has close relationships (Strengthening hypothesis) (Tuominen et al., 2021; Tuominen, Stenberg, et al., 2019), it is interesting to take a closer look at the interaction quality between the dreamer and different persons in the dream (see Table 5.21). Within the context of the Social Simulation Theory, the strengthening of social bonds with close persons is crucial for survival; therefore, training social skills in dreams had had an evolutionary benefit. However, the emotional quality of the interactions between the dreamer and close persons within the dream was more often negative than positive – e.g., for the father, the mother, and the brother (see Table 5.21). This contradicts this proposition of the Social Simulation Theory, as one would expect that positive dream interactions strengthen the waking-life social bonds, but negative interactions might have the opposite effect. For other persons, like male friends, the ratio of positive and negative interactions was balanced; this was also the case for a former partner of the dreamer (Schredl, 2011a). Only for one female friend, the positive interactions clearly outweighed the negative ones (see Table 5.21). It would be very interesting to study the effect of social dream emotions on the closeness of waking-life relationships in a longitudinal design. Selterman et al. (2014), for example, found – using a diary design – that dreams including infidelity and/or jealousy were associated with less intimate feelings and more conflict with their partners on subsequent days. Whether this is unidirectional or not is an open question; that is, these dreams might reflect already-existing conflicts, and recalling such dreams would increase the awareness of the dreamer regarding these issues. In this line of thinking, it's not the dream itself that is responsible for increasing the emotional distance between the partners, but the evaluation of the dream ("Why do I dream bad things about my partner") by the waking consciousness (see Chapter 1.3 regarding the question of why it is so difficult to study the effect of specific dreams on waking life).

The next factor is associated with the type of waking life experience (see Table 11.3); that is, specific types of waking-life experiences have a higher or lower chance of getting incorporated into subsequent dreams than others. So far, the focus was on cognitive activities like reading, writing, and arithmetic (Hartmann, 2000): even though students spent a lot of time every day with these activities (41.6% of the elicited waking-activities were cognitive activities), they rarely dream about them; only 18.6% of the dream activities were reading, writing, working on a computer (Schredl & Hofmann, 2003). On the other hand, social activities like talking with friends comprised 15.2% of the time spent with the activities elicited in the study, but 27.7% of the dreams included talking with friends. That is, in relation to the amount of time spent with this social activity in waking life, it is overrepresented in dreams; dreams preferentially depict social topics. This is in line with the so-called sociality bias, an axiom of the Social Simulation Theory (Revonsuo et al., 2015) that postulates that dreams are beneficial in improving social skills. If so, social interaction should be a prominent dream feature. The analyses of the present dream series support this postulate, as persons known to the dreamer are present in more than 50% of the dreams. Unfortunately, systematic evaluations could not be performed, as exact times spent with social interactions in waking life per day or per week were not available.

A factor that has not been studied systematically yet was termed "ordinariness." As described in Chapter 8.4, the dreamer has to wear glasses because he is severely short-sighted. One of the activities with the glasses he performed most was putting them on or taking them off when going to bed or leaving the bed. But, only two of the 142 glasses dreams included this topic, equaling only 0.016% of all dreams. Neither of these two dreams took place in the dreamer's bedroom. Many of the glasses dreams were related to unusual situations – e.g., glasses are broken. Similarly, mirrors are an everyday object most people use at least once every day, but seeing one's reflection in the mirror or in another reflecting surface (window) is extremely rare (N = 13 dreams; see Table 8.16). The dreamer's bed in the dreamer's bed room is also very rare (N = 22 dreams of N = 1,001 bed dreams; see Table 8.13); most of the beds and bedrooms (if specified) are extraordinary. Even those dreams, including the dreamer's bed in his bedroom, do not reflect the typical sleep setting of the dreamer – e.g., there are animals or someone else who never been in the bedroom of the dreamer in real life (see Table 8.14). These examples clearly indicate that mundane things – activities that are automatized and don't involve much attention (like putting down the glasses prior to going to bed) – are underrepresented in dreams. Thus, dreams do not reflect everything we experience in our waking life in the same manner but select for specific experiences, like social interaction, or omit mundane, ordinary experiences.

The last factor depicted in Table 11.3 was termed "Good, old times." The idea is that, if one looks back on specific phases in one's life, everything or most things were good. Berntsen et al. (2011), for example, reported that, consistent with the notion of a positivity bias in old age, the positive events were judged to be markedly more central to one's life story and identity than were the negative events. In dream research, most studies had focused on the long-lasting effects of negative life events, including traumatic experiences – e.g. war (Sandman et al., 2013; Schredl & Piel, 2004) and childhood abuse (Mathes et al., 2022). In two single case studies, a separation was followed by negatively toned dreams about the ex-partner (Domhoff, 2003; Schredl & Neuhäusler, 2019). The ex-partner dreams were more negatively toned compared to the partner dreams (Schredl, Cadiñanos Echevarria, et al., 2020) – a findings that makes sense, as these dreams reflect the problems that preceded the break-up or occurred during the break-up period. In a student sample (Schredl & Wood, 2021), negative emotions related to the ex-partner in the dream outweighed the positive ones. These findings support the notion that negative life events can have long-lasting effects on dreams. The emotional quality of the dream interactions between the dreamer's true love and the dreamer was balanced during relationship periods and in the phases of separation (Schredl, 2011a); this analysis, however, ended with the third separation in 2005. Eleven years later, in 2016, the emotions of the dreamer toward his true love were more often positive (75%) then negative (25%) (see Table 5.14). Can this be an indicator of a positivity bias, not focusing on the conflicts and problems they had (that are responsible for the three break-ups) but on the positive aspects of their relationship – the intimacy and connectedness the dreamer had enjoyed very much. It would be very interesting to study this possible positivity bias regarding former relationship partners or deceased close persons in larger samples.

Another source of dreams is stimuli that are processed by the person while s/he is asleep and get incorporated into dreams. There is a broad literature (Schredl, 2018b) how different stimulus modalities (acoustic, olfactory, pressure, etc.) are sometimes integrated into the dream plot, often in a creative way. In a lab setting where stimuli were presented during REM sleep, a substantial percentage of dreams were affected – e.g., light flashes (39% incorporation), vibrations applied to the finger (45% incorporation) (Paul et al., 2014), or electrical stimuli applied to the thumb (55% incorporation) (Koulack, 1969). However, in the home setting, dreams that incorporate stimuli that accidentally occurred while the dreamer slept seem to be very rare (see Chapter 6.6). The dreamer identified only 12 cases (0.09% of all dreams) that were associated with stimuli (most often external stimuli like noises [duck quacking] or music). One might speculate that this is an underestimation, as the dreamer would not have been able to connect an external stimulus to the dream if the stimulus were not present anymore during the awakening process. It would be interesting (and time consuming) to monitor external stimuli regularly – for example, auditory stimuli that occur while the person is asleep – and check those recordings for whether unusual stimuli occurred and whether an incorporation of these stimuli into the dream happened. This would require many nights as home sleep settings are typically relatively noise-free and not full of unusual auditory stimuli.

One dream example in the series referred to the incorporation of pain; that is, the incorporation of an internal stimulus. As pointed out in Chapter 6, there was a time when researchers thought that many dream images could be attributed to external or internal stimuli (Weygandt, 1893). Whereas modern dream research clearly supported the idea that external stimuli can be integrated into dreams, it is much more difficult to attribute dream content to internal stimuli, especially those that are always or very often present during sleep – e.g., flying dreams to the movements of the lungs (*"Lungenflügel"* in German) (Schönhammer, 2004) or erotic dreams to sexual arousal (erection or increased vaginal blood flow) (Fisher, 1966). Based on this theory, the question would be why not all dreams are sexual or flying dreams, as this kind of internal stimuli are always present during REM sleep. Another interesting example is the toilet dreams; that is, having the urge to pee in the dream but waking up before this need could be fulfilled, and after waking up, noticing the urge to urinate and use the toilet. The dream is a wake-up call: go to the toilet before you wet the bed. That is, the idea would be that the urge to urinate is integrated into the dream and leads to awakening, so the dreamer can relieve herself/himself and continue her/his sleep (without the danger of wetting the bed). In the present dream series, 2.33% of the dreams included the topic that the dreamer wanted to use or used a toilet, but only a small percentage (7.41%) of those dreams were "classical" toilet dreams; that is, the dreamer feels the urge to urinate but wakes up before he can relieve himself. One can argue in favor of the *"Leibreizttheorie"* that the stimulus (full bladder or bowel pressure) might be integrated into the dream, even without awakening the dreamer, but explaining why about 50% of the dreams include successful urinating or defecating cannot be explained by the *"Leibreiztheorie"*; that is, explaining dream content by incorporation of internal stimuli, as this (urinating/defecating) did not happen. Overall, the closer look at toilet dreams renders it unlikely that the main driving force behind toilet dreams is the urge to urinate (which is, by the way, very often present if one wakes up in the second part of the night); it seems more likely that these dreams are also explained by the continuity hypothesis respective by the extended CDC theory.

Overall, several factors affecting the continuity between waking and dreaming reported in the literature (Schredl, 2003, 2018b) were also found in the analyses of the present dream series. However, taking a closer look, there might be even more factors involved in explaining continuity that have not yet been studied empirically.

11.2 Contribution to theories about dream functions: my personal view

As pointed out in Chapter 1.3, empirical data supporting any of the numerous theories about dream function(s) (see Table 1.3) are still lacking. Not that researcher didn't attempt to solve the mystery; the reason for that is that the current state of available methodology for eliciting dream reports does not allow systematic studies of possible dream functions of un-remembered dreams. As this chapter presents the personal view of the author how remembering and recording so many dreams can contribute to these theories about function, I would like to switch to a more casual writing style.

First, I would like to start with the idea that dreams serve the same function as a specific form of mind-wandering called Imagined Interactions (Eldredge et al., 2015). As pointed out in Chapter 1 (see Table 1.4), there is a considerable overlap, phenomenological and neurophysiological (default mode network), between mind-wandering (daydreaming) and dreaming; that is, between a specific form of subjective experiencing in the waking state when the person doesn't have any tasks at hand and subjective experiencing during sleep. Some researchers (Eeles et al., 2020) even argue that the continuity between waking and dreaming is best explained by the continuity between mind-wandering and dreaming (on an emotional and thematic level). The postulated functions for Imagined Interactions in waking are: (1) relational maintenance, (2) conflict linkage, (3) rehearsal, (4) self-understanding, (5) catharsis, and (6) compensation. These functions can be seen as functions mind-wandering has in keeping the psyche working (for a differentiation between different uses of the word function, see Table 1.4), but in the long run, a healthy psyche is very likely to increase one's chances for reproducing; that is, this function of mind-wandering might also have served an evolutionary function, and thus, has been selected for. The authors (Eldredge et al., 2015) found that 71.7% of the dream reports could be attributed to one of the Imagined Interaction functions; however, they point out that, often, not the dream itself but what the dreamer was thinking about the dream in the waking state fulfilled the specific function. The following dream illustrated this: "I was standing on the rim of the Grand Canyon arguing with my mom when she fell off and died." It is difficult to determine what the function of this dream might be from this alone, and external coders were unable to do so. However, once provided with the dreamer's own interpretation of what the dream meant – in this case, "it helped me remember how much I loved my mom and that I needed to make up with her after the fight we had yesterday" – the functions become clear (p. 252; Eldredge et al., 2015). This part of their findings is interesting, as it stresses the importance of remembering the dream; that is, the dream fulfills its function if it is remembered and reflected on. I was intrigued by this study because I myself do a lot of rehearsing of an important conversation or email that is coming up in the near future, what are the best arguments to present, how the other person could react to this argument, and so on. Thinking about this waking-life phenomenon in relation the possible dream function, I became aware that the rehearsal function of Imagined Interactions is only beneficial if I remember the specific argument I had come up with during mind-wandering. If I forgot, it is gone. The same is valid for ideas that come up spontaneously in times of relaxed wakefulness; for example, during the time between waking up and getting out of the bed. These ideas are often related to current projects of mine, like writing a paper or this book; for example, this reference might be helpful in supporting my arguments, etc. Again, it became clear that, if I forget this idea, then the benefit is gone (therefore, I often write them down as soon as I can). If this is transferred to dreams, it would imply that only remembered dreams serve this particular function, like providing creative insights, good ideas for upcoming waking-life events/tasks. Based on the classification of the dream function theories (see Tables 1.4 and 11.4), one could argue that remembered dreams can stimulate creativity.

One group of dream function theories postulates that we practice skills in dreams that prepare us for the future (see Table 11.4); for example, coping with threats, the Threat Simulation Theory (Revonsuo, 2000b), practicing social skills, the Social Simulation Theory (Revonsuo et al., 2015), or skills in general, like it is the case in children's play (Bulkeley, 1993). In my view, there are some problems with these theories, especially if they are applied to non-remembered dreams (which is the large majority of dreams). The study (Schädlich et al., 2017) in which dart throwing was practiced in the lucid dream-state clearly indicated that skill levels were only improved if the practice in the dream was carried out in a systematic way; just dreaming about darts or the task was not helpful for improving the waking performance. Similarly, mental practice in waking – stressing again the parallel between mind-wandering and dreaming – only improves performance if the skill at hand is practiced diligently and repeatedly within the imagination; just worrying about the skill or upcoming competition isn't helpful (Driskell et al., 1994; Vealey, 2007). If I look at my dreams, the dream reports my participants reported, and dream reports in the literature, this form of systematic practice is not common in the typical non-lucid dream; I would even say completely absent. Another line of thinking is based on the high efficacy of the Imagery Rehearsal Therapy for treating nightmares (Krakow & Zadra, 2006, 2010). Nightmares that have lasted for decades can be reduced in their frequency or even vanish completely if the dreamer practices systematically imagining a successful coping strategy for the unpleasant nightmare scenario – even a single session with homework (practicing the new ending for two weeks once a day) can work wonders (Krakow et al., 1995; Lüth et al., 2021). This raises the question of why normal dreaming cannot fulfill the function of reducing nightmares, whereas a single session of a waking-life imagination can do the trick. The idea that nightmares help improve skills in dealing with threats is also not that convincing for me, as most nightmares end (with awakening) before the dreamer does anything that might help her or his cause. The only message the waking ego can learn from, for example, dreams of being chased is that running away (you can also term this as avoidance behavior) is not helpful. But, to my knowledge, this is not learned in the dream but – if suggested to the dreamer – has been applied in the waking state. In my experience as a dream group leader, I often found that dreams reflect the current status of the person's skills and understanding of the world. After putting the dream scenario in context with the current waking life (Schredl, 2015a), the skills training begins in the waking state by reflecting on the dream; for example, what would have helped me in that situation and so on. This personal observation would favor the theory that dreams reflect, sometimes very clearly and illustratively, what is going on, but dreaming is not mainly related to skills training. As I pointed out in Chapter 1.3, empirical testing of the simulation theories is currently not possible. Lastly, the question of why dreams simulate actions that are definitely not preparing us for the future – e.g., flying dreams, dreams about breaking the law (0.80% in this dream series; Schredl, 2021c), or other bizarre stuff – e.g., elevators that are not working properly (Schredl, 2020c) – is unanswered. These dreams are clearly not compatible with the simulation theories.

In my own experience, having remembered and recorded a large number of dreams and stimulated by the empathy theory of dreaming stating that dream sharing can increase empathy toward the dreamer and facilitate group bonding (Blagrove et al., 2019; Blagrove et al., 2021), I thought about whether dreaming – at least, the remembered dreams – have increased my own skills in empathy and, in a broader sense, my skills regarding Theory of Mind; this is, seeing the world from the perspective of another person. The basis for that argument is that dream experiences, including social interactions, can include experiences the dreamer never had in waking life; for example, experiencing the horror of war. This can help one to empathize with persons who live in war zones. Melanie Rosen (2022) went even further, suggesting that the bizarre and unusual dream experiences can increase empathy toward persons who have problems with cognition – e.g., persons with mental disorders like schizophrenia.

Although, there is some evidence that task-related dreams are correlated with higher increases in performance after sleep (Klepel & Schredl, 2019; Wamsley & Stickgold, 2019; Wamsley et al., 2010), a meta-analysis (Hudachek & Wamsley, 2023) indicated an overall strong association, but the findings are mixed regarding sleep stages; that is, in sleep lab studies, NREM dreams (N = 10 studies) showed an association with post-sleep performance improvement, but for REM dreams (N = 12 studies), the relationship was less clear. From a personal view, I can clearly state that my dreams were not related to any improvements in declarative memory (the memory type that is mainly consolidated in NREM sleep, preferentially in slow wave sleep). So, there was no replay of knowledge or vocabulary in dreams that enhanced my waking-life levels. But also other skills – for example, juggling (the circus-arts hobby) – didn't show up in such a way that I would say I learned something in the dream that improved my waking-life performance; intensive training in waking life was necessary to improve skills in juggling or unicycling. Second, Wamsley et al. (2010) reported that their task-related dreams included only indirect references to the task – for example, the music of the task – but she did not have dreams in which the dreamer was really practicing the maze task. As the lucid dream study of Schädlich et al. (2017) showed that only "real" practicing improves post-sleep performance levels, I agree with Wamsley (2014) that dreams can reflect sleep-dependent memory consolidation (one might even argue that the task-related dreams are recollections of the performing the task, thus explained by the continuity hypothesis) but do not play a crucial role in enhancing the neurophysiological processes that are involved in sleep-dependent memory consolidation.

The fourth group of theories deal with emotions (see Table 11.4). I can remember a dream in which real catharsis occurred. I had a major dispute with two colleagues of mine and dreamed that I really said to them what I think of them (words not repeated in this book), but afterwards, already within the dream and after waking up, the tension had subsided and, being calmer, I did not feel the urge to be verbally aggressive toward these colleagues. But I also remembered recurrent dreams in which the brakes of the car I was driving weren't working properly; I could not fully stop the car. These dreams increased my worries about driving in the waking state (as I am a very infrequent driver) but quickly subsided when I drove again in "real" life – as the brakes were functioning properly. Based on my experience, I would not agree to the theory of emotional regulation based on my dreams, but that might be idiosyncratic, as I also never experienced real

TABLE 11.4 Theories about dream functions

Theory	Arguments in favor and against
Creativity theories	Recalled dreams stimulate waking-life creativity.
Simulation theories	Non-lucid dreams do not include systematic training. Why practice skills that will never be used in waking life?
Memory theories	Dreaming can reflect sleep-dependent memory consolidation, but is not the driving force.
Emotion regulation theories	Dreams help us to regulate (negative) emotions.

nightmares (although it was postulated that nightmares indicate a failure of the mood regulation function).

A problem that bothers me in regard to the question of whether dreaming has an evolutionary function (see Chapter 1.3) is the fact that REM sleep is much older than our *Homo sapiens* species. Michel Jouvet (1979b) found that cats in which he experimentally disabled the REM atonia by brain stem lesions showed "oneiric behavior" during REM sleep, like grooming, chasing something. This suggests that cats might have some form of experiencing during REM sleep. Would these experiences (it would be difficult to call them dreams, as these experiences could never be reported) fulfill similar function(s) postulated for human dreaming? Furthermore, if one argues that only remembered dreams have a function, the question arises whether animals can recall their dream experiences. Given the aforementioned parallel between mind-wandering and dreaming: Do mammals mind-wander? These research question seems difficult to answer, even though a colleague of mine told me that a gorilla acted strangely upon awaking, as if he had experienced something completely different in his sleep.

Another idea that might be worth a look is that dreaming might have a skill-training function in children and adolescents that would fit in with the analogy between dreaming and play (Bulkeley, 2019), but dreaming in adulthood has lost this function.

To conclude the section about my personal view regarding dream function(s): I currently think that dreaming itself, defined as subjective experiences during sleep, do not have an extra function in addition to the functions of sleep, like memory consolidation. Dream experiences reflect what's going on in the mind, like a mirror. That is, unremembered dreams have no specific function; their existence indicates that especially we humans feature a brain that is capable of producing a whole-world experience, even without any input from the outside. Most evolutionists would agree that the human brain, with this extraordinary capacity of producing language, thoughts, emotions, images, etc., has provided humans the edge in the process of natural selection. In the case of dreaming, nature did not bother to turn this skill during sleep.

11.3 Recalled dreams have a function: stimulating creativity and problem solving

Research and anecdotes alike indicate that dreams that are remembered and reflected on in waking life can be very beneficial for the dreamer – e.g., providing creative impulses (Barrett, 2001; Horowitz et al., 2023; Schredl & Erlacher, 2007), providing insights – e.g., improving self-understanding (Hill & Goates, 2004; Malinowski, 2021a, 2021b) – and providing help regarding important decisions in life (Hoss & Gongloff, 2017; Olsen et al.,

2020). On the other hand, robust evidence of a possible function of non-remembered dreams is non-existent. Thus, the model proposed in this chapter focuses on a possible function of remembered dreams. Interestingly, the continuity hypothesis and the broader concept of the Continuity Discontinuity Creativity (CDC) theory, which focuses on explaining why we dream about specific topics and emotions, fits very well in this framework.

In the field of creative problem solving, a two-step process has been proposed (Harms et al., 2018; Isaksen & Gaulin, 2005). The first step is called brainstorming; during this phase, all ideas and associations were collected without evaluating whether they might fit or not fit the situation. The basic idea behind this is that unconstrained thought processes facilitate generating ideas that are unusual, new, and innovative. The second step includes the selection and evaluation process; each of the ideas produced in step 1 are evaluated as to whether they might offer a practical solution to the problem.

Transferring this well-established model to dreaming in order to outline a possible function of dreaming (see Table 11.5), one could argue that the first step of brainstorming is accomplished by dreaming. As can be seen throughout the book, dreams are very creative and, quite often, produce unusual or even bizarre ideas. On the other hand, dream content is not completely random; dreams reflect waking-life issues that are salient for the dreamer, and this adds to the benefit of the brainstorming process, as these ideas are related, in one way or another, with the problems at hand. In contrast to earlier problem-solving theories (e.g., Wright & Koulack, 1987), this theory suggests that the function of problem solving is only fulfilled if the waking consciousness applies the ideas provided by dreams to the actual problem. Thus, the problem solving does not (or only very rarely) take place in the dream itself. In this context, the study of Dement (1974) is interesting. He presented creative problems to a large number of students (they should work on these tasks during the 15 minutes prior to sleep and should record their dreams). One of the problems was as follows: "The letters O, T, T, F, F . . . form the beginning of an infinite sequence. Find a simple rule for determining any or all successive letters. According to your rule, what would be the next two letters of the sequence?" (p. 99). Overall, they collected 1,148 dreams, but only nine included the correct solution, and in two of those cases, the student said s/he had found the solution prior to sleep onset. The correct

TABLE 11.5 Dream function of recalled dreams: a two-step process of problem solving

Step	Provided by
Brainstorming – generating ideas	Dream consciousness
Evaluation process – what solutions are adequate, useful, beneficial	Waking consciousness getting input from remembered dreams

solution was: "The next two letters in the sequence are S, S. The letters represent the first letters used in spelling out the numerical sequence: One, Two, Three, Four, Five, Six, Seven etc." Overall, 87 dreams were related to the problem; thus, not a very strong continuity between the pre-sleep period and dream content, which is to be expected, as dreams can reflect all waking-life experiences of the previous day (and the near and distant past), especially the personally salient ones (Schredl, 2018b). Dement (1974) interpreted this finding that problem solving within a dream is extremely rare and might not be a function of dreaming. A very illustrative example regarding creativity in dreams was recorded by the dreamer:

Dream example:

> *Then I go to my room, throw my things on the table that I took from downstairs. In the process, I discover that I still have tools from my brother. I want to give it back to him soon, a hex wrench, 4 allen wrenches and a strange bottle opener. I have never seen anything like this before. The front part is a beer bottle opener. This part can be removed and a spiral for corks is revealed. At the bottom is a ring, so the cork can be turned on well straight. It is very well thought out and works magnificently. I can see the details clearly.*

After waking up, the dreamer realized that this bottle opener could not work in reality; thus, the dreamer thought in the dream that it was a wonderful innovation, but checking in reality indicated that it was not. This would fit in the proposed theory; an idea produced under unconstrained conditions must not be the solution to the waking-life problem. The proposed theory is supported by the research on dream-stimulated creativity and the beneficial effects of working with dreams (see introduction to this chapter).

However, the postulated model leaves a lot of questions unanswered. First, many researchers – e.g. Zadra and Stickgold (2021) – would argue against a theory focusing on remembered dreams, as most dreams are not recalled. A counterargument would be that we do not know how often our ancestors – for example, those who lived in Africa (early *Homo sapiens*) – recalled their dreams. One might speculate that 12 hrs/night (near the equator) and no artificial light sources might be conducive for high dream recall. On the other hand, one could argue that this beneficial effect of remembered dreams is a side effect or add-on effect but not the main reason why dreaming might be favored by natural selection. The underlying idea would be that dreaming might be a spandrel (having this capability of subjective experiences during waking was the driving force in evolution, and nature didn't bother to turn off subjective experiences during the night) but can still be beneficial for the person.

The summarize, the proposed model does not make any claims about possible functions of unremembered dreams, but rather, focuses on the beneficial effects of remembered dreams, which have been demonstrated and might be valid, even if dreaming itself didn't provide an edge in evolution.

11.4 Future directions

The material presented in the book offered some insights into the question of how dreaming works. As with science in general, every empirical study also raises new questions. The extensive analysis of this long dream series is no exception. One area of suggestions relates to future analyses of long dream series – to tap into their unique potential – and the other area concerns the advancement of dream research in general.

First, it would be very interesting to have similar in-depth analysis of other dream series in order to look at whether, for example, the finding that the frequency of schoolmate dreams did not decrease over time is specific for this dreamer or might point at a not-yet-understood factor that affects the continuity between waking and dreaming. During the book, some of the findings have been compared with empirical studies based on larger samples – e.g., emotional quality of partner and ex-partner dreams. Thus, these in-depth analyses of long dream series can lead to hypotheses that can be tested empirically in larger samples.

Regarding the present dream series, there are a lot of areas unexplored, especially the areas of dream emotions and work-related dreams. For studying dream emotions, it would have been helpful to have ratings of the dreamer's waking life emotions, but to the knowledge of the author, no long-term dream journalist has done such a sophisticated recording of her or his waking-life emotional status. Nevertheless, one might look at dream emotions during stressful periods, as has been done, for example, by Hartmann and Brezler (2008) studying dreams of US Americans after the terrorist attacks in 9/11/01.

A topic that came up while writing the book was the concept of blending (see Chapter 5.3); for example, a woman in the dream that is a composite of different partners. Why do dreams do that? Within this context, the concept of condensation (German: *Verdichtung*), formulated by Sigmund Freud (1900/1991), comes to mind. In his theory, condensation is at work when a single idea (an image, memory, or thought) or dream object stands for several associations related to waking life. But tracking these different associations has been done in waking, analyzing the dream. The blending instances in this series are already perceived as composites within the dream. It would be very interesting to study whether the blending of persons is also a relevant topic in dreams of other people.

Another interesting topic is the change of dream elements over time. As pointed out by Fosse et al. (2003) and Malinowski and Horton (2014b), complex waking-life situations are not replayed in dreams (in this dream series, that was very obvious for topics like money and pain), but often, it is a mixture of memories, even with a splash of creativity. While analyzing the dream series for this book, the author recognized that some dream elements were closer to real life at the beginning of the dream series and changed over time. An example would be the school building (the dreamer spent nine yrs in this building); in the beginning of the dream series, the building in the dream was more or less the building the dreamer knew from waking life, but over time, the school building had special features not present in real life – e.g., another proportion of the entrance hall. Studying this topic in more detail might be helpful to understand how memory sources were incorporated into dreams or, even on a more basic level, how human memory works (not like a hard drive on a computer, where the information is fixed, but like a neural network, where adding new experiences changes the old ones).

As pointed out in Chapter 3.2, it would be very beneficial, for studying the dream series empirically, if new statistical methods that were applicable to time series with gaps (fluctuating dream recall) and often-binary-outcome variables were developed. So far, only one approach for analyzing frequency changes in binary time series with gaps has been published (Klingenberg, 2008).

On a more general level, the analyses presented in this book clearly showed that a simple version of the continuity hypothesis is not sufficient to explain the large variability of dream content, especially the discontinuities and bizarre elements; for example, the question "Why do we dream that we can fly?" A first attempt to formulate a broader model – the CDC model – was undertaken. Concepts like emotional continuity and metaphorical expressions of basic patterns provide a wealth of suggestions for future empirical research.

The review – even though very comprehensive – on the empirical literature on possible dream functions indicates that dream research knows very little about one of the most fundamental questions; that is, "Why do we dream?" In the opinion of the author, this question can only be tackled in a systematic way if technology evolves in the future, especially "dream reading"; that is, using imagining techniques to predict dream content so one does not have to solely rely on dream reports (dream experiences remembered upon awakening). Experimental research would benefit from the method of "Inception," which was the basic storyline of the movie *Inception* (released in 2010) by Christopher Nolan. If one would be able to change dreams without the dreamer being aware of it, systematic studies of possible dream functions would be possible. These technologies, however, also raise ethical issues that should be discussed in the research community as well as in the general public (Carr et al., 2020).

Overall, dream research can help us to understand how consciousness works and hopefully answer the question about why we all dream every night in the near future.

12

EPILOGUE

Needless to say, this book was a lot of work. Recording, typing, and tagging 12,769 dreams was only the first step. Analyzing the different topics, including coding different aspects regarding these topics, was the second, also very labor-intensive, step. Lastly, the writing-up and relating the present findings with the current literature completed the project. Although the motivation had its ups and downs, especially regarding the third step, I still had fun in doing all this. At the end of the book, I would like to address the question "What did I learn about how dreaming works?"

Being a proponent of the continuity hypothesis of dreaming, the intensive analysis carried out and presented in this book made it very clear to me that continuity is not everything; the creativity of dreams has no proper place in this theoretical framework. This led to a first draft of the CDC theory, which hopefully stimulates future empirical research.

The re-reading of the literature on possible dream functions (with a lot of very recently published papers) and discussion with colleagues made it very clear how limited our understanding regarding the basic question "Why do we dream?" is. My conclusion, being a cautious person, was to focus on the function of remembered dreams and leave the question whether unremembered dreams had an evolutionary function to future researchers.

The intensive study of the dream series also made me aware of how limited our understanding about the interaction between brain and consciousness is. How are these two different domains related? How do they interact? How can the brain "produce" the whole-world experience of dreaming without any input from the outside? This question is not that different from the question of how the waking brain can "produce" the experience of a world based on a few sensory stimuli. Some researchers even say "magic factor" because

DOI: 10.4324/9781003300373-12

we don't know how the brain is "producing" the world of subjective experiences (therefore, I write "produce" in quotation marks). Despite knowing so little or just because of that, I am still fascinated by dreams. This fascination is on top of the personal meaning dreams do have for me, reflecting my psychological issues in very creative and illustrative ways.

To summarize, even though I am very relieved that the book project is complete, I will continue recording, typing, and analyzing my dream series, first, based on my personal motivation as a dreamer, as I am still fascinated by the creativity of dreaming and, second, based on my motivation as a researcher, as there are so many interesting and unanswered questions in the field of dreams.

REFERENCES

Alperstein, N. M., & Vann, B. H. (1997). Star gazing: A socio-cultural approach to the study of dreaming about media figures. *Communication Quarterly*, *45*, 142–152.

Arnulf, I., Grosliere, L., Le Corvec, T., Golmard, J.-L., Lascols, O., & Duguet, A. (2014). Will students pass a competitive exam that they failed in their dreams? *Consciousness and Cognition*, *29*, 36–47. https://doi.org/10.1016/j.concog.2014.06.010

Baird, B., Tononi, G., & LaBerge, S. (2022). Lucid dreaming occurs in activated rapid eye movement sleep, not a mixture of sleep and wakefulness. *Sleep*, *45*(4), zsab294. https://doi.org/10.1093/sleep/zsab294

Bakan, P. (1978). Two streams of consciousness: A typological approach. In K. S. Pope & J. L. Singer (Eds.), *The stream of consciousness* (pp. 159–184). Springer.

Barrett, D. (1991). Flying dreams and lucidity: An empirical study of their relationship. *Dreaming*, *1*, 129–134. http://dx.doi.org/10.1037/h0094325

Barrett, D. (2001). *The committee of sleep: How artists, scientists, and athletes use dreams for creative problem-solving–and how you can too.* Crown.

Bautista, J., Lawrence, J., Pass, K., & Hicks, R. A. (1992). The language of dreaming for college students who learned English as their second language. *Sleep Research*, *21*, 125.

Belicki, K., Gulko, N., Ruzycki, K., & Aristotle, J. (2003). Sixteen years of dreams following spousal bereavement. *OMEGA – Journal of Death and Dying*, *47*(2), 93–106. http://ome.sagepub.com/cgi/content/abstract/47/2/93

Bell, A. P., & Hall, C. S. (1971). *The personality of a child molester: An analysis of dreams.* Aldine-Atherton.

Bender, H., & Mischo, J. (1960). Präkognition in Traumserien: Dokumentation und Strukturanalyse sinnvoller Koinzidenzen im "Fall Gotenhafen" – Erster Teil. *Zeitschrift für Parapsychologie und Grenzgebiete der Psychologie*, *4*, 114–198.

Bender, H., & Mischo, J. (1961). Präkognition in Traumserien: Dokumentation und Strukturanalyse sinnvoller Koinzidenzen im "Fall Gotenhafen". *Zeitschrift für Parapsychologie und Grenzgebiete der Psychologie*, *5*, 10–47.

Bentley, M. (1915). The study of dreams. *American Journal of Psychology, 26,* 196–210.

Bergquist, P., & Warshaw, C. (2019). Does global warming increase public concern about climate change? *The Journal of Politics, 81*(2), 686–691. https://doi.org/10.1086/701766

Berman, L. E. (1985). Rearview-mirror dreams. *Psychoanalytic Inquiry, 5,* 257–269.

Berntsen, D., Rubin, D. C., & Siegler, I. C. (2011). Two versions of life: Emotionally negative and positive life events have different roles in the organization of life story and identity. *Emotion, 11*(5), 1190–1201. https://doi.org/10.1037/a0024940

Berres, S., & Erdfelder, E. (2021). The sleep benefit in episodic memory: An integrative review and a meta-analysis. *Psychological Bulletin, 147*(12), 1309–1353. https://doi.org/10.1037/bul0000350

Beuerle, F., & Schredl, M. (2017). Dreaming in Vienna: Analyzing dreams of Arthur Schnitzler and Sigmund Freud [Electronic]. *International Journal of Dream Research, 10*(2), 164–172. https://doi.org/10.11588/ijodr.2017.2.40686

Blagrove, M., Hale, S., Lockheart, J., Carr, M., Jones, A., & Valli, K. (2019). Testing the empathy theory of dreaming: The relationships between dream sharing and trait and state empathy. *Frontiers in Psychology, 10,* 1351. www.frontiersin.org/article/10.3389/fpsyg.2019.01351

Blagrove, M., Henley-Einion, J., Barnett, A., Edwards, D., & Seage, C. H. (2011). A replication of the 5–7 day dream-lag effect with comparison of dreams to future events as control for baseline matching. *Consciousness and Cognition, 20*(2), 384–391. https://doi.org/10.1016/j.concog.2010.07.006

Blagrove, M., Lockheart, J., Carr, M., Basra, S., Graham, H., Lewis, H., Murphy, E., Sakalauskaite, A., Trotman, C., & Valli, K. (2021). Dream sharing and the enhancement of empathy: Theoretical and applied implications. *Dreaming, 31*(2), 128–139. https://doi.org/10.1037/drm0000165

Bleske-Rechek, A., Somers, E., Micke, C., Erickson, L., Matteson, L., Stocco, C., Schumacher, B., & Ritchie, L. (2012). Benefit or burden? Attraction in cross-sex friendship. *Journal of Social and Personal Relationships, 29*(5), 569–596. https://doi.org/10.1177/0265407512443611

Bohlman, P. V. (2013). *The Cambridge history of world music.* Cambridge University Press. https://doi.org/10.1017/CHO9781139029476

Bortz, J. (1999). *Statistik für Sozialwissenschaftler.* Springer.

Botman, H. I., & Crovitz, H. F. (1989). Dream reports and autobiographical memory. *Imagination, Cognition and Personality, 9,* 213–224.

Bown, J., & Gackenbach, J. (2019). The influence of media understood through video game play. In R. J. Hoss & R. P. Gongloff (Eds.), *Dreams: Understanding biology, psychology, and culture* (Vol. 2, pp. 712–715). Greenwood.

Brush, L. C. (1993). A classification system for longitudinal analysis of dream patterns. *Dreaming, 3,* 33–48.

Bulkeley, K. (1993). Dreaming is play. *Psychoanalytic Psychology, 10,* 501–514.

Bulkeley, K. (2018). The meaningful continuities between dreaming and waking: Results of a blind analysis of a woman's 30-year dream journal. *Dreaming, 28*(4), 337–350. https://doi.org/10.1037/drm0000083

Bulkeley, K. (2019). Dreaming is imaginative play in sleep: A theory of the function of dreams. *Dreaming, 29*(1), 1–21. https://doi.org/10.1037/drm0000099

Calkins, M. W. (1893). Statistics of dream. *American Journal of Psychology, 5,* 311–343.

Capps, D., & Carlin, N. (2011). Sublimation and symbolization: The case of dental anxiety and the symbolic meaning of teeth. *Pastoral Psychology, 60*(6), 773–789. https://doi.org/10.1007/s11089-011-0368-1

Carlson, D. A. (1977). Dream mirrors. *Psychoanalytic Quarterly, 46,* 38–70.

Carr, M., Haar, A., Amores, J., Lopes, P., Bernal, G., Vega, T., Rosello, O., Jain, A., & Maes, P. (2020). Dream engineering: Simulating worlds through sensory stimulation. *Consciousness and Cognition, 83,* 102955. https://doi.org/10.1016/j.concog.2020.102955

Cartwright, R. D., Lloyd, S., Knight, S., & Trenholm, I. (1984). Broken dreams: A study of the effects of divorce and depression on dream content. *Psychiatry, 47,* 251–259.

Cohen, J. (1988). *Statistical power analysis for the behavioral sciences.* Lawrence Erlbaum.

Corriere, R., Hart, J., Karle, W., Jerry, B., Stephen, G., & Lee, W. (1977). Toward a new theory of dreaming. *Journal of Clinical Psychology, 33,* 807–820.

Crick, F., & Mitchison, G. (1983). The function of dream sleep. *Nature, 304,* 111–114.

Curci, A., & Rime, B. (2008). Dreams, emotions, and social sharing of dreams. *Cognition and Emotion, 22*(1), 155–167. https://doi.org/10.1080/02699930701274102

Davies, G. (2002). *A history of money.* University of Wales Press.

De Koninck, J., Christ, G., Rinfret, N., & Proulx, G. (1988). Dreams during language learning: When and how is the new language integrated. *Psychiatric Journal of the University of Ottawa, 13,* 72–74.

Dement, W. C. (1960). The effect of dream deprivation. *Science, 131,* 1705–1707.

Dement, W. C. (1974). *Some must watch while some must sleep.* W. H. Freeman.

Deserno, H., & Kächele, H. (2013). Traumserien – Ihre Verwendung in Psychotherapie und Therapieforschung. In B. Janta, B. Unruh, & S. Walz-Pawlita (Eds.), *Der Traum* (pp. 233–244). Psychosozial-Verlag.

Deutsches Klima-Konsortium. (2020). *Was wir heute übers Klima wissen: Basisfakten zum Klimawandel, die in der Wissenschaft unumstritten sind.* Retrieved January 11, 2021, from www.klimafakten.de/meldung/was-wir-heute-uebers-klima-wissen-basisfakten-zum-klimawandel-die-der-wissenschaft

Diekelmann, S., Wilhelm, I., & Born, J. (2009). The whats and whens of sleep-dependent memory consolidation. *Sleep Medicine Reviews, 13,* 309–321. https://doi.org/10.1016/j.smrv.2008.08.002

Domhoff, G. W. (1996). *Finding meaning in dreams: A quantitative approach.* Plenum Press.

Domhoff, G. W. (2003). *The scientific study of dreams: Neural networks, cognitive development and content analysis.* American Psychological Association.

Domhoff, G. W. (2015). Dreaming as embodied simulation: A widower's dreams of his deceased wife. *Dreaming, 25*(3), 232–256. https://doi.org/10.1037/a0039291

Domhoff, G. W. (2017a). The invasion of the concept snatchers: The origins, distortions, and future of the continuity hypothesis. *Dreaming, 27*(1), 14–39. https://doi.org/10.1037/drm0000047

Domhoff, G. W. (2017b). Now an invasion by a Freudian concept-snatcher: Reply to Erdelyi. *Dreaming, 27*(4), 345–350. https://doi.org/10.1037/drm0000068

Domhoff, G. W. (2018a). Can stimulus-incorporation and emotion-assimilation theorists revive the continuity hypothesis they deprived of cognitive meaning? A reply to Jenkins. *Dreaming, 28*(4), 356–359. https://doi.org/10.1037/drm0000091

Domhoff, G. W. (2018b). Dreaming is an intensified form of mind-wandering, based in an augmented portion of the default network. In K. C. R. Fox (Ed.), *The Oxford handbook of spontaneous thought: Mind-wandering, creativity, and dreaming* (pp. 355–370). Oxford University Press.

Domhoff, G. W. (2018c). *The emergence of dreaming: Mind-wandering, embodied simulation, and the default network*. Oxford University Press.

Domhoff, G. W. (2022). *The neurocognitive theory of dreaming: The where, how, when, what, and why of dreams*. MIT Press.

Domhoff, G. W., Meyer-Gomes, K., & Schredl, M. (2005–2006). Dreams as the expression of conceptions and concerns: A comparison of German and American college students. *Imagination, Cognition & Personality, 25*, 269–282.

Domhoff, G. W., & Schneider, A. (2008a). Similarities and differences in dream content at the cross-cultural, gender, and individual levels. *Consciousness and Cognition, 17*, 1257–1265.

Domhoff, G. W., & Schneider, A. (2008b). Studying dream content using the archive and search engine on DreamBank.net. *Consciousness and Cognition, 17*, 1238–1247.

Domhoff, G. W., & Schneider, A. (2015). Assessing autocorrelation in studies using the Hall and Van de Castle coding system to study individual dream series. *Dreaming, 25*(1), 70–79. https://doi.org/10.1037/a0038791

Dresler, M., Baird, B., Erlacher, D., Czisch, M., Spoormaker, V. I., & LaBerge, S. (2022). Lucid dreaming. In M. Kryger, T. Roth, & W. C. Dement (Eds.), *Principles and practice of sleep medicine* (6th ed., pp. 579–585). Elsevier.

Dresler, M., Wehrle, R., Spoormaker, V. I., Koch, S. P., Holsboer, F., Steiger, A., Obrig, H., Samann, P. G., & Czisch, M. (2012). Neural correlates of dream lucidity obtained from contrasting lucid versus non-lucid REM sleep: A combined EEG/fMRI case study. *Sleep, 35*, 1017–1020. https://doi.org/10.5665/sleep.1974

Driskell, J. E., Copper, C., & Moran, A. (1994). Does mental practice enhance performance? *Journal of Applied Psychology, 79*(4), 481–492. https://doi.org/10.1037/0021-9010.79.4.481

Edwards, C. L., Malinowski, J., Ruby, P. M., Bennett, P., McGee, S. L., & Blagrove, M. (2015). Comparing personal insight gains due to consideration of a recent dream and consideration of a recent event using the Ullman and Schredl dream group methods. *Frontiers in Psychology, 6*. https://doi.org/10.3389/fpsyg.2015.00831

Eeles, E., Pinsker, D., Burianova, H., & Ray, J. (2020). Dreams and the daydream retrieval hypothesis. *Dreaming, 30*(1), 68–78. https://doi.org/10.1037/drm0000123

Eisnitz, A. J. (1961). Mirror dreams. *Journal of the American Psychoanalytic Association, 9*, 461–479.

Ekeh, P. P. (1972). Examination dreams in Nigeria: A sociological study. *Psychiatry, 35*, 352–365.

Eldredge, J. H., Honeycutt, J. M., White, R. C., & Standige, M. (2015). On the functions of imagined interactions in night dreams. *Imagination, Cognition and Personality, 35*(3), 244–257. https://doi.org/10.1177/0276236615595231

Ellman, S. J., Spielman, A. J., Luck, D., Steiner, S. S., & Halperin, R. (1991). REM deprivation: A review. In S. J. Ellman & J. S. Antrobus (Eds.), *The mind in sleep – Psychology and psychophysiology* (pp. 327–376). John Wiley.

Erdelyi, M. H. (2017). The continuity hypothesis. *Dreaming, 27*(4), 334–344. https://doi.org/10.1037/drm0000063

Erlacher, D., Ehrlenspiel, F., & Schredl, M. (2011). Frequency of nightmares and gender significantly predict distressing dreams of German athletes before competitions or games. *Journal of Psychology, 145*, 331–342.

Erlacher, D., Furrer, V., Ineichen, M., Braillard, J., & Schmid, D. (2022). Combining wake-up-back-to-bed with cognitive induction techniques: Does earlier sleep interruption reduce lucid dream induction rate? *Clocks & Sleep, 4*(2), 230–239. https://doi.org/10.3390/clockssleep4020021

Erlacher, D., Schädlich, M., Stumbrys, T., & Schredl, M. (2014). Time for actions in lucid dreams: Effects of task modality, length, and complexity. *Frontiers in Psychology, 4*. https://doi.org/10.3389/fpsyg.2013.01013

Erlacher, D., Schmid, D., Schuler, S., & Rasch, B. (2020). Inducing lucid dreams by olfactory-cued reactivation of reality testing during early-morning sleep: A proof of concept. *Consciousness and Cognition, 83*, 102975. https://doi.org/10.1016/j.concog.2020.102975

Erlacher, D., & Schredl, M. (2010). Practicing a motor task in a lucid dream enhances subsequent performance: A pilot study. *Sport Psychologist, 24*, 157–167.

Erlacher, D., Schredl, M., & LaBerge, S. (2003). Motor area activation during dreamed hand clenching: A pilot study on EEG alpha band. *Sleep and Hypnosis, 5*, 182–187.

Faraday, A. (1976). *The dream game: Discover yourself through your dreams.* Penguin Books. http://gateway-bayern.de/BV042401405

Faraday, A. (1985). *Deine Träume – Schlüssel zur Selbsterkenntnis (Org.: The dreamgame 1974)* Fischer Taschenbuch.

Fazekas, P., & Nemeth, G. (2020). Dreaming, mind-wandering, and hypnotic dreams [perspective]. *Frontiers in Neurology, 11*(1203). https://doi.org/10.3389/fneur.2020.565673

Feigelson, C. (1975). The mirror dream. *Psychoanalytic Study of the Child, 30*, 341–355.

Fierz, M. (1987). Die Traumserie des Girolane Cardano aus dem Jahr 1561. *Analytische Psychologie, 18*, 235–265.

Fisher, C. (1966). Dreaming and sexuality. In R. M. Loewenstein, L. M. Newman, M. Schur, & A. J. Solnit (Eds.), *Psychoanalysis – A general psychology* (pp. 537–569). International Universities Press.

Fleming, S. (2012). Review of 'Inception'. *Journal of Feminist Family Therapy: An International Forum, 24*(2), 165–166. https://doi.org/10.1080/08952833.2012.648128

Fosse, M. J., Fosse, R., Hobson, J. A., & Stickgold, R. J. (2003). Dreaming and episodic memory: A functional dissociation? *Journal of Cognitive Neuroscience, 15*, 1–9.

Foulkes, D. (1962). Dream reports from different stages of sleep. *Journal of Abnormal and Social Psychology, 65*, 14–25.

Foulkes, D. (1982). *Children's dreams: Longitudinal studies.* John Wiley and Sons.

Foulkes, D., Meier, B., Strauch, I., Kerr, N., Bradley, L., & Hollifield, M. (1993). Linguistic phenomena and language selection in the REM dreams of German-English bilinguals. *International Journal of Psychology, 28*, 871–891.

Fox, K. C. R. (2018). Neural correlates of self-generated imagery and cognition throughout the sleep cycle. In K. C. R. Fox (Ed.), *The Oxford handbook of spontaneous thought: Mind-wandering, creativity, and dreaming* (pp. 371–384). Oxford University Press.

Freud, S. (1900/1991). *The interpretation of dreams (Org.: Die Traumdeutung).* Penguin Books.

Fromm, E. (1980). *Märchen, Mythen, Träume (The forgotten language 1951).* Bertelsmann.

Funkhouser, A. T., & Schredl, M. (2010). The frequency of déjà vu (déjà rêve) and the effects of age, dream recall frequency and personality factors. *International Journal of Dream Research, 3*, 60–64.

Gabryś-Barker, D. (2015). What the languages of our dreams tell us about our multilinguality. In E. Piechurska-Kuciel & M. Szyszka (Eds.), *The ecosystem of the foreign language learner, second language learning and teaching* (pp. 3–17). Springer International Publishing. https://doi.org/10.1007/978-3-319-14334-7_1

Gackenbach, J., & Bown, J. (2019). The effects of media on dreaming. In K. Valli & R. J. Hoss (Eds.), *Dreams: Understanding biology, psychology, and culture* (Vol. 1, pp. 219–224). Greenwood.

Gackenbach, J., & Gahr, S. (2015). Media use and dream associations between Canadians of differing cultural backgrounds. *International Journal of Dream Research, 8*(1), 2–9. https://doi.org/10.11588/ijodr.2015.1.15857

Gackenbach, J., Rosie, M., Bown, J., & Sample, T. (2011). Dream incorporation of video-game play as a function of interactivity and fidelity. *Dreaming, 21*(1), 32–50. https://doi.org/10.1037/a0022868

Gackenbach, J., Sample, T., Mandel, G., & Tomashewsky, M. (2011). Dream and blog content analysis of a long term diary of a video game player with obsessive compulsive disorder. *Dreaming, 21*(2), 124–147. https://doi.org/10.1037/a0023058

Gahagan, L. (1936). Sex differences in recall of stereotyped dreams, sleep-talking and sleep-walking. *Pedical Seminary and Journal of Genetic Psychology, 48*, 227–236.

Garcia, C. (2000). *Differences in dreams in a bilingual college population* [Master thesis]. https://scholarworks.sjsu.edu

Garfield, P. L. (1973). Keeping a longitudinal dream record. *Psychotherapy: Theory, Research and Practice, 10*, 223–228.

Garfield, P. L. (1974). *Creative dreaming.* Simon and Schuster.

Garfield, P. L. (1976). Dream content – Does it reflect changes in self-concept? *Sleep Research, 5*, 136.

Garfield, P. L. (2001). *The universal dream key: The twelve most common dream themes around the world.* Cliff Street Books.

Gastaut, H., & Broughton, R. (1964). A clinical and polygraphic study of episodic phenomena during sleep. *Recent Advances in Biological Psychiatry, 7*, 197–221.

Gazzaniga, M. S., Ivry, R., & Mangun, G. R. (2019). *Cognitive neuroscience: The biology of the mind.* W.W. Norton & Company. http://gateway-bayern.de/BV046272051

Geißler, C., & Schredl, M. (2020). College students' erotic dreams: Analysis of content and emotional tone. *Sexologies, 29*(1), e11–e17. https://doi.org/10.1016/j.sexol.2019.08.003

Geoffroy, P. A., & Palagini, L. (2021). Biological rhythms and chronotherapeutics in depression. *Progress in Neuro-Psychopharmacology and Biological Psychiatry*, *106*, 110158. https://doi.org/10.1016/j.pnpbp.2020.110158

Gerne, M. (1987). *Problemlösung im Traum am Beispiel der Trauerverarbeitung* [Dissertation an der Philosophischen Fakultät].

Ghorayeb, I., Napias, A., Denechere, E., & Mayo, W. (2019). Validation of the French version of the Mannheim Dream Questionnaire in a French adult sample. *International Journal of Dream Research*, *12*(2), 23–34. https://doi.org/10.11588/ijodr.2019.2.61611

Giguere, B., & LaBerge, S. (1995). To touch a dream: An experiment in touch, pain, and pleasure. *NightLight: Lucitity Institute Newsletter*, *7*(1), 1–6, 11.

Goblot, E. (1896). Le souvenir des rêves. *Revue Philosophique de la France et de l'étranger*, *42*, 288–290. www.jstor.org/stable/41079842

Gottfried, J. A. (2006). Smell: Central nervous processing. *Advances in Oto-Rhino-Laryngology*, *63*, 44–69. https://doi.org/10.1159/000093750

Graf, D., Schredl, M., & Göritz, A. S. (2021). Frequency and motives of sharing dreams: Personality correlates. *Personality and Individual Differences*, *175*, 110699. https://doi.org/10.1016/j.paid.2021.110699

Griffith, R. M., Miyagi, O., & Tago, A. (1958). The universality of typical dreams: Japanese vs. Americans. *American Anthropologist*, *60*, 1173–1179. https://doi.org/10.1525/aa.1958.60.6.02a00110

Guénolé, F., & Nicolas, A. (2010). Le rêve est un état hypnique de la conscience: pour en finir avec l'hypothèse de Goblot et ses avatars contemporains. *Neurophysiologie Clinique/Clinical Neurophysiology*, *40*(4), 193–199. https://doi.org/10.1016/j.neucli.2010.04.001

Güll, R. (2015). Vom Fräulein vom Amt zum Handy (From female operators to cell phones). *Statistisches Monatsheft Baden-Württemberg*, (3), 45–48.

Hacker, F. (1911). Systematische Traumbeobachtungen unter der besonderen Berücksichtigung der Gedanken. *Archiv für Die Gesamte Psychologie*, *21*, 1–130.

Hall, C. S. (1947). Diagnosting personality by the analysis of dreams. *Journal of Abnormal and Social Psychology*, *42*, 68–79.

Hall, C. S. (1948). Frequencies in certain categories of manifest content and their stability in long dream series. *American Psychologist*, *3*, 274.

Hall, C. S. (1967). Representation of the laboratory setting in dreams. *Journal of Nervous and Mental Disease*, *144*, 198–206.

Hall, C. S. (1981). Do we dream during sleep? Evidence for the Goblot hypothesis. *Perceptual and Motor Skills*, *53*, 239–246.

Hall, C. S. (1984). "A ubiquitous sex difference in dreams" revisited. *Journal of Personality and Social Psychology*, *46*, 1109–1117.

Hall, C. S., & Domhoff, B. J. (1963). Aggression in dreams. *International Journal of Social Psychiatry*, *9*, 259–267. https://doi.org/10.1177/002076406300900403

Hall, C. S., & Domhoff, B. J. (1968). The dreams of Freud and Jung. *Psychology Today*, 42–45, 64–65.

Hall, C. S., Domhoff, G. W., Blick, K. A., & Weesner, K. E. (1982). The dreams of college men and women in 1959 and 1980: A comparison of dream contents and sex differences. *Sleep*, *5*, 188–194. https://doi.org/10.1093/sleep/5.2.188

Hall, C. S., & Nordby, V. J. (1972). *The individual and his dreams*. New American Library.

Hall, C. S., & Van de Castle, R. L. (1966). *The content analysis of dreams.* Appleton-Century-Crofts.

Han, H. J., & Schweickert, R. (2016). Continuity: Knowing each other, emotional closeness, and appearing together in dreams. *Dreaming, 26*(4), 299–307. https://doi.org/10.1037/drm0000038

Han, H. J., Schweickert, R., Xi, Z., & Viau-Quesnel, C. (2016). The cognitive social network in dreams: Transitivity, assortativity, and giant component proportion are monotonic. *Cognitive Science, 40*(3), 671–696. https://doi.org/10.1111/cogs.12244

Harms, M., Kennel, V., & Reiter-Palmon, R. (2018). Team creativity: Cognitive processes underlying problem solving. In R. Reiter-Palmon (Ed.), *Team creativity and innovation.* (pp. 61–86). Oxford University Press.

Harris, J. C. (2010). The red book: Liber novus. *Archives of General Psychiatry, 67*(6), 554–556. https://doi.org/10.1001/archgenpsychiatry.2010.68

Hartmann, E. (1991). *Boundaries in the mind.* Basic Books.

Hartmann, E. (1996). We do not dream of the three "R"s: A study and its implications. *Sleep Research, 25,* 136.

Hartmann, E. (2000). We do not dream of the 3 R's: Implications for the nature of dream mentation. *Dreaming, 10,* 103–110. https://doi.org/10.1023/A:1009400805830

Hartmann, E. (2007). The nature and functions of dreaming. In D. Barrett & P. McNamara (Eds.), *The new science of dreaming – Volume 3: Cultural and theoretical perspectives* (pp. 171–192). Praeger.

Hartmann, E. (2011). *The nature and functions of dreaming.* Oxford University Press.

Hartmann, E., & Brezler, T. (2008). A systematic change in dreams after 9/11/01. *Sleep, 31,* 213–218.

Hearne, K. M. T. (1978). *Lucid dreams: An electrophysiological and psychological study* [Doctoral dissertation].

Herman, J. H., Taylor, M. E., Furman, B., & Roffwarg, H. P. (1979). The influence of tunnel vision goggles on dream content. *Sleep Research, 8,* 161.

Hess, G., Schredl, M., Gierens, A., & Domes, G. (2020). Effects of nightmares on the cortisol awakening response: An ambulatory assessment pilot study. *Psychoneuroendocrinology, 122,* 104900. https://doi.org/10.1016/j.psyneuen.2020.104900

Hess, G., Schredl, M., & Goritz, A. S. (2017). Lucid dreaming frequency and the Big Five personality factors. *Imagination, Cognition and Personality, 36*(3), 240–253. https://doi.org/10.1177/0276236616648653

Hill, C. E., & Goates, M. K. (2004). Research on the Hill cognitive-experiential dream model. In C. E. Hill (Ed.), *Dream work in therapy: Facilitating exploration, insight, and action* (pp. 245–288). American Psychological Association.

Hitschmann, E. (1931). Wandlungen der Traumsymbolik beim Fortschritt der Behandlung. *Internationale Zeitschrift für Psychoanalyse, 17,* 140–142.

Hobson, J. A. (2009). REM sleep and dreaming: Towards a theory of protoconsciousness. *Nature Reviews Neuroscience, 10*(11), 803–813. https://doi.org/10.1038/nrn2716

Hobson, J. A., & McCarley, R. W. (1977). The brain as a dream state generator: An activation-synthesis hypothesis of the dream process. *American Journal of Psychiatry, 134,* 1335–1348.

Hobson, J. A., Pace-Schott, E. F., & Stickgold, R. (2000). Dreaming and the brain: Toward a cognitive neuroscience of conscious states. *Behavioral and Brain Sciences, 23,* 793–842.

Hobson, J. A., & Schredl, M. (2011). The continuity and discontinuity between waking and dreaming: A dialogue between Michael Schredl and Allan Hobson concerning the adequacy and completeness of these notions. *International Journal of Dream Research*, *4*, 3–7. https://doi.org/10.11588/ijodr.2011.1.9087

Hoche, A. (1927). *Das träumende Ich*. Gustav Fischer.

Hoel, E. (2021). The overfitted brain: Dreams evolved to assist generalization. *Patterns*, *2*(5), 100244. https://doi.org/10.1016/j.patter.2021.100244

Hong, C. C., Jin, Y., Potkin, S. G., Buchsbaum, M., Wu, J. C., Callagham, G., Nudleman, K., & Gillin, J. C. (1996). Language in dreaming and regional EEG alpha power. *Sleep*, *19*, 232–235.

Horikawa, T., Tamaki, M., Miyawaki, Y., & Kamitani, Y. (2013). Neural decoding of visual imagery during sleep. *Science*, *340*(6132), 639–642. https://doi.org/10.1126/science.1234330

Horowitz, A. H., Esfahany, K., Gálvez, T. V., Maes, P., & Stickgold, R. (2023). Targeted dream incubation at sleep onset increases post-sleep creative performance. *Scientific Reports*, *13*(1), 7319. https://doi.org/10.1038/s41598-023-31361-w

Hoss, R. J. (2010). Content analysis of the potential significance of color in dreams: A preliminary investigation. *International Journal of Dream Research*, *3*, 80–90.

Hoss, R. J. (2020). Trauma and PTSD nightmare content. In J. F. Pagel (Ed.), *Parasomnia dreaming: Exploring other forms of sleep consciousness* (pp. 111–174). Nova Science.

Hoss, R. J., & Gongloff, R. P. (2017). *Dreams that change our lives*. Chiron Publications.

Howell, T. J., & Bennett, P. C. (2011). Can dogs (Canis familiaris) use a mirror to solve a problem? *Journal of Veterinary Behavior: Clinical Applications and Research*, *6*(6), 306–312. https://doi.org/10.1016/j.jveb.2011.03.002

Hudachek, L., & Wamsley, E. J. (2023). A meta-analysis of the relation between dream content and memory consolidation. *Sleep*, zsad111. https://doi.org/10.1093/sleep/zsad111

Husband, R. W. (1936). Sex differences in dream contents. *Journal of Abnormal and Social Psychology*, *30*, 513–521.

Ibanez, A. M., Martin, R. S., Hurtado, E., & Lopez, V. (2009). ERPs studies of cognitive processing during sleep. *International Journal of Psychology*, *44*(4), 290–304. https://doi.org/10.1080/00207590802194234

Idir, Y., Oudiette, D., & Arnulf, I. (2022). Sleepwalking, sleep terrors, sexsomnia and other disorders of arousal: The old and the new. *Journal of Sleep Research*, e13596. https://doi.org/10.1111/jsr.13596

Isaksen, S. G., & Gaulin, J. P. (2005). A reexamination of brainstorming research: Implications for research and practice. *Gifted Child Quarterly*, *49*(4), 315–329. https://doi.org/10.1177/001698620504900405

Jenkins, D. (2018). When is a continuity hypothesis not a continuity hypothesis? Why continuity is now a problematic name for a continuity hypothesis. *Dreaming*, *28*(4), 351–355. https://doi.org/10.1037/drm0000089

Jouvet, M. (1979a). Memoires et "cerveau dedoube" au cours du reve: A propos de 2525 souvenirs de reve. *Revue du Practicien*, *29*, 29–32.

Jouvet, M. (1979b). What does a cat dream about? *Trends in Neurosciences*, *2*, 280–282. https://doi.org/10.1016/0166-2236(79)90110-3

Jouvet, M. (1994). *Die Nachtseite des Bewußtseins – Warum wir träumen*. Rowohlt.

Jouvet, M. (1999). *The paradox of sleep – The story of dreaming*. MIT Press.

Jung, C. G. (1979). Allgemeine Gesichtspunkte zur Psychologie des Traumes. In C. G. Jung (Ed.), *Gesammelte Werke Band 8: Die Dynamik des Unbewußten* (pp. 268–308). Walter.

Jung, C. G., & Jaffé, A. (1967). *Erinnerungen, Träume, Gedanken*. Rascher. http://gateway-bayern.de/BV000921427

Junger, G. (1955). Der Traumrhythmus: Ergebnisse einer statistischen Untersuchung. *Schweizerische Zeitschrift fur Psychologie und Ihre Anwendungen, 14*, 297–308.

Kahan, T. L. (2012). Cognitive expertise and dreams. In D. Barrett & P. McNamara (Eds.), *Encyclopedia of sleep and dreams: The evolution, function, nature, and mysteries of slumber* (pp. 135–139). Greenwood.

Kahan, T. L., & Sullivan, K. T. (2012). Assessing metacognitive skills in waking and sleep: A psychometric analysis of the Metacognitive, Affective, Cognitive Experience (MACE) questionnaire. *Consciousness and Cognition, 21*, 340–352. https://doi.org/10.1016/j.concog.2010.09.002

Kern, S., Auer, A., Gutsche, M., Otto, A., Preuß, K., & Schredl, M. (2014). Relation between waking politic, music and sports related tasks and dream content in students of politics and psychology students. *International Journal of Dream Research, 7*, 80–84. https://doi.org/10.11588/ijodr.2014.1.13124

Kinsey, A. C. (1953). *Sexual behavior in the human female*. Saunders.

Kinsey, A. C., Pomeroy, W. B., & Martin, C. E. (1948). *Sexual behavior in the human male* (11. print. ed.). Saunders.

Kipphardt, H. (1986). *Traumprotokolle*. Rororo Taschenbuch.

Kirtley, D. D., & Hall, C. S. (1975). Prospero: A study of personality through dreams. In D. D. Kirtley (Ed.), *The psychology of blindness* (pp. 221–298). Nelson-Hall.

Klepel, F., & Schredl, M. (2019). Correlation of task-related dream content with memory performance of a film task – A pilot study. *International Journal of Dream Research, 12*(1), 112–118. https://doi.org/10.11588/ijodr.2019.1.59320

Klepel, F., Schredl, M., & Göritz, A. S. (2019). Dreams stimulate waking-life creativity and problem solving: Effects of personality traits. *International Journal of Dream Research, 12*(1), 95–102.

Klingenberg, B. (2008). Regression models for binary time series with gaps. *Computational Statistics and Data Analysis, 52*(8), 4076–4090. https://doi.org/10.1016/j.csda.2008.01.019

Knight, C., Studdert-Kennedy, M., & Hurford, J. R. (2000). *The evolutionary emergence of language: Social function and the origins of linguistic form*. Cambridge University Press.

Knoth, I. S., & Schredl, M. (2011). Physical pain, mental pain and malaise in dreams. *International Journal of Dream Research, 4*, 17–23. https://doi.org/10.11588/ijodr.2011.1.9074

Köhler, P. (1912). Beiträge zur systematischen Traumbeobachtung. *Archiv fur Die Gesamte Psychologie, 23*, 415–483.

König, N., Fischer, N., Friedemann, M., Pfeiffer, T., Göritz, A. S., & Schredl, M. (2018). Music in dreams and music in waking: An online study. *Psychomusicology: Music, Mind, and Brain, 28*(2), 65–70. https://doi.org/10.1037/pmu0000208

König, N., Heizmann, L. M., Göritz, A. S., & Schredl, M. (2017). Colors in dreams and the introduction of color TV in Germany: An online study. *International Journal of Dream Research, 10*, 59–64. https://doi.org/10.11588/ijodr.2017.1.34577

König, N., & Schredl, M. (2021). Music in dreams: A diary study. *Psychology of Music*, *49*(3), 351–359. https://doi.org/10.1177/0305735619854533

Köthe, M., & Pietrowsky, R. (2001). Behavioral effects of nightmares and their correlations to personality patterns. *Dreaming*, *11*, 43–52.

Koulack, D. (1969). Effects of somatosensory stimulation on dream content. *Archives of General Psychiatry*, *20*, 718–725.

Kraepelin, E. (1906). *Über Sprachstörungen im Traum*. Wilhelm Engelmann.

Kraepelin, E. (1910). Über Sprachstörungen im Traum. *Psychologische Arbeiten (Leipzig)*, *5*, 1–104.

Krakow, B., Kellner, R., Pathak, D., & Lambert, L. (1995). Imagery rehearsal treatment for chronic nightmares. *Behavior Research and Therapy*, *33*, 837–843.

Krakow, B., & Zadra, A. L. (2006). Clinical management of chronic nightmares: Imagery rehearsal therapy. *Behavioral Sleep Medicine*, *4*, 45–70.

Krakow, B., & Zadra, A. L. (2010). Imagery rehearsal therapy: Principles and practice. *Sleep Medicine Clinics*, *5*, 289–298. https://doi.org/10.1016/j.jsmc.2010.01.004

Kramer, M. (2007). *The dream experience: A systematic exploration*. Routledge.

Kramer, M., & Glucksman, M. L. (2006). Changes in manifest dream affect during psychoanalytic treatment. *Journal of the American Academy of Psychoanalysis & Dynamic Psychiatry*, *34*, 249–260.

Kramer, M., & Roth, T. (1979). The stability and variability of dreaming. *Sleep*, *1*, 319–325.

Krone, L. B., & Vyazovskiy, V. V. (2019). The function of sleep. In K. Valli & R. J. Hoss (Eds.), *Dreams: Understanding biology, psychology, and culture* (Vol. 1, pp. 42–54). Greenwood.

Kunzendorf, R. G., Hartmann, E., Cohen, R., & Cutler, J. (1997). Bizarreness of the dreams and daydreams reported by individuals with thin and thick boundaries. *Dreaming*, *7*, 265–271.

LaBerge, S. (1989). Welcome to the world of lucid dreaming. *NightLight: Lucitity Institute Newsletter*, *1*(1), 1–2.

LaBerge, S. P. (1980a). Lucid dreaming as a learnable skill: A case study. *Perceptual and Motor Skills*, *51*, 1039–1042.

LaBerge, S. P. (1980b). *Lucid dreaming: An exploratory study of consciousness during sleep* [Doctoral dissertation].

LaBerge, S. P. (1985). *Lucid dreaming*. Jeremy P. Tarcher.

Lal, S., & Whorwell, P. J. (2002). What do patients with irritable bowel syndrome dream about? A comparison with inflammatory bowel disease. *Digestive and Liver Disease*, *34*, 506–509.

Lambrecht, S., Schredl, M., Henley-Einion, J., & Blagrove, M. (2013). Self-rated effects of reading, TV viewing and daily activities on dreaming in adolescents and adults: The UK library study. *International Journal of Dream Research*, *6*, 41–44. https://doi.org/10.11588/ijodr.2013.1.9724

Lange, B. P., Wühr, P., & Schwarz, S. (2021). Of time gals and mega men: Empirical findings on gender differences in digital game genre preferences and the accuracy of respective gender stereotypes. *Frontiers in Psychology*, *12*, 1–12. https://doi.org/10.3389/fpsyg.2021.657430

Lehmiller, J. J. (2018). *The psychology of human sexuality*. Wiley Blackwell.

Leischner, A. (1965). Über Träume in fremden Sprachen bei Gesunden und Aphasischen. *Neuropsychologia*, *3*, 191–204.

Levitan, L., & LaBerge, S. (1993). Through the glass lightly: Testing the limits of dream control – The light and mirror experiment. *NightLight: Lucidity Institute Newsletter, 5*(2), 5–10.

Liljeström, S., Juslin, P. N., & Västfjäll, D. (2013). Experimental evidence of the roles of music choice, social context, and listener personality in emotional reactions to music. *Psychology of Music, 41*(5), 579–599. https://doi.org/10.1177/0305735612440615

Lindorff, D. (1995). One thousand dreams: The spiritual awakening of Wolfgang Pauli. *Journal of Analytical Psychology, 40*, 555–569.

Lortie-Lussier, M., Cote, L., & Vachon, J. (2000). The consistency and continuity hypothesis revisited through the dreams of women at two periods of their lives. *Dreaming, 10*, 67–76.

Lüth, K., Schmitt, J., & Schredl, M. (2021). Conquering nightmares on the phone: One-session counseling using imagery rehearsal therapy. *Somnologie, 25*(3), 197–204. https://doi.org/10.1007/s11818-021-00320-w

Maeder, A. (1912). Über die Funktion des Traumes. *Jahrbuch für Psychoanalytische und Psychopathologische Forschungen, 4*, 692–702.

Mageo, J. M. (2021). Defining new directions in the anthropology of dreaming. In J. M. Mageo & R. E. Sheriff (Eds.), *New directions in the anthropology of dreaming* (pp. 3–22). Routledge.

Maggiolini, A., Cagnin, C., Crippa, F., Persico, A., & Rizzi, P. (2010). Content analysis of dreams and waking narratives. *Dreaming, 20*, 60–76. https://doi.org/10.1037/a0018824

Malinowski, J. E. (2021a). Insight from dream and event discussions using the Schredl method of dreamwork in experienced and inexperienced dreamworkers. *International Journal of Dream Research, 14*(1), 52–60. https://doi.org/10.11588/ijodr.2021.1.75451

Malinowski, J. E. (2021b). *The psychology of dreaming*. Routledge.

Malinowski, J. E., & Horton, C. L. (2014a). Evidence for the preferential incorporation of emotional waking-life experiences into dreams. *Dreaming, 24*(1), 18–31. https://doi.org/10.1037/a0036017

Malinowski, J. E., & Horton, C. L. (2014b). Memory sources of dreams: The incorporation of autobiographical rather than episodic experiences. *Journal of Sleep Research, 23*, 441–447. https://doi.org/10.1111/jsr.12134

Malinowski, J. E., & Horton, C. L. (2015). Metaphor and hyperassociativity: The imagination mechanisms behind emotion assimilation in sleep and dreaming. *Frontiers in Psychology, 6*, 1132. https://doi.org/10.3389/fpsyg.2015.01132

Malinowski, J. E., & Horton, C. L. (2021). Dreams reflect nocturnal cognitive processes: Early-night dreams are more continuous with waking life, and late-night dreams are more emotional and hyperassociative. *Consciousness and Cognition, 88*, 103071. https://doi.org/10.1016/j.concog.2020.103071

Mallett, R., Carr, M., Freegard, M., Konkoly, K., Bradshaw, C., & Schredl, M. (2021). Exploring the range of reported dream lucidity. *Philosophy and the Mind Sciences, 2*, 1–23. https://doi.org/10.33735/phimisci.2021.63

Maquet, P., Peters, J.-M., Aerts, J., Delfiore, G., Deguelde, C., Luxen, A., & Franck, G. (1996). Functional neuroanatomy of human rapid-eye-movement sleep and dreaming. *Nature, 383*, 163–166.

Mashour, G. A. (2011). Dreaming during anesthesia and sedation. *Anesthesia and Analgesia, 112*(5), 1008–1010. http://ovidsp.ovid.com/ovidweb.cgi?

T=JS&CSC=Y&NEWS=N&PAGE=fulltext&D=ovftl&AN=000005
39-201105000-00004

Mathes, J., & Schredl, M. (2013). Gender differences in dream content: Are they related to personality? *International Journal of Dream Research*, 6, 104–109. https://doi.org/10.11588/ijodr.2013.2.10954

Mathes, J., & Schredl, M. (2014). Analyzing a large sample of diary dreams – How typical are typical dreams? *Somnologie*, 18, 107–112. https://doi.org/10.1007/s11818-013-0653-6

Mathes, J., Schredl, M., & Göritz, A. S. (2014). Frequency of typical dream themes in most recent dreams: An online study. *Dreaming*, 24(1), 57–66. https://doi.org/10.1037/a0035857

Mathes, J., Schuffelen, J., Gieselmann, A., & Pietrowsky, R. (2022). Nightmare distress is related to traumatic childhood experiences, critical life events and emotional appraisal of a dream rather than to its content. *Journal of Sleep Research*, e13779. https://doi.org/10.1111/jsr.13779

Matthews, M. L. (2016). Dreams: Fifty years and counting. *Psychological Perspectives*, 59(3), 365–375. www.redi-bw.de/db/ebsco.php/search.ebscohost.com/login. aspx%3fdirect%3dtrue%26db%3dpsyh%26AN%3d2016-44047-006%26site% 3dehost-live

Maury, A. (1861). *Le sommeil et les reves*. Didier.

McCarley, R. W., & Hoffman, E. (1981). REM sleep dreams and the activation-synthesis hypothesis. *American Journal of Psychiatry*, 138, 904–912.

McCutcheon, L., Shabahang, R., Williams, J., Aruguete, M., & Huynh, H. (2021). Dreaming about favorite celebrities in two different cultures. *International Journal of Dream Research*, 14(1). https://doi.org/10.11588/ijodr.2021.1.76309

McNamara, P., Pae, V., Teed, B., Tripodis, Y., & Sebastian, A. (2016). Longitudinal studies of gender differences in cognitional process in dream content. *International Journal of Dream Research*, 9, 40–45. https://doi.org/10.11588/ijodr.2016.1.26552

Mediano, M., Montoro, P. R., Contreras, M. J., & Mayas, J. (2022). Assessment of a Spanish version of the Mannheim Dream questionnaire (MADRE) in a young adult Spanish sample. *International Journal of Dream Research*, 15(2), 184–197. https://doi.org/10.11588/ijodr.2022.2.84172

Meier, B. (1993). Speech and thinking in dream. In C. Cavallero & D. Foulkes (Eds.), *Dreaming as cognition* (pp. 58–76). Harvester Wheatsheaf.

Merei, F. (1965). Our interpersonal relations in the manifest dream content. *Pszichologiai Tanulmanyok*, 8, 49–70.

Merei, F. (1994). Social relationships in manifest dream content. *Journal of Russian and East European Psychology*, 32, 46–68.

Middleton, W. C. (1933). Nocturnal dreams. *Scientific Monthly*, 37, 460–464.

Middleton, W. C. (1942). The frequency with which a group of unselected college students experiences colored dreaming and colored hearing. *Journal of General Psychology*, 27, 221–229.

Morley, I. (2013). *The prehistory of music: Human evolution, archeology and the origins of musicality*. Oxford University Press.

Moverley, M., Schredl, M., & Göritz, A. S. (2018). Media dreaming and media consumption – An online study. *International Journal of Dream Research*, 11(2), 127–134. https://doi.org/10.11588/ijodr.2018.2.46416

Myers, W. A. (1976). Imagery companions, fantasy twins, mirror dreams and depersonalization. *Psychoanalytic Quarterly*, 45, 503–524.

Nasser, L., & Bulkeley, K. (2009). The typical dreams of Jordanian college students. In K. Bulkeley, K. Adams, & P. M. Davis (Eds.), *Dreaming in Christianity and Islam: Culture, conflict, and creativity* (pp. 200–216). Rutgers University Press.

Nelson, J. (1888a). Der Traum als Naturnothwendigkeit erklärt, W. Robert; Das Leben im Traum. Eine Studie, Paul Schwartzkopff; Schlaf und Traum. Eine populäre wissenschaftliche Darstellung, Friedrich Scholz. *American Journal of Psychology, 1*(2), 330–332. https://doi.org/10.2307/1411355

Nelson, J. (1888b). A study of dreams. *American Journal of Psychology, 1*, 367–401.

Nielsen, T. A., & Powell, R. A. (1989). The 'dream-lag' effect: A 6-day temporal delay in dream content incorporation. *Psychiatric Journal of the University of Ottawa, 14*, 561–565.

Nielsen, T. A., Zadra, A. L., Simard, V., Saucier, S., Stenstrom, P., Smith, C., & Kuiken, D. (2003). The typical dreams of Canadian university students. *Dreaming, 13*, 211–235. https://doi.org/10.1023/B:DREM.0000003144.40929.0b

Noble, D. (1950). A study of dreams in schizophrenia and allied states. *American Journal of Psychiatry, 107*, 612–616.

Nöltner, S., & Schredl, M. (2023). Interactions with family members in students' dreams. *Dreaming, 33*, 19–31. https://doi.org/10.1037/drm0000212

North, A. C., Hargreaves, D. J., & O'Neill, S. A. (2000). The importance of music to adolescents. *British Journal of Educational Psychology, 70*(2), 255–272. https://doi.org/10.1348/000709900158083

Oberlerchner, H. (2006). Die Burg – Bearbeitung eines zentralen Konflikts in einer Traumserie. *Forum der Psychoanalyse, 22*(4), 386–393.

Okabe, S., Fukuda, K., Mochizuki-Kawai, H., & Yamada, K. (2018). Favorite odor induces negative dream emotion during rapid eye movement sleep. *Sleep Medicine, 47*, 72–76. https://doi.org/10.1016/j.sleep.2018.03.026

Olsen, M. R., Schredl, M., & Carlsson, I. (2020). Conscious use of dreams in waking life (nontherapy setting) for decision-making, problem-solving, attitude formation, and behavioral change. *Dreaming, 30*(3), 257–266. https://doi.org/10.1037/drm0000138

Oudiette, D., Leu, S., Pottier, M., Buzare, M.-A., Brion, A., & Arnulf, I. (2009). Dreamlike mentations during sleepwalking and sleep terrors in adults. *Sleep, 32*, 1621–1627.

Pagel, J. F., Blagrove, M., Levin, R., States, B. O., Stickgold, R., & White, S. (2001). Definitions of dream: A paradigm for comparing field descriptive specific studies of dream. *Dreaming, 11*, 195–202. https://doi.org/10.1023/A:1012240307661

Pagel, J. F., & Kwiatkowski, C. F. (2003). Creativity and dreaming: Correlation of reported dream incorporation into waking behavior with level and type of creative interest. *Creativity Research Journal, 15*(2/3), 199. https://doi.org/10.1080/10400419.2003.9651412

Paquette, A. (2018). The interpretation of independent agents and spiritual content in dreams. *International Journal of Dream Research, 11*(2), 86–105. https://doi.org/10.11588/ijodr.2018.2.41217

Paul, F., Alpers, G. W., Reinhard, I., & Schredl, M. (2019). Nightmares do result in psychophysiological arousal: A multimeasure ambulatory assessment study. *Psychophysiology, 56*(7), e13366. https://doi.org/10.1111/psyp.13366

Paul, F., Schädlich, M., & Erlacher, D. (2014). Lucid dream induction by visual and tactile stimulation: An exploratory sleep laboratory study. *International*

Journal of Dream Research, 7(1), 61–66. https://doi.org/10.11588/ijodr.2014.1.13044

Paul, F., & Schredl, M. (2012). Male-female ratio in waking-life contacts and dream characters. *International Journal of Dream Research*, 5, 119–124. https://doi.org/10.11588/ijodr.2012.2.9406

Perlis, M. L., & Nielsen, T. A. (1993). Mood regulation, dreaming and nightmares: Evaluation of a desensitization function for REM sleep. *Dreaming*, 3, 243–257.

Pierce, C. M. (1963). Dream studies in enuresis research. *Canadian Psychiatric Association Journal*, 8, 415–419.

Pierce, C. M., Whitman, R. M., Maas, J. W., & Gay, M. L. (1961). Enuresis and dreaming: Experimental studies. *Archives of General Psychiatry*, 4, 166–170.

Plailly, J., Villalba, M., Vallat, R., Nicolas, A., & Ruby, P. (2019). Incorporation of fragmented visuo-olfactory episodic memory into dreams and its association with memory performance. *Scientific Reports*, 9(1), 15687. https://doi.org/10.1038/s41598-019-51497-y

Purcell, S., Mullington, J., Moffit, A., Hoffmann, R., & Pigeau, R. (1986). Dream self-reflectiveness as a learned cognitive skill. *Sleep*, 9(3), 423–437.

Radestock, P. (1879). *Schlaf und Traum: Eine physiologisch-psychologische Untersuchung*. Breitkopf und Härtel.

Rainville, R. E., & Rush, L. L. (2009). A contemporary view of college-aged students' dreams. *Dreaming*, 19, 152–171.

Raymond, I., Nielsen, T. A., Lavigne, G., & Choiniere, M. (2002). Incorporation of pain in dreams of hospitalized burn victims. *Sleep*, 25, 765–770.

Rechtschaffen, A., & Buchignani, C. (1992). The visual appearance of dreams. In J. S. Antrobus & M. Bertini (Eds.), *The neuropsychology of sleep and dreaming* (pp. 143–155). Lawrence Erlbaum.

Reed, H. (1978). Meditation and lucid dreaming: A statistical relationship. *Sundance Community Dream Journal*, 2, 237–238.

Revonsuo, A. (2000a). Did ancestral humans dream for their lives? *Behavioral and Brain Sciences*, 23, 1063–1082.

Revonsuo, A. (2000b). The reinterpretation of dreams: An evolutionary hypothesis of the function of dreaming. *Behavioral and Brain Sciences*, 23, 877–901. https://doi.org/10.1017/s0140525x00004015

Revonsuo, A., Tuominen, J., & Valli, K. (2015). The avatars in the machine. In T. K. Metzinger & J. M. Windt (Eds.), *Open MIND* (pp. 1–28). MIND Group. https://doi.org/10.15502/9783958570375

Rizzolo, A. (1922). A study of 100 consecutively recorded dreams. *American Journal of Psychology*, 35, 244–254. https://doi.org/10.2307/1413827

Rosen, M. (2022). Dreaming as a virtual reality delusion simulator: Gaining empathy whilst we sleep. *International Journal of Dream Research*, 15(1), 73–85. https://doi.org/10.11588/ijodr.2022.1.83147

Roussy, F., Raymond, I., Gonthier, I., Grenier, J., & De Koninck, J. (1998). Temporal references in manifest dream content: Confirmation of increased remoteness as the night progresses. *Sleep Supplement*, 21, 285.

Saint-Denys, H. d. (1982). *Dreams and how to guide them (Original: 1867)*. Duckworth.

Sandman, N., Valli, K., Kronholm, E., Ollila, H. M., Revonsuo, A., Laatikainen, T., & Paunio, T. (2013). Nightmares: Prevalence among the Finnish general adult population and war veterans during 1972–2007. *Sleep*, *36*, 1041–1050. https://doi.org/10.5665/sleep.2806

Saunders, D. T., Roe, C. A., Smith, G., & Clegg, H. (2016). Lucid dreaming incidence: A quality effects meta-analysis of 50 years of research. *Consciousness and Cognition*, *43*, 197–215. http://dx.doi.org/10.1016/j.concog.2016.06.002

Sausgruber, H. (1988). Analyse langer Traumserien. *Ärztliche Praxis und Psychotherapie*, *10*, 29–36.

Sausgruber, H. (1989). Analyse langer Traumserien – II. Teil: Beschreibung von Häufigkeiten. *Ärztliche Praxis und Psychotherapie*, *11*, 31–40.

Scapin, F., Dehon, H., & Englebert, J. (2018). Assessment of a French version of the Mannheim Dream questionnaire (MADRE) in a Belgian sample. *International Journal of Dream Research*, *11*(1), 46–53. https://doi.org/10.11588/ijodr.2018.1.42597

Schädlich, M., Erlacher, D., & Schredl, M. (2017). Improvement of darts performance following lucid dream practice depends on the number of distractions while rehearsing within the dream – A sleep laboratory pilot study. *Journal of Sports Sciences*, *35*(23), 2365–2372. https://doi.org/10.1080/02640414.2016.1267387

Schechter, N., Schmeidler, G. R., & Staal, M. (1965). Dream reports and creative tendencies in students of the arts, sciences and engineering. *Journal of Consulting Psychology*, *29*, 415–421.

Schenck, C. H., Hurwitz, T. D., & Mahowald, M. W. (1993). REM sleep behavior disorder: An update on a series of 96 patients and a review of the world literature. *Journal of Sleep Research*, *2*, 224–231.

Schenck, C. H., Scott, R., Ettinger, M. G., & Mahowald, M. W. (1986). Chronic behavioral disorders of human REM sleep: A new category of parasomnia. *Sleep*, *9*, 293–308.

Schmidt, D. (1999). Stretched dream science: The essential contribution of long-term naturalistic studies. *Dreaming*, *9*, 43–69.

Schneck, J. M. (1956). Total loss of teeth in dreams. *American Journal of Psychiatry*, *112*, 939.

Schnitzler, A. (2012). *Träume – Das Traumtagebuch 1875–1931*. Wallstein.

Schönhammer, R. (2004). *Fliegen, Fallen, Flüchten: Psychologie intensiver Träume*. dgvt.

Schredl, M. (1998). The stability and variability of dream content. *Perceptual and Motor Skills*, *86*, 733–734.

Schredl, M. (2000). Time series analysis in dream research. *Perceptual and Motor Skills*, *91*, 915–916.

Schredl, M. (2002). Questionnaire and diaries as research instruments in dream research: Methodological issues. *Dreaming*, *12*, 17–26. http://dx.doi.org/10.1023/A:1013890421674

Schredl, M. (2003). Continuity between waking and dreaming: A proposal for a mathematical model. *Sleep and Hypnosis*, *5*, 38–52.

Schredl, M. (2004). Seasons in dreams. *Perceptual and Motor Skills*, *98*, 1438–1440.

Schredl, M. (2006). Factors affecting the continuity between waking and dreaming: Emotional intensity and emotional tone of the waking-life event. *Sleep and Hypnosis*, *8*, 1–5.

Schredl, M. (2007). Gender differences in dreaming. In D. Barrett & P. McNamara (Eds.), *The new science of dreaming – Volume 2: Content, recall, and personality correlates* (pp. 29–47). Praeger.

Schredl, M. (2008a). Dream recall frequency in a representative German sample. *Perceptual and Motor Skills*, *106*, 699–702. https://doi.org/10.2466/pms.106.3.699-702

Schredl, M. (2008b). Laboratory references in dreams: Methodological problem and/or evidence for the continuity hypothesis of dreaming? *International Journal of Dream Research*, *1*, 3–6.

Schredl, M. (2008c). Personality correlates of flying dreams. *Imagination, Cognition and Personality*, *27*, 129–137. https://doi.org/10.2190/IC.27.2.d

Schredl, M. (2008d). Spontaneously reported colors in dreams: Correlations with attitude towards creativity, personality and memory. *Sleep and Hypnosis*, *10*, 54–60.

Schredl, M. (2010a). Nightmare frequency and nightmare topics in a representative German sample. *European Archives of Psychiatry and Clinical Neuroscience*, *260*, 565–570. https://doi.org/10.1007/s00406-010-0112-3

Schredl, M. (2010b). Reading books about dream interpretation: Gender differences. *Dreaming*, *20*(4), 248–253. https://doi.org/10.1037/a0020901

Schredl, M. (2010c). History of dream research: The dissertation "Entstehung der Träume (Origin of dreams)" of Wilhelm Weygandt published in 1893. *International Journal of Dream Research*, *3*, 95–97. https://doi.org/10.11588/ijodr.2010.1.507

Schredl, M. (2011a). Dreams of a romantic partner in a dream series: Comparing relationship periods with periods of being separated. *International Journal of Dream Research*, *4*, 127–131. https://doi.org/10.11588/ijodr.2011.2.9150

Schredl, M. (2011b). Frequency and nature of pain in a long dream series. *Sleep and Hypnosis*, *13*, 1–6.

Schredl, M. (2011c). Toilet dreams: Incorporation of waking-life memories? *International Journal of Dream Research*, *4*, 41–44.

Schredl, M. (2012a). Continuity hypothesis and color in dreams. In D. Barrett & P. McNamara (Eds.), *Encyclopedia of sleep and dreams: The evolution, function, nature, and mysteries of slumber* (pp. 164–165). Greenwood.

Schredl, M. (2012b). Continuity in studying the continuity hypothesis of dreaming is needed. *International Journal of Dream Research*, *5*, 1–8. http://archiv.ub.uni-heidelberg.de/ojs/index.php/IJoDR/article/view/9306

Schredl, M. (2012c). Dreaming about wearing glasses: Analyzing a long dream series of a short-sighted person. *International Journal of Dream Research*, *5*, 99–101.

Schredl, M. (2012d). Old school friends: Former social relationship patterns in a long dream series. *International Journal of Dream Research*, *5*, 143–147.

Schredl, M. (2013a). Animal dreams in a long dream series. *International Journal of Dream Research*, *6*, 59–64.

Schredl, M. (2013b). Dreams of core family members in a long dream series. *International Journal of Dream Research*, *6*, 114–118. https://doi.org/10.11588/ijodr.2013.2.11055

Schredl, M. (2013c). Nightmare frequency in a representative German sample. *International Journal of Dream Research*, *6*, 119–122. https://doi.org/10.11588/ijodr.2013.2.11127

Schredl, M. (2014). Smoking dreams in the dream series of a non-smoker. *International Journal of Dream Research*, *7*, 76–79. https://doi.org/10.11588/ijodr.2014.1.12059

Schredl, M. (2015a). The continuity between waking and dreaming: Empirical research and clinical implications. In M. Kramer & M. Glucksman (Eds.), *Dream research – Contributions to clinical practice* (pp. 27–37). Routledge.

Schredl, M. (2015b). Dreaming about dreaming: Analysis of a long dream series. *International Journal of Dream Research*, 8, 142–145.

Schredl, M. (2015c). Time specifications in dream of a long series: Time of day and day of the week. *International Journal of Dream Research*, 8, 62–66.

Schredl, M. (2016). Temperature perception in dreams: Analysis of a long dream series. *International Journal of Dream Research*, 9, 79–81. https://doi.org/10.11588/ijodr.2016.1.26627

Schredl, M. (2017a). Is dreaming related to sleep-dependent memory consolidation? In N. Axmacher & B. Rasch (Eds.), *Cognitive neuroscience of memory consolidation* (pp. 161–172). Springer.

Schredl, M. (2017b). Pass or fail? Examination dreams in a long dream series [Electronic]. *International Journal of Dream Research*, 10(1), 69–74. https://doi.org/10.11588/ijodr.2017.1.34578

Schredl, M. (2017c). Theorizing about the continuity between waking and dreaming: Comment on Domhoff (2017). *Dreaming*, 27(4), 351–359. https://doi.org/10.1037/drm0000062

Schredl, M. (2018a). Reminiscences of love: Former romantic partners in dreams. *International Journal of Dream Research*, 11(1), 69–73. https://doi.org/10.11588/ijodr.2018.1.43842

Schredl, M. (2018b). *Researching dreams: The fundamentals*. Palgrave Macmillan.

Schredl, M. (2019a). Sport dreams in a long dream series. *International Journal of Dream Research*, 12(2), 85–88. https://doi.org/10.11588/ijodr.2019.2.64732

Schredl, M. (2019b). Typical dream themes. In K. Valli & R. J. Hoss (Eds.), *Dreams: Understanding biology, psychology, and culture* (Vol. 1, pp. 180–188). Greenwood.

Schredl, M. (2020a). "Baby, you can drive my car" – Means of transportation in a long dream series. *International Journal of Dream Research*, 13(1), 56–61. https://doi.org/10.11588/ijodr.2020.1.67601

Schredl, M. (2020b). Dream recording frequency in psychology students. *International Journal of Dream Research*, 13(2), 306–308. https://doi.org/10.11588/ijodr.2020.2.75354

Schredl, M. (2020c). "What goes up must come down" – Elevators in a long dream series. *Imagination, Cognition and Personality*, 40(2), 143–153. https://doi.org/10.1177/0276236620926486

Schredl, M. (2021a). Animals in a long dream series. *International Journal of Dream Research*, 14(1), 151–155. https://doi.org/10.11588/ijodr.2021.1.79436

Schredl, M. (2021b). Being naked in dreams: Analysis of a long dream series. *International Journal of Dream Research*, 14(2), 327–331. https://doi.org/10.11588/ijodr.2021.2.82663

Schredl, M. (2021c). "Breaking the law" in dreams: Analysis of a long dream series. *International Journal of Dream Research*, 14(1), 147–150. https://doi.org/10.11588/ijodr.2021.1.78797

Schredl, M. (2021d). Clocks in dreams: Analysis of a long dream series. *Clocks & Sleep*, 3(4), 609–614. www.mdpi.com/2624-5175/3/4/43

Schredl, M. (2021e). Family members in a long dream series. *International Journal of Dream Research*, 14(2), 323–326. https://doi.org/10.11588/ijodr.2021.2.82662

Schredl, M. (2021f). The percentage of male and female dream characters in a long dream series. *International Journal of Dream Research*, 14(1), 141–143. https://doi.org/10.11588/ijodr.2021.1.77526

Schredl, M. (2021g). The recording of one's dreams in children, adolescents, and adults: The UK library study. *International Journal of Dream Research*, *14*(1), 114–120. https://doi.org/10.11588/ijodr.2021.1.77247

Schredl, M. (2022). Music topics in a long dream series. *International Journal of Dream Research*, *15*(1). https://doi.org/10.11588/ijodr.2022.1.83829

Schredl, M., Anderson, L. M., Kahlert, L. K., & Kumpf, C. S. (2020). Work-related dreams: An online survey. *Clocks & Sleep*, *2*(3), 273–281. https://doi.org/10.3390/clockssleep2030021

Schredl, M., Atanasova, D., Hörmann, K., Maurer, J. T., Hummel, T., & Stuck, B. A. (2009). Information processing during sleep: The effect of olfactory stimuli on dream content and dream emotions. *Journal of Sleep Research*, *18*, 285–290.

Schredl, M., Bailer, C., Weigel, M. S., & Welt, M. S. (2020). Dreaming about dogs: An online survey. *Animals*, *10*(10), 1915. https://doi.org/10.3390/ani10101915

Schredl, M., Berres, S., Klingauf, A., Schellhaas, S., & Göritz, A. S. (2014a). The Mannheim Dream questionnaire (MADRE): German and English versions. *International Journal of Dream Research*, *7*(2). https://doi.org/10.11588/ijodr.12014.11582.16798.

Schredl, M., Berres, S., Klingauf, A., Schellhaas, S., & Göritz, A. S. (2014b). The Mannheim Dream questionnaire (MADRE): Retest reliability, age and gender effects. *International Journal of Dream Research*, *7*, 141–147. https://doi.org/10.11588/ijodr.2014.2.16675

Schredl, M., Berres, S., Klingauf, A., Schellhaas, S., & Göritz, A. S. (2015). Factors affecting the frequency of music dreams: An online study. *International Journal of Dream Research*, *8*(2), 139–141. https://doi.org/10.11588/ijodr.2015.2.23473

Schredl, M., & Bulkeley, K. (2019). Dream sharing frequency: Associations with sociodemographic variables and attitudes toward dreams in an American sample. *Dreaming*, *29*(3), 211–219. https://doi.org/10.1037/drm0000107

Schredl, M., & Bulkeley, K. (2020). Lucid nightmares: An exploratory online study. *International Journal of Dream Research*, *13*(2), 215–219. https://doi.org/10.11588/ijodr.2020.2.72364

Schredl, M., Buscher, A., Haaß, C., Scheuermann, M., & Uhrig, K. (2015). Gender differences in dream socialisation in children and adolescents. *International Journal of Adolescence and Youth*, *20*(1), 61–68. https://doi.org/10.1080/02673843.2013.767211

Schredl, M., Cadiñanos Echevarria, N., Saint Macary, L., & Weiss, A. F. (2020). Partners and ex-partners in dreams: An online survey. *International Journal of Dream Research*, *13*(2), 274–280. https://doi.org/10.11588/ijodr.2020.2.75338

Schredl, M., Ciric, P., Götz, S., & Wittmann, L. (2004). Typical dreams: Stability and gender differences. *Journal of Psychology*, *138*, 485–494. https://doi.org/10.3200/JRLP.138.6.485-494

Schredl, M., Coors, J., Anderson, L. M., Kahlert, L. K., & Kumpf, C. S. (2022). Work–life balance in dreams: Frequency and emotional tone of work-related and hobby-related dreams. *Journal of Sleep Research*, *n/a*(n/a), e13674. https://doi.org/10.1111/jsr.13674

Schredl, M., Desch, S., Röming, F., & Spachmann, A. (2009). Erotic dreams and their relationship to waking-life sexuality. *Sexologies*, *18*, 38–43. https://doi.org/10.1016/j.sexol.2008.05.001

Schredl, M., & Doll, E. (1998). Emotions in diary dreams. *Consciousness and Cognition, 7*, 634–646. https://doi.org/10.1006/ccog.1998.0356

Schredl, M., Dyck, S., & Kühnel, A. (2020). Inducing lucid dreams: The wake-up-back-to-bed technique in the home setting. *Dreaming, 30*(4), 287–296. https://doi.org/10.1037/drm0000152

Schredl, M., Ebert, K., Riede, M., & Störkel, L. (2015). How much information about the dreamer is in one dream report? An experimental study and its clinical implications. *International Journal of Dream Research, 8*, 58–61.

Schredl, M., & Engelhardt, H. (2001). Dreaming and psychopathology: Dream recall and dream content of psychiatric inpatients. *Sleep and Hypnosis, 3*, 44–54.

Schredl, M., & Erlacher, D. (2003). The problem of dream content analysis validity as shown by a bizarreness scale. *Sleep and Hypnosis, 5*, 129–135.

Schredl, M., & Erlacher, D. (2004). Lucid dreaming frequency and personality. *Personality and Individual Differences, 37*(7), 1463–1473. https://doi.org/10.1016/j.paid.2004.02.003

Schredl, M., & Erlacher, D. (2007). Self-reported effects of dreams on waking-life creativity: An empirical study. *Journal of Psychology, 141*, 35–46. https://doi.org/10.3200/JRLP.141.1.35-46

Schredl, M., & Erlacher, D. (2008). Relationship between waking sport activities, reading and dream content in sport and psychology students. *Journal of Psychology, 142*, 267–275. https://doi.org/10.3200/JRLP.142.3.267-276

Schredl, M., & Erlacher, D. (2011). Frequency of lucid dreaming in a representative German sample. *Perceptual and Motor Skills, 111*, 60–64. https://doi.org/10.2466/09.PMS.112.1.104-108

Schredl, M., & Erlacher, D. (2020). Fever dreams: An online study. *Frontiers in Psychology, 11*, 53. https://doi.org/10.3389/fpsyg.2020.00053

Schredl, M., Fröhlich, S., Schlenke, S., Stregemann, M., Voß, C., & De Gioia, S. (2015). Emotional responses to dream sharing: A field study. *International Journal of Dream Research, 8*, 135–138. https://doi.org/10.11588/ijodr.2015.2.23052

Schredl, M., Fuchedzhieva, A., Hämig, H., & Schindele, V. (2008). Do we think dreams are in black and white due to memory problems? *Dreaming, 18*, 175–180.

Schredl, M., Fulda, S., & Reinhard, I. (2006). Dream recall and the full moon. *Perceptual and Motor Skills, 102*, 17–18.

Schredl, M., Funkhouser, A., & Göritz, A. S. (2017). Frequency of déjà rêvé: Effects of age, gender, dream recall, and personality. *Journal of Consciousness Studies, 24*(7–8), 155–162.

Schredl, M., Geißler, C., & Göritz, A. S. (2019). Factors influencing the frequency of erotic dreams: An online study. *Psychology & Sexuality, 10*(4), 316–324. https://doi.org/10.1080/19419899.2019.1638297

Schredl, M., & Göritz, A. S. (2014). Umgang mit Alpträumen in der Allgemeinbevölkerung: Eine Online-Studie [Coping with nightmares in the general population: An online study]. *Psychotherapie, Psychosomatik und Medizinische Psychologie, 64*(5), 192–196. https://doi.org/10.1055/s-0033-1357131

Schredl, M., & Göritz, A. S. (2019a). Social media, dreaming, and personality: An online study. *CyberPsychology, Behavior & Social Networking, 22*(10), 657–661. https://doi.org/10.1089/cyber.2019.0385

Schredl, M., & Göritz, A. S. (2019b). Who keeps a dream journal? Sociodemographic and personality factors. *Imagination, Cognition and Personality, 39*(2), 211–220. https://doi.org/10.1177/0276236619837699

Schredl, M., & Göritz, A. S. (2020). Dream journaling: Stability and relation to personality factors. *Dreaming, 30*(3), 278–286. https://doi.org/10.1037/drm0000137

Schredl, M., Henley-Einion, J., & Blagrove, M. (2016). Lucid dreaming and personality in children/adolescents and adults: The UK library study. *International Journal of Dream Research, 9*, 75–78. https://doi.org/10.11588/ijodr.2016.1.26454

Schredl, M., Hoffmann, L., Sommer, J. U., & Stuck, B. A. (2014). Olfactory stimulation during sleep can reactivate odor-associated images. *Chemosensory Perception, 7*, 140–146. https://doi.org/10.1007/s12078-014-9173-4

Schredl, M., & Hofmann, F. (2003). Continuity between waking activities and dream activities. *Consciousness and Cognition, 12*, 298–308. https://doi.org/10.1016/S1053-8100(02)00072-7

Schredl, M., & Jacob, S. (1998). Ratio of male and female characters in a dream series. *Perceptual and Motor Skills, 86*, 198–200. https://doi.org/10.2466/pms.1998.86.1.198

Schredl, M., Kälberer, A., Zacharowski, K., & Zimmermann, M. (2017). Pain dreams and dream emotions in patients with chronic back pain and healthy controls. *Open Pain Journal, 10*, 65–72.

Schredl, M., Kleinferchner, P., & Gell, T. (1996). Dreaming and personality: Thick vs. thin boundaries. *Dreaming, 6*, 219–223. https://doi.org/10.1037/h0094456

Schredl, M., & Knoth, I. S. (2012). Nighttime in dreams. *Perceptual and Motor Skills, 114*, 457–460.

Schredl, M., & König, N. (2016). Beds in dreams. *International Journal of Dream Research, 9*(2), 134–136. https://doi.org/10.11588/ijodr.2016.2.30894

Schredl, M., Loßnitzer, T., & Vetter, S. (1998). Is the ratio of male and female dream characters related to the waking-life pattern of social contacts? *Perceptual and Motor Skills, 87*, 513–514.

Schredl, M., & Neuhäusler, A. (2019). With or without you? Dreaming about the romantic partner – A case study. *International Journal of Dream Research, 12*(1), 141–146. https://doi.org/10.11588/ijodr.2019.1.59638

Schredl, M., & Noveski, A. (2018). Lucid dreaming: A diary study. *Imagination, Cognition & Personality, 38*(1), 5–17.

Schredl, M., Paul, F., Lahl, O., & Göritz, A. S. (2010–2011). Gender differences in dream content: Related to biological sex or sex role orientation? *Imagination, Cognition, and Personality, 30*, 171–183. https://doi.org/10.2190/IC.30.2.e

Schredl, M., & Piel, E. (2004). War-related dream themes in Germany from 1956 to 2000. *Journal of Sleep Research Supplement, 13*(1), 658.

Schredl, M., & Piel, E. (2006). War-related dream themes in Germany from 1956 to 2000. *Political Psychology, 27*, 299–307.

Schredl, M., & Piel, E. (2008). Interest in dream interpretation: A gender difference. *Dreaming, 18*, 11–15.

Schredl, M., & Reinhard, I. (2008). Gender differences in dream recall: A meta-analysis. *Journal of Sleep Research, 17*, 125–131. https://doi.org/10.1111/j.1365-2869.2008.00626.x

Schredl, M., & Reinhard, I. (2009–2010). The continuity between waking mood and dream emotions: Direct and second-order effects. *Imagination, Cognition and Personality, 29*, 271–282. https://doi.org/10.2190/IC.29.3.f

Schredl, M., & Reinhard, I. (2012). Frequency of a romantic partner in a dream series. *Dreaming, 22*(4), 223–229. https://doi.org/10.1037/a0030252

Schredl, M., Rieger, J., & Göritz, A. S. (2018). Measuring lucid dreaming skills: A new questionnaire (LUSK). *International Journal of Dream Research*, *11*(1), 54–61. http://journals.ub.uni-heidelberg.de/index.php/IJoDR/article/view/44040

Schredl, M., Sahin, V., & Schäfer, G. (1998). Gender differences in dreams: Do they reflect gender differences in waking life? *Personality and Individual Differences*, *25*, 433–442. https://doi.org/10.1016/S0191-8869(98)00035-X

Schredl, M., Samaras, A., Henley-Einion, J., & Blagrove, M. (2018). Book preferences and nightmares: The U.K. library study. *Dreaming*, *28*(1), 24–32. https://doi.org/10.1037/drm0000074

Schredl, M., & Schmitt, J. (2019). Dream recall frequency, nightmare frequency, attitude towards dreams, and other dream variables in patients with sleep-related breathing disorders. *Somnologie*, *23*(2), 109–115. https://doi.org/10.1007/s11818-019-0199-3

Schredl, M., & Schweickert, R. (2022). Social network in the 2015 dreams of a male dreamer. *International Journal of Dream Research*, *15*(1), 118–125. https://doi.org/10.11588/ijodr.2022.1.85607

Schredl, M., Struck, V. S., Schwert, C., Blei, M., Henley-Einion, J., & Blagrove, M. (2019). Gender differences in the dream content of children and adolescents: The UK library study. *American Journal of Psychology*, *132*(3), 315–324. www.jstor.org/stable/10.5406/amerjpsyc.132.3.0315

Schredl, M., & Wood, L. C. (2021). Partners and ex-partners in dreams: A diary study. *Clocks & Sleep*, *3*(2), 289–297. https://doi.org/10.3390/clockssleep3020018

Schredl, M., Zumstein, J., Baumann, S., & Schmidt, M. (2022). Lucid dreaming frequency and sensory-processing sensitivity. *Imagination, Cognition and Personality*, 02762366221094245. https://doi.org/10.1177/02762366221094245

Schwitzgebel, E. (2002). Why did we think we dreamed in black and white? *Studies in History and Philosophy of Science*, *33*, 649–660.

Schwitzgebel, E. (2003). Do people still report dreaming in black and white? An attempt to replicate a questionnaire from 1942. *Perceptual and Motor Skills*, *96*, 25–29.

Selterman, D., Apetroaia, A. I., Riela, S., & Aron, A. (2014). Dreaming of you: Behavior and emotion in dreams of significant others predict subsequent relational behavior. *Social Psychological and Personality Science*, *5*(1), 111–118. https://doi.org/10.1177/1948550613486678

Settineri, S., Frisone, F., Alibrandi, A., & Merlo, E. M. (2019). Italian adaptation of the Mannheim Dream Questionnaire (MADRE): Age, gender and dream recall effects. *International Journal of Dream Research*, *12*(1), 119–129.

Sharpless, B. A., & Barber, J. P. (2011). Lifetime prevalence rates of sleep paralysis: A systematic review. *Sleep Medicine Reviews*, *15*(5), 311–315. https://doi.org/10.1016/j.smrv.2011.01.007

Shumway, R. H., & Stoffer, D. S. (2017). *Time series analysis and its applications: With R examples* (4th ed.). Springer.

Sicard, J., & de Bot, K. (2013). Multilingual dreaming. *International Journal of Multilingualism*, *10*(3), 331–354. https://doi.org/10.1080/14790718.2012.755187

Siclari, F., Baird, B., Perogamvros, L., Bernardi, G., LaRocque, J. J., Riedner, B., Boly, M., Postle, B. R., & Tononi, G. (2017). The neural correlates of dreaming. *Nature Neuroscience*, *20*, 872–878 https://doi.org/10.1038/nn.4545

Sierra-Siegert, M., Jay, E.-L., Florez, C., & Garcia, A. E. (2019). Minding the dreamer within: An experimental study on the effects of enhanced dream recall on creative thinking. *The Journal of Creative Behavior, 53*(1), 83–96. https://doi.org/10.1002/jocb.168

Sikka, P., Feilhauer, D., Valli, K., & Revonsuo, A. (2017). How you measure is what you get: Differences in self- and external ratings of emotional experiences in home dreams. *American Journal of Psychology, 130*(3), 367–384. https://doi.org/10.5406/amerjpsyc.130.3.0367

Sikka, P., Valli, K., Virta, T., & Revonsuo, A. (2014). I know how you felt last night, or do I? Self- and external ratings of emotions in REM sleep dreams. *Consciousness and Cognition: An International Journal, 25*, 51–66. http://dx.doi.org/10.1016/j.concog.2014.01.011

Silber, M. H., St. Louis, E. K., & Boeve, B. F. (2022). Rapid eye movement sleep parasomnias. In M. Kryger, T. Roth, & W. C. Dement (Eds.), *Principles and practice of sleep medicine* (6th ed., pp. 1093–1101). Elsevier.

Silver, D. (1985). Mirror in dreams: Symbol of the mother's face. *Psychoanalytic Inquiry, 5*, 253–256.

Sladen, D., & Frings, P. (1990). Dreams of a life-time reveal the personality of the dreamer. *Association for the Study of Dreams Newsletter, 7(1)*, 8–9.

Smith, M. E., & Hall, C. S. (1964). An investigation of regression in a long dream series. *Journals of Gerontology, 19*, 66–71.

Snyder, F. (1970). The phenomenology of dreaming. In L. Madow & L. H. Snow (Eds.), *The psychodynamic implications of the physiological studies on dreams* (pp. 124–151). Charles C. Thomas.

States, B. O. (1992). The meaning of dreams. *Dreaming, 2*, 249–262.

Stekel, W. (1911). *Die Sprache des Traumes.* J. F. Bergmann.

Stephan, J., Schredl, M., Henley-Einion, J., & Blagrove, M. (2012). TV viewing and dreaming in children: The UK library study. *International Journal of Dream Research, 5*, 130–133.

Stocks, A., Carr, M., Mallett, R., Konkoly, K., Hicks, A., Crawford, M., Schredl, M., & Bradshaw, C. (2020). Dream lucidity is associated with positive waking mood. *Consciousness and Cognition, 83*, 102971. https://doi.org/10.1016/j.concog.2020.102971

Strauch, I., Kaiser, N., Lederbogen, S., Pütz, P., & Traber, Y. (1997). *Träume und Wachphantasien von der späten Kindheit bis zur Adoleszenz – Ergebnisse einer Längsschnittuntersuchung.* Abschlußbericht (Auszug).

Strauch, I., & Meier, B. (1996). *In search of dreams: Results of experimental dream research.* State University of New York Press.

Stumbrys, T. (2011). Lucid dreaming: Discontinuity or continuity in consciousness? *International Journal of Dream Research, 4*, 93–97. http://archiv.ub.uni-heidelberg.de/ojs/index.php/IJoDR/article/view/9146

Stumbrys, T. (2018). Lucid nightmares: A survey of their frequency, features, and factors in lucid dreamers. *Dreaming, 28*(3), 193–204. https://doi.org/10.1037/drm0000090

Stumbrys, T., Erlacher, D., Johnson, M., & Schredl, M. (2014). The phenomenology of lucid dreaming: An online survey. *American Journal of Psychology, 127*(2), 191–204. https://doi.org/10.5406/amerjpsyc.127.2.0191

Stumbrys, T., Erlacher, D., & Malinowski, P. (2015). Meta-awareness during day and night: The relationship between mindfulness and lucid dreaming. *Imagination, Cognition and Personality, 34*(4), 415–433. http://ica.sagepub.com/content/34/4/415.abstract

Stumbrys, T., Erlacher, D., Schädlich, M., & Schredl, M. (2012). Induction of lucid dreams: A systematic review of evidence. *Consciousness and Cognition, 21*(3), 1456–1475. https://doi.org/10.1016/j.concog.2012.07.003

Sturzenacker, G., & Pearson, C. (2012). Journaling of dreams. In D. Barrett & P. McNamara (Eds.), *Encyclopedia of sleep and dreams: The evolution, function, nature, and mysteries of slumber* (pp. 373–377). Greenwood.

Symons, D. (1993). The stuff that dreams aren't made of: Why wake-state and dream-state sensory experiments differ. *Cognition, 47*, 181–217.

Takahara, M., Nittono, H., & Hori, T. (2006). Effect of voluntary attention on auditory processing during REM sleep. *Sleep, 29*, 975–982.

Tan, S., & Fan, J. (2022). A systematic review of new empirical data on lucid dream induction techniques. *Journal of Sleep Research, 32*(3), e13786. https://doi.org/10.1111/jsr.13786

Tedlock, B. (1991). The new anthropology of dreaming. *Dreaming, 1*, 161–178.

Tuominen, J., Olkoniemi, H., Revonsuo, A., & Valli, K. (2021). 'No man is an island': Effects of social seclusion on social dream content and REM sleep. *British Journal of Psychology, 113*, 84–104. https://doi.org/10.1111/bjop.12515

Tuominen, J., Revonsuo, A., & Valli, K. (2019). The social simulation theory. In K. Valli & R. J. Hoss (Eds.), *Dreams: Understanding biology, psychology, and culture* (Vol. 1, pp. 132–137). Greenwood.

Tuominen, J., Stenberg, T., Revonsuo, A., & Valli, K. (2019). Social contents in dreams: An empirical test of the Social Simulation Theory. *Consciousness and Cognition, 69*, 133–145. https://doi.org/10.1016/j.concog.2019.01.017

Uga, V., Lemut, M. C., Zampi, C., Zilli, I., & Salzarulo, P. (2006). Music in dreams. *Consciousness and Cognition, 15*, 351–357.

Uslar, D. v. (2003). *Tagebuch des Unbewussten. Abenteuer im Reich der Träume.* Königshausen & Neumann.

Vaillancourt-Morel, M.-P., Daspe, M.-È., Lussier, Y., & Zadra, A. (2021). Targets of erotic dreams and their associations with waking couple and sexual life. *Dreaming, 31*(1), 44–56. https://doi.org/10.1037/drm0000160

Vallat, R., Chatard, B., Blagrove, M., & Ruby, P. (2017). Characteristics of the memory sources of dreams: A new version of the content-matching paradigm to take mundane and remote memories into account. *PLoS ONE, 12*(10), e0185262. https://doi.org/10.1371/journal.pone.0185262

Valli, K., Frauscher, B., Gschliesser, V., Wolf, E., Falkenstetter, T., Schönwald, S. V., Ehrmann, L., Zangerl, A., Marti, I., Boesch, S. M., Revonsuo, A., Poewe, W., & Högl, B. (2012). Can observers link dream content to behaviours in rapid eye movement sleep behaviour disorder? A cross-sectional experimental pilot study. *Journal of Sleep Research, 21*, 21–29. http://dx.doi.org/10.1111/j.1365-2869.2011.00938.x

Van den Bulck, J. (2004). Media use and dreaming: The relationship among television viewing, computer game play, and nightmares or pleasant dreams. *Dreaming, 14*, 43–49. https://doi.org/10.1037/1053-0797.14.1.43

Van den Bulck, J., Çetin, Y., Terzi, Ö., & Bushman, B. J. (2016). Violence, sex, and dreams: Violent and sexual media content infiltrate our dreams at night. *Dreaming, 26*(4), 271–279. https://doi.org/10.1037/drm0000036

Van Eeden, F. (1913). A study of dreams. *Proceedings of the Society for Psychical Research, 26*, 431–461.

Vealey, R. S. (2007). Mental skills training in sport. In *Handbook of sport psychology* (3rd ed., pp. 287–309). John Wiley & Sons, Inc.

Verdone, P. (1965). Temporal reference of manifest dream content. *Perceptual and Motor Skills, 20,* 1253–1268.

Vogel, G. W., Thurmond, A., Gibbons, P., Sloan, K., Boyd, M., & Walker, M. P. (1975). REM sleep reduction effects on depression syndromes. *Archives of General Psychiatry, 32,* 765–777.

Vogelsang, L., Anold, S., Schormann, J., Wübbelmann, S., & Schredl, M. (2016). The continuity between waking-life musical activities and music dreams. *Dreaming, 26*(2), 132–141. https://doi.org/10.1037/drm0000018

Wald, A., & Wolfowitz, J. (1940). On a test whether two samples are from the same population. *Annals of Mathematical Statistics, 11*(2), 147–162. https://doi.org/10.1214/aoms/1177731909

Walker, M. P., & van der Helm, E. (2009). Overnight therapy? The role of sleep in emotional brain processing. *Psychological Bulletin, 135*(5), 731–748. https://doi.org/10.1037/a0016570

Wamsley, E. J. (2014). Dreaming and offline memory consolidation. *Current Neurology and Neuroscience Reports, 14*(3), 1–7. https://doi.org/10.1007/s11910-013-0433-5

Wamsley, E. J. (2018). Dreaming and waking thought as a reflection of memory consolidation. In K. C. R. Fox (Ed.), *The Oxford handbook of spontaneous thought: Mind-wandering, creativity, and dreaming* (pp. 457–468). Oxford University Press.

Wamsley, E. J. (2022). Constructive episodic simulation in dreams. *PLoS ONE, 17*(3), e0264574. https://doi.org/10.1371/journal.pone.0264574

Wamsley, E. J., & Stickgold, R. (2019). Dreaming of a learning task is associated with enhanced memory consolidation: Replication in an overnight sleep study. *Journal of Sleep Research, 28*(1), 1–8. https://doi.org/10.1111/jsr.12749

Wamsley, E. J., Tucker, M., Payne, J. D., Benavides, J. A., & Stickgold, R. (2010). Dreaming of a learning task is associated with enhanced sleep-dependent memory consolidation. *Current Biology, 20,* 850–855. https://doi.org/10.1016/j.cub.2010.03.027

Ward, C. H., Beck, A. T., & Rascoe, E. (1961). Typical dreams incidence among psychiatric patients. *Archives of General Psychiatry, 5,* 606–615.

Webb, C. S. (2017). *The music behind the dreams: Learn creative dreaming as 100+ top artists reveal their breakthrough inspirations.* Craig Sim Webb.

Weygandt, W. (1893). *Entstehung der Träume.* Grübel & Sommerlatte.

Whitman, R. M., Kramer, M., & Baldridge, B. J. (1963). Which dream does the patient tell? *Archives of General Psychiatry, 8,* 277–282.

Woman. (1915). Aspects of dream life. *Journal of Abnormal Psychology, 10,* 100–119.

Wright, J., & Koulack, D. (1987). Dreams and contemporary stress: A disruption-avoidance-adaptation model. *Sleep, 10,* 172–179. https://doi.org/10.1093/sleep/10.2.172

Yoshimura, K., Terada, N., Matsui, Y., Terai, A., Kinukawa, N., & Arai, Y. (2004). Prevalence of and risk factors for nocturia: Analysis of a health screening program. *International Journal of Urology, 11*(5), 282–287. https://doi.org/10.1111/j.1442-2042.2004.00791.x

Younis, I., Abdelrahman, S. H., Ibrahim, A., Hasan, S., & Mostafa, T. (2017). Sex dreams in married women: Prevalence, frequency, content, and drives. *Dreaming, 27*(3), 251–259. https://doi.org/10.1037/drm0000058

Yu, C. K.-C. (2008). Typical dreams experienced by Chinese people. *Dreaming, 18,* 1–10. https://doi.org/10.1037/1053-0797.18.1.1

Zadra, A., & Gervais, J. (2011). Sexual content of men and women's dreams. *Sleep and Biological Rhythms, 9*(4), 372.

Zadra, A., & Stickgold, R. (2021). *When brains dream: Exploring the science and mystery of sleep.* W. W. Norton.

Zadra, A. L., Nielsen, T. A., & Donderi, D. C. (1998). Prevalence of auditory, olfactory and gustatory experiences in home dreams. *Perceptual and Motor Skills, 87,* 819–826.

Zadra, A. L., Nielsen, T. A., Germain, A., Lavigne, G., & Donderi, D. C. (1998). The nature and prevalence of pain in dreams. *Pain Research and Management, 3,* 155–161.

Zadra, A. L., & Robert, G. (2012). Dream recall frequency: Impact of prospective measures and motivational factors. *Consciousness and Cognition, 21,* 1695–1702.

INDEX